stain on edges
2·19·19 vmc

Natural Baby
and Childcare

SECOND EDITION

Natural Baby and Childcare

SECOND EDITION

Lauren Feder, M.D.

Updated by LeTrinh Hoang, D.O.
Author of *Osteopathy for Children*

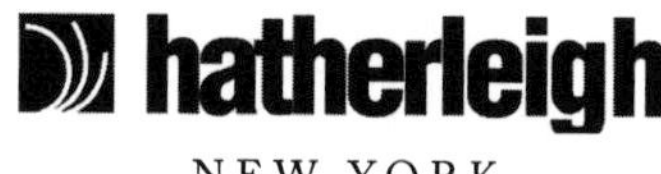

NEW YORK

hatherleigh

Hatherleigh Press is committed to preserving and protecting the natural resources of the earth. Environmentally responsible and sustainable practices are embraced within the company's mission statement.

Visit us at www.hatherleighpress.com and register online for free offers, discounts, special events, and more.

Natural Baby and Childcare, Second Edition

This book does not give legal or medical advice. Always consult your doctor, lawyer, and other professionals. Names of medications and products are typically followed by TM or ® symbols, but these symbols are not stated in this book.

The ideas and suggestions contained in this book are not intended as a substitute for consulting with a physician. All matters regarding your health require medical supervision.

Library of Congress Cataloging-in-Publication Data is available upon request.
ISBN: 978-1-57826-701-9

Printed in the United States

10 9 8 7 6 5 4 3 2 1

ACKNOWLEDGMENTS

Writing a book is like giving birth to a child; it is a labor intensive experience whose success is made possible by the expertise, support, and patience of others. Many thanks to my agent, Jessica Faust, who was instrumental in the conception of the book; my editor, Andrea Au; the production team, including Deborah Miller, Alyssa Smith, Eugenie Delaney, Jacinta Monniere, and Ann Marie Kalajian; and the publicity/marketing team, including Kevin Moran and Erin Byram, for their dedication to the project. In addition, my gratitude extends to Jennifer Jahner, Wiep de Vries, R.N., and the Wellness Nurses of the Los Angeles Alliance for Childhood, and homeopaths Mary Grace, DHM, RsHom (NA), CCH and Julie Mann, RsHom (NA), CCH.

To my family and friends, especially my mother, Ellie Davis, a wonderful role model who has always taken pride and pleasure in being a mother. To my father, Dr. Robert J. Feder, whose footsteps I follow, albeit along my own path. I now know what he meant when he wrote to me the day I became a doctor, "To the beginning of a fabulous and rewarding career which I hope will bring as much enjoyment, enrichment, and fulfillment as I have experienced." This is all made possible thanks to my patients, young and old, who share a common belief in homeopathy, holistic medicine, and natural parenting for a healthier generation.

And my love and appreciation for my sons, Étienne and Quentin, and my husband and partner, Dr. René Haarpaintner, who walks this path beside me. He has been a pillar of strength who keeps our house a home.

To the philosopher Mervyn Brady and the students of the Academy of European Arts and Culture, whose light and energy fill my soul. My cup runneth over.

Lauren Feder, M.D.
Los Angeles

To my inspirations,
Étienne
and
Quentin
who guided me through every chapter of this book . . .
and beyond

In 2014, the world lost a holistic physician, homeopath, teacher, and faithful advocate for natural health and healing. Dr. Lauren Feder passed away on November 28, 2014 of bone cancer surrounded by her loving family. It was her wish that our office continues to provide a safe haven for parents and families seeking a kind and gentle medical holism. She brought homeopathy to patients and parents by teaching through her books, lectures, articles, and website.

Dr. Feder and I were colleagues who knew of each other and of our distinct holistic specialties. She called me in to help her in her time of need and we found that our philosophies were compatible and quite synergistic. She chose me to continue her office to provide a safe harbor for patients and families seeking refuge from the conventional medical system that would only offer antibiotics, steroids, and strong prescriptions medications as a first line of treatment.

In updating this book, Dr. Feder's legacy of teaching continues. In addition, I hope to share my version of a medical holism which is a slightly different but parallel philosophical path. Osteopathy, like homeopathy, shares the common vision that the human body has the capacity for self recovery; that in helping patients get better, we look to support their health and not just finding and treating disease.

I wish to thank my parents for encouraging my early interest in medicine. I wish to thank my mentor, Herb Miller, D.O., for helping me to understand the mechanical human body from its earliest formation to how it bears the gravitational weight load as it ages. I tell patients that I will be a pediatrician until I retire, and I will be an osteopath until the day I die.

—LeTrinh Hoang, D.O., Los Angeles

Man is at his highest when nature is his teacher.

–Mervyn Brady

CONTENTS

INTRODUCTION: Optimal Health for Your Child 1

PART I. Holistic Health and Natural Therapies for Children 8

CHAPTER 1
Even Healthy Children Get Sick: 11
Thinking Holistically About Pediatric Health and Illness
*The Natural Perspective on Health and Disease ✿ What Is Natural Parenting?
Knowing When to Call the Doctor: Acute and Chronic Diseases*

CHAPTER 2
Straddling the Fence: 19
Bridging Conventional and Holistic Medicine
Antibiotics: The Promise and the Problem of Conventional Medicine ✿ Incorporating Conventional with Holistic Medicine ✿ Choosing Conventional and Holistic Practitioners

CHAPTER 3
Overview of Natural Therapies for Children 26
*Homeopathy ✿ Herbal Medicine ✿ Gemmotherapy ✿ Bach Flower Essences
Aromatherapy ✿ Naturopathy ✿ Chiropractic ✿ Osteopathy ✿ Craniosacral Therapy
Anthroposophical Medicine ✿ Acupuncture and Chinese Medicine ✿ Ayurvedic Medicine*

PART II. Stages and Ages 36

CHAPTER 4
Newborns (Birth to One Month) 39
Developmental Milestones ✿ Forty-Day Period ✿ Doulas ✿ Tests and Procedures Following Birth: Apgar Score, Eye Drops for Newborns, Vitamin K, Newborn Screening Blood Test, Umbilical Cord Care, Circumcision ✿ Jaundice ✿ Diapers: Disposable versus Cloth ✿ Swaddling ✿ Babywearing and Carrying ✿ Bonding and Attachment Parenting

CHAPTER 5
Infants (One Month to One Year) 66
Developmental Milestones ✿ Colic ✿ Crawling ✿ Your Baby's Teeth ✿ Introducing Solids ✿ Pacifiers and Thumbsucking ✿ Cribs, Playpens, and Walkers ✿ Sudden Infant Death Syndrome (SIDS) ✿ Working Parents and Caregivers

CHAPTER 6
Toddlers (Ages 1 to 4) 91
Developmental Milestones ✿ Babyproofing ✿ Tantrums ✿ Toilet Training Daycare and Preschool Germs ✿ Learning Disabilities ✿ Birth Order

CHAPTER 7
Children (Ages 5 to 10) 109
Developmental Milestones ✿ Growing Pains ✿ Bedwetting, Sleepwalking, and Nightmares Teething in Older Children ✿ Childhood Obesity and Exercise ✿ Childrearing Approaches and Education

CHAPTER 8
Preteens (Ages 11 to 13) 123
Developmental Milestones ✿ Menstruation ✿ Acne ✿ Competitive Sports Eating Disorders ✿ Junk Food ✿ Television and Video Games ✿ The Internet and Cell Phones

PART III. Natural Parenting Basics 144

CHAPTER 9
Applying Natural Remedies 147
The ABCs of Case-Taking ✿ Buying Homeopathic and Natural Medicines ✿ Administering Homeopathic Medicines ✿ Administering Gemmotherapy ✿ Administering Essential Oils ✿ External Healing Applications: Making a Compress, Poultice, Bath, or Inhalation ✿ Common Home Remedies ✿ Infant and Child Massage

CHAPTER 10
Decorating, Clothing, and Bathing 168
Creating a Nontoxic Environment for Your Baby ✿ Dressing Your Child The Family Bath ✿ Sun Safety

CHAPTER 11
Sleep 183
Your Baby's Sleep Patterns ✿ Napping ✿ The Bedtime Ritual ✿ Poor Sleep ✿ Conventional Sleep Training Methods ✿ The Family Bed ✿ Sleeping Tips for Parents

CHAPTER 12
Breastfeeding: Nursing Your Newborn . . . and Beyond 199
What Is In Breastmilk? ✿ Benefits of Breastfeeding ✿ The Best Diet for Nursing Mothers ✿ How to Breastfeed ✿ Breastfeeding Positions ✿ Breastfeeding for Special Needs: Cesarean Birth, Premature Baby, Twins, and Augmentation ✿ When You Should Not Breastfeed ✿ Difficulties with Breastfeeding ✿ Relactation, Adoptive Nursing, and Donor Milk ✿ Breastpumping and Storing Milk ✿ Breastfeeding in Public ✿ Weaning ✿ Formula Feeding

CHAPTER 13
Healthy Nutrition 233
The Standard American Diet ✿ Nutritional Building Blocks 101 ✿ How to Prepare Natural Foods for Kids ✿ Meal Planning ✿ Food Allergies and Sensitivities ✿ Foods and Additives to Avoid ✿ Vegetarian Diet

CHAPTER 14
Vaccines 278
The Immune System ✿ Pros and Cons of Vaccinations ✿ Standard Vaccinations Alternatives to the Standard Vaccination Schedule ✿ The Safe Shot Strategy

CHAPTER 15
Bonding, Mind, and Spirit 305
The Spiritual Life of Children: The Philosophy of Childhood ✿ The Arts: Fairy Tales, Music, and Math ✿ Popular Culture, Recreation, and Creative Play ✿ Adoption, Assisted Reproduction Technology, and the Changing Family

PART IV. A to Z Guide to Common Childhood Conditions 318
Acne ✿ Allergies and Allergic Reactions ✿ Anxiety ✿ Appendicitis ✿ Asthma ✿ Bee Stings ✿ Bladder Infections ✿ Boils ✿ Broken Bones ✿ Bronchitis ✿ Bruises ✿ Burns ✿ Canker Sores ✿ Chickenpox ✿ Circumcision ✿ Cold Sores ✿ Colic ✿ Common Cold ✿ Conjunctivitis (Pinkeye) ✿ Constipation ✿ Cough ✿ Cradle Cap ✿ Cramps ✿ Croup ✿ Dental Procedures ✿ Diaper Rash ✿ Diarrhea ✿ Drug Allergies ✿ Ear Infections (Otitis Media) ✿ Emotional Upset ✿ Fever ✿ Fifth Disease ✿ Flu ✿ Food Allergies ✿ Food Poisoning ✿ Gastroesophageal Reflux ✿ Grief and Sorrow ✿ Growing Pains ✿ Hand-Foot-Mouth Disease ✿ Hay Fever ✿ Headaches ✿ Hives and Allergic Reactions ✿ Indigestion ✿ Injuries ✿ Insect Bites and Stings ✿ Insomnia ✿ Jaundice ✿ Lead Poisoning ✿ Lice (Pediculus Capitis) ✿ Lyme Disease ✿ Mastitis ✿ Measles ✿ Menstrual Cramps and PMS ✿ Milk Supply ✿ Motion Sickness ✿ Mouth Sores ✿ Mumps ✿ Nausea ✿ Nosebleeds ✿ Osgood-Schlatter Disease ✿ Pinkeye ✿ Pinworm ✿ PMS ✿ Pneumonia ✿ Poison Ivy, Poison Oak, and Poison Sumac ✿ Rash ✿ Roseola and Fifth Disease ✿ Respiratory Syncytial Virus (RSV) ✿ Rubella (German Measles) ✿ Sever's Disease ✿ Sinus Infection ✿ Sore Throat (Pharyngitis) ✿ Sprain ✿ Stomachache ✿ Strep Throat ✿ Stuffed Nose ✿ Sunburn ✿ Surgery ✿ Teething ✿ Tetanus ✿ Thrush ✿ Vaccine Safety ✿ Vomiting ✿ Warts ✿ Whooping Cough

PART V. Natural Medicine Chest 456

Homeopathic Medicines 459

Aconitum napellus ✿ *Allium cepa* ✿ *Antimonium tartaricum* ✿ *Apis mellifica* ✿ *Arnica montana* ✿ *Arsenicum album* ✿ *Belladonna* ✿ *Bryonia alba* ✿ *Calcarea carbonica* ✿ *Calcarea phosphorica* ✿ *Cantharis* ✿ *Chamomilla* ✿ *Colocynthis* ✿ *Drosera* ✿ *Euphrasia officinalis* ✿ *Ferrum phosphoricum* ✿ *Gelsemium* ✿ *Hepar sulphuris calcareum* ✿ *Hypericum perforatum* ✿ *Ignatia amara* ✿ *Ipecacuanha* ✿ *Kali bichromicum* ✿ *Ledum palustre* ✿ *Magnesia phosphorica* ✿ *Mercurius* ✿ *Natrum muriaticum* ✿ *Nux vomica* ✿ *Oscillococcinum* ✿ *Pulsatilla nigricans* ✿ *Rhus toxicodendron* ✿ *Ruta graveolens* ✿ *Spongia tosta*

Gemmotherapy 486

Black Currant ✿ *Black Honeysuckle* ✿ *Briar Rose* ✿ *Common Birch* ✿ *English Elm* ✿ *European Alder* ✿ *European Grapevine* ✿ *European Hornbean* ✿ *European Walnut* ✿ *Fig Tree* ✿ *Hedge Maple* ✿ *Lemon Bark* ✿ *Lime Tree* ✿ *Lithy Tree* ✿ *Oriental Plane Tree* ✿ *Prim Wort* ✿ *Raspberry* ✿ *Red Spruce* ✿ *Rosemary* ✿ *Wineberry*

Natural Essentials 492

Calendula officinalis ✿ *Hot Water Bottle* ✿ *Hydrogen Peroxide* ✿ *Lavender* ✿ *Mullein-Garlic Ear Drops Saline*

Your Natural First Aid Kit 495

CASE-TAKING WITH THE SOAP CHART 497

GUIDE TO COMMON SYMPTOMS AND REMEDIES 499

RESOURCES AND FURTHER READINGS 503

INDEX 515

INTRODUCTION

Optimal Health for Your Child

> Of all nature's gifts to the human race, what is sweeter to a man than his children?
>
> —Cicero

As a doctor specializing in natural medicine, I see hundreds of patients every year, all with different ideas and expectations of what natural medicine has to offer. Some see me because they have tried conventional medicine without success and need a new treatment philosophy; others have used natural treatments successfully for years and find little reason to visit a standard physician. Still others are curious, interested in natural health but unsure how to incorporate it into their lives. Whatever the individual paths to my office, nearly all my patients come seeking a form of healthcare that honors both the body and the spirit, and that goes beyond treating surface-level symptoms to address wellbeing and health on more fundamental levels.

I have had tremendous success with natural medicine, both in my practice and at home with my children, and in this book will share the proven remedies and parenting techniques I have used and prescribed for years. Whether you are new to natural health or very much experienced in it, this book is a comprehensive, user-friendly guide to incorporating holistic wisdom and natural medicine into your family life. It focuses on all stages of infant and childhood development, and suggests ways that natural parenting and healthcare techniques can work alongside the routines you have already established with your children. If you are a new parent wondering about issues like breastfeeding or vaccination, or are raising older children and looking for more effective and natural ways to treat their cuts, scrapes, colds, and earaches, this book can be a valuable resource in finding out how to make natural methodologies a part of your family. It is based on insights I've gleaned both as a physician and a parent, and reflects the many years I have spent researching, teaching, and working in the area of natural health and parenting.

For me, health has always been the most personal of subjects. It is central to how we feel, how we live, and how we relate to the world around us. What I strive for with my children and patients is optimal health—health that encompasses our physical and emotional selves, and provides us the energy to live vitally and courageously. Holistic forms of healthcare share this commitment to optimal health. They tend to the body, but also offer a more natural way of living in relationship with our environment. For children, this means remedies that are nontoxic and that work without side effects, and parenting options that allow for greater bonding and stronger development. Natural healthcare does not require that you give up your conventional doctor, or put away the decongestants and antihistamines forever. Rather, this book is meant to offer you a wide array of natural choices that you can use in conjunction with standard practices, or on their own as your primary routine. The choice is yours.

My Path to Natural Medicine

As the daughter of a renowned Los Angeles ear, nose, and throat doctor, medicine and healthcare have been parts of my life since I can remember. From an early age, I was interested in alternative medicine and healthy living, but it wasn't until I was training to be a physician myself that I began to understand how powerfully effective natural forms of medicine could be. During my residency at UCLA/Veterans Administration Wadsworth, I started employing therapies such as homeopathy, acupuncture, and osteopathy for my own basic healthcare. The results amazed me. Not only did these approaches heal both chronic and acute symptoms fully, they gave me a way to marry my passion for medicine with my sincere desire to "do no harm."

I decided to specialize in homeopathy. It had worked so well for my own needs, I wanted to share my knowledge, and began a path of study that took me around the world and allowed me to learn from many of the foremost homeopaths internationally. I opened my own practice in Los Angeles, and in the nearly ten years since, have watched interest in homeopathy and other natural forms of medicine grow along with recognition that conventional medicine does not hold all of the answers. Our children need more than "standard" healthcare, and homeopathy and other natural therapies offer the alternative: individualized attention, non-toxic treatments, and a focus on optimal health.

My interest in and knowledge of natural parenting has been honed in raising my two sons. When I learned I was pregnant with my oldest child, I faced a choice: Have the baby in the hospital under the supervision of an obstetrician, or plan for a homebirth with the help of a midwife. Initially, I decided to go with the obstetrician. But in my prenatal visits, many of my questions went unanswered. I felt rushed and overwhelmed, and pregnancy, rather than the most exciting and beautiful experience I could imagine, started to seem more and more like a health hazard. I remembered from my medical rotations the IVs, bright lights, and sterile rooms of the labor and delivery wards, as well as the rushed attitudes and lack of warmth. It wasn't appealing, and felt at odds with my hopes for the delivery.

I began to explore the possibility of delivering with a midwife. A few years before, a friend had had her first child at home and I recalled my incredulity. What about the pain? I thought. What if there is a medical problem? Now I found myself pregnant, and saw the option of homebirth entirely different. Rather than a sterile and impersonal environment, I could deliver my baby in my own home, supported by people who knew me. I researched midwives, and discovered that, contrary to my assumptions, they were experienced clinicians, provided excellent prenatal care, and trained to handle emergencies during birth. The offices I visited were professional, warm, and comfortable, and I felt for the first time that I was being listened to as an individual rather than a patient.

As I prepared for my homebirth, I began to explore other aspects of natural parenting, weighing choices about the crib versus the family bed, whether to circumcise, and if and when to vaccinate. Many of these alternative views on parenting were strange to my Western upbringing, but I was attracted to the "back to basics" approach. If certain ways of parenting had worked for generations, why fix them? And if simpler methods gave me more energy to parent and resulted in a happier baby, I could see no reason to complicate my approach.

My experiences in pregnancy, during birth, and with my babies were superb, and I have made it one of my priorities to educate people about these little-known options to standard delivery. But whether you go with homebirth or the hospital, natural parenting is a philosophy that will fit your comfort level and lifestyle no matter the age of your children. It encompasses wisdom that has been passed on through generations by mothers, fathers, healers, and midwives, and has been tried and tested in my own life and many others. Most importantly, natural parenting is about trusting your instincts. We know how to parent naturally, but what we are taught about parenting often flies in the face of our initial instincts. This book will, among other things, encourage you to trust your own judgment and learn for yourself how to ward off and heal the most common ailments your child will encounter.

How to Use This Book

This book is not meant to replace your doctor, but to expand your home medicine cabinet and widen your parenting philosophy with a multitude of simple, practical, and time-honored homeopathic remedies and natural treatments. Knowing when and how to use homeopathic remedies can help shorten the duration of certain illnesses and head others off before they start—all by employing natural, non-toxic substances. One such remedy is *Aconitum napellus* or *Aconite.* I call *Aconite* the ultimate "SOS" (sudden onset of symptoms) remedy. When my ten-year-old son, Étienne, awoke one night with a fever and cough after an exhausting day of play, I administered a dose of *Aconite* which helped him get back to sleep. Although I kept him home the next day and gave him several more doses of *Aconite,* he missed only one day of school and made a speedy and full recovery. *Aconite* also helped my other son, Quentin, when he had a bike accident riding with his cousins. When I arrived on the scene he and Grandmother were crying and shaking; I gave them both *Aconite* to counter the anxiety. By the time we arrived at the emergency room, Quentin calmly allowed doctors to take x-rays and stitch him up.

Many homeopathic medicines are similarly effective and versatile, and the key to using them is knowing that they are available. Part I gives you an overview of natural therapies for children and shows you how to combine them with conventional treatments. Parts II and III will introduce you to basic natural parenting techniques, Part II by age and Part III by topic. If you are a new parent, the sections on birthing options, breastfeeding, sleeping arrangements, and the first week will be of particular interest. Parents of toddlers and older children will find information on vaccinations, nutrition, and developmental milestones such as speaking and walking. And all parents can make use of the A to Z compendium of treatments for common infant and childhood ailments in Part IV. Whether your concern is diaper rash or the flu, the book presents natural remedies that are easy to administer at home, and often safer, more practical, and less expensive options than another trip to the doctor's office. In cases where conventional treatments are particularly well-known or popular, I weigh the pros and cons, offering information on natural remedies side by side with their conventional counterparts. Finally, Part V gives you a "Natural Medicine Chest" of common, everyday remedies safe for home use. Most basically, the book is meant to expand your healthcare options as a parent, and introduce you to the remedies and solutions I have seen make profound differences in people's lives—my own and my family's included.

Nothing matters more to us than the health of our children, but often hectic schedules and busy lives mean we stick to the same routines and reach for the same medications, even if we know the side effects or results are not ideal. The underlying message of this book is that natural medicine is easy medicine—it can mean fewer trips to the doctor, fewer trips to the pharmacy, and more quality time with your child. While incorporating new habits always requires initial adjustments to schedules and routines, in the long run, natural health and parenting allow for better time spent as a family. This book provides simple, step-by-step advice on working natural health into "regular" parenting habits, and in the process, will also give you a means of thinking about your child's health holistically—not as an absence of symptoms, but as an abundance of vitality, joy, and curiosity.

Note to Readers

Female pronouns are used throughout this book, as its writing took as much focus and energy as having a child. In this case, as the mother of two boys, I've decided that this is my baby girl!

Dr. Hoang's Path to Natural Healing

In practicing conventional pediatrics, I found that there were many children who got sick, were given a prescription, and got better only to come back with the same problems. They were not cured. They received only a temporary solution until the next time they got sick again. We were not really figuring out why they were getting sick. When I started studying Osteopathy, I found that kids I treated got better and would remain healthy over longer periods of time. I soon came to understand that mechanical contraints within the human body could lead to later problems. In infants and children, the primary causes of mechanical constraints can come from as early as a difficult pregnancy, difficult delivery, or injuries acquired in the normal process of growing up. It now made sense that chronic ear infections and chronic congestion could be a result of a stuck ear bone that can't rhythmically move in symphony with its counterpart to allow drainage of the sinuses and ear (eustachian) tubes. For more information on this topic, read my book *Osteopathy for Children*.

As I leaned more into a medical holism, I sought more natural approaches to helping children with their symptoms. Homeopathy offers a safe, drug-free alternative that parents can use as a first line that they can feel comfortable about. The patients I saw that took homeopathics and gemmotherapies were not sick as often, and when they did get sick, their sicknesses were not as severe compared to kids that didn't use either. For my family, with a good diet and healthy lifestyle, along with Osteopathy and Homeopathy when needed, we hardly ever get sick.

My path also lead me to learn about EHS (electrohypersensitive syndrome) medicine and understanding the EMF around us. As the world becomes more industrialized, digitized, and techonologically advanced, the many modern conveniences that make life easier also contribute to and alter the electromagnetic fields (EMF) around us. Increasingly, we hear of individuals who develop nonspecific symptoms of headache, dizziness, mental fog, and fatigue which they attribute to being in these artificial EMFs. Those reporting severe symptoms find relief by making dramatic changes in their work and lifestyle. These people are diagnosed as "electromagnetic hypersenstitive" (EHS). This is an exciting new field of study for me after having suffered with EHS for two years and ultimately finding a cure for myself. What I have learned, I have applied in my practice to inform my families and help them improve the health of their children in an excessively wired world. This new understanding of how electricity affects human health, combined with Osteopathy and Homeopathy, makes for extraordinary treatment sessions.

This is my main contribution in this new edition of Natural Baby and Childcare. In addition to updating the existing material, I am pleased to add practical advice from a general pediatric perspective and an osteopathic mechanical philosophy. I hope that the sections on “Our Wired World” and “Digital Addiction” provide valuable insight as well as easy practical solutions in the hopes that new families can incorporate this information to protect themselves and optimize their and their children’s health.

PART I

Holistic Health and Natural Therapies

If one way be better than another, that you may be sure is Nature's way.

–*Aristotle*

I AM PART OF A GROWING NUMBER OF HEALTH-care practitioners who have integrated holistic and complementary medicine into their medical practices. Originally, many of these alternative ways of thinking were foreign to my medical training, which discouraged interest in non-pharmaceutical therapies. My feelings changed, however, during my residency, when I was successfully treated by a holistic doctor for a thyroid condition. I was so impressed with the results, I decided to specialize in holistic medicine, and over ten years later, I have cultivated a medical practice that treats people of all ages and backgrounds—many of them patients who have found conventional medical treatments ineffective or disappointing. My philosophy is "back-to-basics," emphasizing alternative treatments for health-related issues and natural preventative methods. I realize that choosing the best health care for your child is overwhelming and sometimes even anxiety-producing, and I try—in my practice and in my articles and lectures—to advocate for a simpler and more naturally effective approach to treating illness and nurturing health.

This approach is known as natural parenting. While natural parenting encompasses a wide range of practices, from preparing organic foods to breastfeeding, I focus in this book on specific ways to integrate alternative and homeopathic healthcare into your home and the lives of your family. Natural parenting is regular parenting; it speaks to the innate, wise, and practical traditions that have been passed on through generations. Furthermore, it empowers parents; knowing how to act as the first line of defense against illness for your child is the best way to keep them active, happy, and healthy.

chapter 1

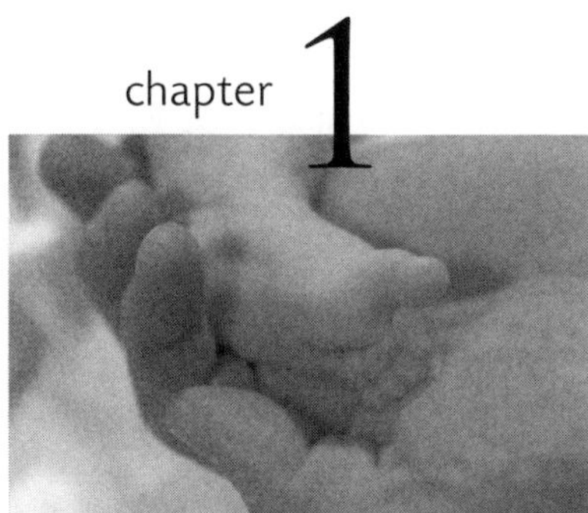

Even Healthy Children Get Sick: Thinking Holistically About Pediatric Health and Illness

I am sorry to say that Peter was not very well during the evening. His mother put him to bed and made some chamomile tea; and she gave a dose of it to Peter!

"One table-spoonful to be taken at bed-time."

–*The Tale of Peter Rabbit* by Beatrix Potter

FROM OUR FIRST FEVER to our latest bout of the flu, we humans are fluent in the language of illness—we know exactly what it feels like to be sick, and we employ a complex vocabulary to describe our symptoms. But while we can label that scratchy throat or aching head with precision, we are less able to describe what it means to be healthy. We tend, in fact, to think of health as the state of "not being sick." This applies to our children's health as well. Pediatric wellness is measured according to a number of guidelines, from height to weight to social skills to sleep habits. But what the numbers cannot tell us is how children feel when they are healthy, and why even the healthiest kids get sick.

As a physician trained in both standard and holistic medicine, I am privy to two ways of thinking about pediatric health. Conventional medicine regards health as an absence of symptoms: when nothing is wrong with us, we are well. On one hand, this definition seems self-evident, however, it does not help us develop a more complex vocabulary for human health and wellness.

The truth is, even healthy children get sick. They get colds, flus, earaches, rashes, sore throats, and coughs. In conventional pediatrics, it is typically expected that a child in daycare or school will get sick once a month. However, in our practice we find that normal healthy children may get sick once a year with the illness "challenging" the child's immune system and acting as a natural "booster." Many of these illnesses are self-limiting, meaning they will heal on their own if untreated, and are signs, moreover, of a strong immune response. In the long run, your child's cold can mean better resistance to more severe illnesses and chronic diseases. Furthermore, it is not uncommon for children to get sick at times of growth, including developmental phases such as teething, walking, and speaking.

All parents know the distress of a sick child—the fever in the middle of the night, the earache that sends them home from school, the cold passed from playmate to playmate. These illnesses are so much part of everyday family life that we often hardly stop to think about how we treat them. As parents and doctors, we want to be able to offer relief at these times, to alleviate our child's discomfort or pain. When symptoms surface, we likely reach for whatever remedy will suppress them most effectively: cough syrup, acetoaminophen, cortisone cream. But while antibiotics, antihistamines, anti-inflammatories, antacids and related medications relieve the outward signs of illness, they do not point to the underlying causes. They do not tell us why a child is getting sick in the first place. And it is no coincidence that so many of the most common over-the-counter medications begin with the prefix "anti"—they work by working against the body.

These conventional medications, also known as allopathic medicine, are designed to alleviate symptoms by manifesting the opposite condition. A runny nose is treated by drying out the nasal passages; diarrhea may be relieved by a medication that causes constipation. These drugs do make us feel better, generally by suppressing whatever symptoms are causing discomfort. However, suppressing symptoms is not always the best strategy for ensuring children's health, particularly when the medications prescribed may have unexpected side effects. If a child is taken to a pediatrician for an itchy rash, the doctor, in many cases, will prescribe cortisone cream. This may not seem like a big deal: a simple cream for a simple rash. A holistic practitioner, however, would see the issue differently. Presented with the same child, I would never prescribe cortisone cream. Not only is cortisone absorbed into the bloodstream with potentially harmful side effects, it can thin the skin, and, more importantly, doesn't address why the child has the skin problem in the first place. Rather than treating the source of the symptom, the cream suppresses the symptom itself.

The medical advancements of the last century are stunning in their achievements: we are treating disease with ever more refined techniques, targeting illness with complex drugs and extensive therapeutic regimes. We understand the mechanics of the body better than at any time in history. But even as we are told we are healthier and living longer, more children every year are on daily medications for chronic conditions like asthma, allergies, and attention deficit disorder. And more parents every year confront the limits of conventional medicine in treating and addressing the causes of chronic illnesses like these.

The stakes are high when it comes to children's health, and unfortunately, healthcare in the U.S. has far to go before it is adequate to the task. In 2000, according the Journal of the American Medical Association (JAMA), the U.S. ranked 12th out of a group of 13 countries when measured against a number of health indicators. The author identifies the third leading cause of death in the nation as iatrogenic, doctor or medication induced. While the study indicates that treatment can, in some cases, be as risky as the condition, this is no reason to avoid the doctor's office. On the contrary, there has never been a better time to demand treatments that go beyond "the standard." Practitioners of natural medicine have, for more than a century, augmented the discoveries of standard medicine with treatments derived from the natural world rather than the laboratory. Unlike conventional medicines, these approaches do not "combat" symptoms because they are not at war with the body. They work, instead, to restore a body to its healthy balance, and to build up the immune system to better resist illness in the future.

When I say that healthy children get sick, I do not mean that all sickness is healthy, or that using medications to suppress symptoms is necessarily poor practice. Rather, I want to emphasize a holistic perspective on health and illness—one that honors the natural remedies healers, physicians, midwives, and herbalists have been using effectively for centuries. This book will offer you practical, natural ways to incorporate holistic wisdom into your home—expanding the options available to you when your child does get sick and suggesting simple ways to cultivate wellness and prevent illnesses in the future.

The Natural Perspective on Health and Disease

As a medical student, I learned that health was the absence of disease. In anatomy and physiology labs, we studied the functioning of the body, its chemical and biological processes, and in classrooms we absorbed the myriad information needed to diagnosis diseases and treat them effectively. We focused primarily on bodies and what could go wrong with them. As a result, we learned to think about our patients as bodies, too. During my residency, it wasn't uncommon for the residents and attending physicians alike to refer to patients by their chief complaint: "Room 255 is the gallbladder," or "144 is the ulcer."

Like many other conventionally trained physicians, I felt I was not getting "the big picture" when it came to human health and wellness. If our job as doctors was to make people well, why did some of our most common medications make patients sicker? And was health really nothing more than not being ill? These questions, along with a condition of my own, led me to explore holistic medicine. During my teens I underwent thyroid surgery twice. I was prescribed thyroid medication, and was told I would need to take it indefinitely. While working with a holistic practitioner in my twenties, I no longer required thyroid medicine, discontinued it, and have not been on any medication since. What I discovered was a vital and important way of thinking about the body—not as a machine at war with disease, but as part of a whole person, inseparable from the thoughts, emotions, and experiences that make up our personalities and histories.

Holistic medicine encompasses a wide variety of practices, including homeopathy, herbs, Chinese medicine and acupuncture, Ayurveda, osteopathy, naturopathy, and chiropractic medicine. What unites these different methodologies is a common belief that bodies are more than a sum of their parts, and that medicine should account for the whole person—mind as well as body. The word holistic derives, of course, from "whole," and holistic medicine takes an integrated approach to treatment, asking not only what is happening symptomatically to the body, but what emotional, psychological, or environmental factors may be contributing to the issue. Also crucial to holistic medicine is the emphasis on natural, non-toxic remedies and procedures. Holistic practitioners generally believe that natural products are safer and more effective means of treating illness than conventional medicines, with fewer side effects and less wear and tear to the body.

Holistic philosophy sees the human being comprised of three interacting planes: the mental, emotional, and physical. In a healthy individual, all three planes are in balance. This is called homeostasis. Notice, however, that the physical plane is not first on the list. In contrast to standard medicine, which generally is solely preoccupied with the physical plane, holistic medicine views health and illness as products of the spirit as much as the body. If our minds are distressed, our emotions in turmoil, and our environment toxic or stressful, our bodies will let us know.

Forms of treatment like homeopathy are considered energy medicine, because they works not only on physical processes, but on the deeper forces that balance body, mind, and emotions. Energy medicines conceive of health as influenced by what is called the vital force, the fundamental animating energy in living beings. While conventional medicine tends to rely on chemical and mechanical explanations for illness, holistic practices understand it in terms of balance. A body seeks balance, or homeostasis, but occasionally, due to a variety of factors, it is not strong enough to ward off disease. Homeopathy and other forms of natural medicine seek to restore balance by strengthening the whole person's ability to resist illness. Conventional medicine, in contrast, seeks to combat illness by combating primarily its symptoms.

By taking into account the mental and emotional state of a patient as well as their physical symptoms, holistic treatment can be much more personal and individually suited. If two children came into my office with the same diagnosis of eczema, in all likelihood they could walk out with completely different prescriptions. Perhaps the first child is happy-go-lucky and extroverted, and has eczema that itches tremendously and is worse after bathing, at night, or with heat. I would prescribe her homeopathic *Sulphur. Sulphur* is indicated for children who tend to be outgoing, but at the same time can be critical and opinionated (and more so with age). These children are affectionate and energetic, but can also be lazy and messy, and they often procrastinate. They don't mind getting dirty outside, and they hate bathing! *Sulphur* is a strong remedy for skin problems in general, and is especially suited to children with this disposition.

Imagine, however, that the second child exhibits a different profile. She is restless and more introverted, and has a tendency to worry a lot—about germs, getting dirty, robbers, or health. Skin conditions for this type of child tend to itch, but often with a burning sensation, which can be relieved with a warm bath. Children with this profile frequently feel chilly, and prefer heat and a warm bath over cool temperatures (*Sulphur* children, on the other hand, tend to be more warm-blooded. For them, heat only aggravates symptoms). For this child, I would prescribe *Arsenicum album,* a remedy also useful in treating nausea, diarrhea, and food poisoning.

Because each child is different in symptoms, thoughts, and feelings, each gets the treatment best suited to his or her needs. At the conventional pediatrician's office, both would have been prescribed the same cortisone cream, but in homeopathy, there are over 600 remedies for eczema, and we prescribe one remedy at a time, one person at a time.

What Is Natural Parenting?

Natural implies accordance with nature, and natural parenting, by extension, focuses on non-artificial remedies and preventative methods. It differs from "standard" parenting advice in crucial ways. Natural parenting:

- Recognizes the importance of many age-old traditions that have been used successfully for generations.
- Reassures parents that they are the best family doctor for first-line defense, while acknowledging the benefits of doctors for serious illnesses.
- Encourages parents to trust commonsense instead of immediately seeking medical advice.
- Discourages blind faith in the medical profession, which is preoccupied with intervention rather than prevention.
- Meets the needs and well being of babies, children, and family in a way that is as natural as possible.
- For simple, self-limiting complaints, relies on remedies and medicines that are safe, non-toxic, and natural with no side effects, rather than on potentially harmful over-the-counter drugs and antibiotics.
- Offers tips and suggestions that are easy to use with practical applications.
- Requires no formal training.

Natural medicine is simple, practical, and easy to incorporate into already existing home rituals. If you are a busy parent worried that natural approaches will demand more time and energy than you have, you will likely find that natural parenting proves to be more time and cost efficient than your current habits. In addition, natural remedies are often safer and just, if not more, as effective than conventional prescription drugs. They are safe for use by newborns, nursing mothers, and mothers-to-be and can be bought over-the-counter at a reasonable cost. Homeopathic and natural medicines are not a replacement for standard medicine, but an empowering alternative for parents who want to play a larger role in their children's health.

Knowing When to Call the Doctor: Acute and Chronic Diseases

We know our children are getting sick because they begin to show symptoms. They get a runny nose, they are tired and irritable, they run a fever. As a physician, these symptoms indicate to me various underlying causes and treatment methods. As a holistic practitioner, I consider them a signal that the person, on a core level, is out of balance. Dr. George Vithoulkas, one on the world's foremost authorities on homeopathic medicine, also defines sickness as a state of imbalance, in which "stimuli are stronger than the organism's natural resistance."

There are three main factors that predispose us to getting sick:

- Heredity or family history
- The strength of a stimulus. If a stimulus, whether a flu virus or a car accident, is stronger than a person's resistance to it, signs and symptoms will occur
- Iatrogenic treatments; medications and their side effects along with other medical treatments can disturb a person's state of balance and lead to illness

In most instances, illness is a natural process for the body. It is part of what are called the "Six Processes of Life," basic rules governing all living organisms. The six processes are growth, digestion, elimination, disease, healing, and regeneration, and they help keep us in balance, physically, mentally, and emotionally. Disease (dis-ease) manifests when there is a change in the functioning of the organism and one experiences "lack of ease." Historically, conventional medicine has treated all disease with the same logic: eliminate the "lack of ease" and you have eliminated the problem. Disease, however, is not so black and white. Certain illnesses are healthy, natural challenges for our immune systems; others signal a chronic imbalance. The challenge for parents and doctors is determining which illnesses are part of a child's expected growth and development, and which indicate a serious problem.

Self-limiting illnesses like flus, colds, and earaches are considered acute illnesses. They will heal if left alone, but require remedies to alleviate discomfort and to shorten their duration. The majority of patients I treat in my practice are seeking help with acute illnesses. I have come to expect a healthy child will experience these self-limiting conditions as often as several times a year. With proper treatments, they recover with increased strength and vitality.

Unfortunately, more children than ever are suffering from chronic illnesses, which are ongoing and unable to heal naturally with time. In recent years I have witnessed a dramatic increase in these sorts of conditions—children who suffer from monthly ear infections, severe asthma, allergies, or eczema, or even behavioral problems like Attention Deficit Hyperactivity Disorder. The explanations for the increase in chronic childhood illnesses are complex and often contradictory; the effects on children and families, however, are profound and evident.

Homeopathy and other forms of natural medicine have proven effective in treating both acute and chronic illnesses. For chronic illnesses in particular, the time and attention natural physicians give to emotional, psychological, and environmental factors results in a more individualized course of treatment without the debilitating side effects associated with drugs like Ritalin or Paxil. Acute illnesses also respond well to homeopathy, and this book will guide you in the remedies that are most effective for the common ailments and health issues of infants and children. While parents can act as the first defense in preventing and treating these acute illnesses, chronic infections, illnesses, or emotional/behavioral issues need the expertise of a professional homeopath or other physician. For a large number of everyday illnesses, however, parents should feel empowered to "think naturally" when it comes to treatment options and prevention. This book will start you on your way.

chapter 2

Straddling the Fence: Bridging Conventional and Holistic Medicine

The physician's highest and only calling is to make the sick healthy, to cure, as it is called.

It is 7:30 in the Davis household and time for the evening ritual. Suzie bathes her 9-month-old son, Alec, and following a night-night book and a long hug, she nurses him to sleep. At 2:00 A.M. Alec wakes up screaming in pain with a fever. After a fitful night, Suzie automatically reaches for the phone to call the pediatrician, but stops herself. "After four courses of antibiotics, Alec keeps getting sick. I can't do this anymore."

THIS WAS THE STORY Suzie told me in my office the following day. She is not alone in her frustration with chronic illness and antibiotics. As antibiotic usage has increased, so too has widespread resistance to its effectiveness. Chronic illness among children has increased substantially since the 1970s, despite advancements in medical treatment and the highly publicized new generation of drug therapies and antibiotics. According to Gary B. Huffnagle, Ph.D., an associate professor of internal medicine and of microbiology and immunology in the University of Michigan Medical School, "Antibiotics knock out bacteria in the gut, allowing fungi to take over temporarily until the bacteria grow back after the antibiotics are stopped. Our research indicates that altering intestinal microflora this way can lead to changes in the entire immune system, which may produce symptoms elsewhere in the body." If confirmed in human clinical studies, Huffnagle believes his research findings could help explain why cases of chronic inflammatory diseases, like asthma and allergies, have been increasing rapidly over the last 40 years—a time period that corresponds with widespread use of antibiotics.

As a result, parents like Suzie are beginning to explore different options in healthcare, looking to homeopathy and other forms of alternative medicine to answer their children's health needs. During Suzie's visit, we determined that Alec's fever and pain resulted from an ear infection. Rather than prescribing another course of antibiotics, I recommended *Chamomilla*, a homeopathic medicine for his fever and illness. A year has passed since Suzie's visit, and Alec is a healthy toddler. He no longer needs antibiotics, and the Davis family and their pediatrician get better nights' sleep.

Antibiotics: The Promise and the Problem of Conventional Medicine

Antibiotics, once touted as wonder drugs, are used to treat bacterial infections. Antibiotics have been around since 1928, when Sir Alexander Fleming, noted by accident that a common mold, Penicillium notatum, was capable of destroying bacteria. Scientists found that strains of penicillin could be produced in large quantities, and batches were made and given to thousands of people with war wounds in World War II. It saved many lives and became known as the miracle cure. Common bacterial infections in children are strep throat, bladder infections (UTI), some sinus infections, and most ear infections. Most coughs, colds, and sore throats are viral, so they usually don't respond to antibiotics. But, sometimes complications from viral infections lead to a secondary bacterial infection.

Although antibiotics have been credited with saving many people, success has led to excessive use. The frequent use of antibiotics for a variety of infections (including viral infections), has led to antibiotic resistance, which has resulted in the decreasing effectiveness of antibiotics. Unfortunately, some people are allergic to some antibiotics and experience hives, shock, and other allergic reactions. Certain antibiotics have specific side effects. For example, Augmentin, a penicillin-like antibiotic commonly used to treat sinus, ear and urinary tract infections in children may cause diarrhea, sore mouth, headache, dizziness, thrush, and more rarely, inflammation of liver, kidney, and colon (colitis), and blood disorders.

Antibiotics also affect the friendly bacteria that normally reside in the digestive system. This leads to fungal superinfections, which cause yeast overgrowth and candida infections that might cause diaper rashes or thrush in the mouth. After taking an antibiotic, many people experience relief from their symptoms. This results in a weaker immune system, which leads to a child becoming more vulnerable to illness soon after finishing a course of antibiotics. Not uncommonly, this can set up a cycle of a child becoming sick again and taking an antibiotic month after month.

Antibiotic use has extended beyond the doctors' office. Standard milk, eggs, and farmed fish contain antibiotics that are given to animals to prevent infections and enhance production. Antibiotics have also been used to treat plant diseases in commercial apple and pear orchards, for instance, many consumers are unaware that their children are receiving antibiotics without ever visiting a doctor! For this reason, many families prefer organic food, without pesticides and antibiotics.

Since I've become more aware about general health and natural medicine, I rarely need to prescribe antibiotics, because the holistic approach to treating illness, strengthening a child's constitution and use of remedies usually offers a complete course of treatment. Without any side effects!

Incorporating Conventional with Holistic Medicine

Despite the various approaches and sometimes difference of opinion, parents can incorporate both conventional and holistic medicine in their children's lives. They are not mutually exclusive. Some families employ two practitioners—the conventional pediatrician or family doctor for the well-child visits and regular check-ups, and the holistic practitioner for treating common illnesses, like colds and ear infections, and chronic conditions, like asthma and allergies, so that they can lessen the need for conventional medicine. However, chronic conditions can often become life-threatening; any life-threatening illness is an emergency and should be addressed with conventional medication immediately. In my practice, I insist that all children who have a history of asthma have inhalers and other forms of standard treatment available to them, even though the natural medicines I prescribe are intended to reduce the use of those treatments. Natural and allopathic medicines can also be combined. For instance, natural medicines can be taken before and after a vaccine to prevent side effects.

Patients who are diagnosed with a chronic condition like asthma can incorporate holistic medicine to heal themselves so that they can get off their long-term medications. Homeopathy can be used to control the early symptoms, while osteopathic treatments can free up the chest wall and ribs so that their breathing is easier and more efficient. Over time, they feel that their chest is no longer tight and consequently do not need medications. This philosophical approach can be used for any system of the body: the gut with chronic abdominal pain, diarrhea, or constipation; the neurologic system for headaches and seizures; the endocrine/hormone system for irregular periods and PMS; and the musculoskeletal system for scoliosis, posture, muscle spasms, and sciatica. For any chronic condition, we maintain a safety net of continuing conventional medication while we work to support the patient's constitution, immune function, and structural framework of the body.

Choosing Conventional and Holistic Practitioners

Changes in healthcare in recent decades have transformed the ways Americans both relate to and decide upon their practitioners. With insurance companies taking a greater role in determining available doctors, and doctors themselves specializing in a wider array of fields, many families find they are "shopping" for a practitioner in ways their parents' and grandparents' generations never had to. The situation has its advantages and disadvantages for parents looking for their first pediatrician: On one hand, options abound; on the other, many feel that their doctor rarely has the time to get to know them and their child personally.

Increasingly, parents are turning to holistic practitioners to provide the kind of personal attention and natural therapies that conventional medicine frequently cannot offer. This does not necessarily mean they are giving up their conventional doctor, but rather taking full advantage of the benefits of both standard and holistic medicine. Whether your inclination is toward the conventional or natural or both, the patient-doctor relationship ideally marks the beginning of long and trusted relationship. Your doctor should be able to address your child's changing needs over many years, and come to know your family as people as well as patients. Still, many people choose a practitioner that meets their needs, and with time realize those needs have changed and move on to other doctors. Remember that a doctor-patient relationship should be flexible, able to accommodate your child's growth and development over a number of years.

If you are looking for your first pediatrician, general practitioner, or family doctor, or seeking a new one, your best resource is word-of-mouth: most parents find out about practitioners from people they know, be it friends, coworkers, family, or through local pharmacies, pregnancy and baby classes, the internet, and insurance companies. The process of choosing a conventional or holistic practitioner involves many of the same concerns regarding specialties, methods of treatment, insurance and hours, and availability. When you are inquiring at a doctor's office, don't be afraid to ask questions on the following topics:

Area of Expertise: We seek out professionals because we have expectations that they are knowledgeable in a certain area. Sometimes, I hear my patients complain that their pediatrician prescribed antibiotics and a decongestant, and nothing natural. Be realistic about your expectations. When you go the baker, you get bread. The same is true with the pediatrician—they are trained in pediatrics and prescribe treatments that they know. If you are interviewing someone who is trained in more than one field, such as an acupuncturist who also practices homeopathy, it is important to find out what modalities they would use and when. A common question I hear from prospective patients who want to avoid antibiotics and other standard medications when possible is, "How often do you prescribe antibiotics?"

Attitudes, Opinions, and Bedside Manner: Bedside manner ranks in equal (if not greater) importance as area of expertise. Warmth, a caring attitude, and the ability to listen are important to patients. Patients want to know that their family is viewed as individual human beings, and not just numbers on a chart. A doctor's office staff is an extension of the doctor herself. Oftentimes, the first impression that a patient receives comes from contact with the doctor's front desk assistants. If the practitioner has an extensive office staff, realize that many of your communications, especially on the phone, may be with the staff and not the doctor.

My patients report that one of the most sensitive topics revolves around the vaccination controversies. Some patients report their doctor made them feel stupid for asking about shots, worthless and irresponsible as a parent, or they faced such skepticism that the parent was uncomfortable asking at all. A physician friend of mine recently confided that being put on a pedestal all day and treated like a god makes one tempted to act in kind. Some physicians can be condescending, haughty, and unable to consider other opinions. I encourage you to choose a practitioner that you like as a person, and feel comfortable with: even if he or she may not agree with your opinions, it is important that the practitioner be respectful.

The Office Visit: Doctors are notorious for making you wait and wait and wait—and they get away with it! If your time is limited, try to schedule your appointments at the beginning of the morning or afternoon if you are able to, so that you are one of the first people seen. As much as I try to be timely, sometimes my schedule is held back, and it may even be because a patient has arrived late and I am waiting for them. It is not uncommon, in some doctors' offices, that the wait is longer than the office visit itself. Depending upon the specialty and the physician, most conventional medical offices are set up to maximize the number of patients seen in one hour. Of course, patients are still able to establish a connection with their doctor, but the rush makes it more difficult. Although all holistic practitioners have different approaches, I've found in my experience that holistic practitioners spend more time with patients. In my own office, it is not unusual for my first visit to last nearly two hours—the time is greatly appreciated by patients.

The Office: It is important to know about hours of operation, as some doctors may work twice a week, others six days. The on-call schedule is important as you want to know if and when you can contact your doctor. Especially when it comes to a child's healthcare, parents want to have a reliable practitioner. A general list of concerns include:

- Hours of operation
- Phone availability
- On-call schedule
- Plan B: What do I do in case of emergency?
- Hospital privileges (important for primary care physicians)

Payment: Insurance companies are beginning to acknowledge and reimburse for holistic forms of medicine, and some modalities are now increasingly covered by insurance companies: these commonly include acupuncture, chiropractic, and massage. If your practitioner practices holistic medicine and is a medical doctor (M.D.) or osteopath (D.O.), your insurance may cover part of the visit. Avoid surprises: discuss the financial arrangements ahead of time to make sure the treatments are within your budget. Depending on your complaint and the type of practitioner, the scheduled visits vary greatly. Initially a visit to a homeopath may be every six weeks (and spaced out thereafter), while a visit to an osteopath may be once a week for a month.

Insurance Companies: As a result of rising medical costs, insurance can be costly in the United States. There are different types of insurance to consider. Some families pay out of pocket for insurance and others are given insurance by their employer. There are plans that allow you to see any doctor (in and out of network), and there are other insurances such as health maintenance organizations (HMOs) where you are given a particular set of doctors, and no flexibility. Some HMOs are beginning to employ some holistic practitioners, but this is still rare. Many people interested in complementary and alternative medicine (CAM) usually pay extra for these visits in order to complement their standard doctor's protocols.

chapter 3

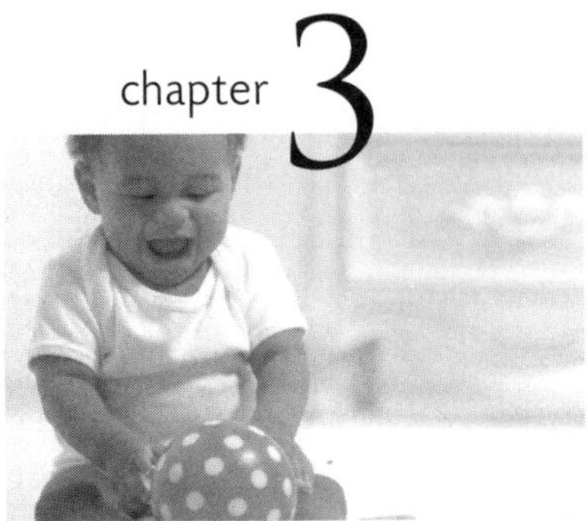

Overview of Natural Therapies for Children

"It is more important to know what sort of person has a disease than to know what sort of disease a person has."

–*Aristotle*

DOCTORS, WHETHER THEY PRACTICE conventional or holistic medicine, agree that maintaining and cultivating health demands more than simply medication. Wellbeing extends from the mind and spirit as well as the body and requires a multi-faceted approach, including:

- Healthy nutrition
- Exercise
- Healthy lifestyle
- Natural medicine and treatments when needed
- Harmony in relationships (work, family, personal)

Although my specialty is homeopathy, I have had the pleasure of learning about and benefiting from every natural therapy presented in this chapter. When I realized that my calling was the holistic health field, I seriously considered many of these fields for a specialty. I was drawn to these therapies because I realized they share a respect for the body's innate wisdom and strive to balance and strengthen the body's own ability to heal. They also recognize the patient as a whole person—body, mind, and emotion—rather than as simply a localized body part, a problem to be treated. This distinction—between the whole health and localized treatment—is one of primary differences between holistic and conventional medicine. From the conventional viewpoint, the child with asthma is ill because of her asthma, while in the holistic thinking, she has asthma because she is ill. Natural therapies look to treat underlying causes as well as manifest symptoms, understanding that those causes may be as much emotional and environmental as they are physical.

Different forms of holistic medicine are not mutually exclusive, and can be used at different periods in your child's growing years. When considering your child's healthcare, keep in mind that some therapies may be more "child-friendly" or appropriate at certain ages. If your child is squirmy and refuses to be touched by a practitioner, then a form of hands-on healing such as chiropractic, osteopathy, or cranial sacral therapy may not be an appropriate treatment at that stage of development. Later, your child may feel more comfortable being touched, as which point these therapies can be revisited.

Homeopathy

When I met five-year-old Sandro, he was covered in hives, a reaction to an antibiotic he had been administered. He was irritable, uncomfortable, and itchy, and while antihistamines, calamine lotion, and oatmeal baths gave temporary relief, they did not solve the underlying problem, his reaction to the drug. I gave Sandro *Apis mellifica* (*Apis* for short), a great remedy for hives as well as bee stings, and he recovered completely—without needing additional medication or suffering side effects.

Apis is derived from honeybees—in fact, from the very venom that causes us to react to their sting—and is a good example of how homeopathy works. Homeopathy is based on the administration of minute doses of drugs, which are capable (in their natural state) of producing symptoms like those of the disease being treated. This principle is known as "the law of similars." In other words, a substance that could cause symptoms in large amounts can heal you in minute homeopathic doses. A common homeopathic remedy, for example, is *Allium cepa* (Red Onion), used to treat runny nose and red eyes from a cold or hay fever—the very symptoms red onion would cause if you were cutting it in the kitchen.

There are over 2,000 homeopathic remedies derived from various plant, mineral, and animal substances. Through a series of dilutions and successions, natural substances are distilled until all that is left in the medicine is their "print," or essence. Just as if you were to touch a pane of glass and leave your fingerprint, so in homeopathy the active agents of the substance remain while potential toxicity is diluted out. The homeopathic process renders natural products non-toxic while increasing their potency, producing a safe and effective treatment for children and adults.

Homeopathy has a long history of treating both acute and chronic illnesses naturally. The scope of this book focuses on providing you with information on how to treat simple acute problems at home. In contrast, the treatment of chronic problems, called constitutional treatment, is based on an in-depth interview in which a homeopath gathers a great many details about your child's current condition, medical complaints, past history, lifestyle, mental and emotional attitudes, past traumas, character, and other relevant information. This information helps a homeopath find an appropriate remedy aimed at treating chronic conditions on a mental, emotional and physical level. Common childhood conditions I treat in my office include:

- Colic
- Thrush
- Teething
- Diaper Rash
- Ear Infection
- Colds/Flu
- Fevers
- Attention Deficit Hyperactivity Disorder
- Skin Rashes

Many people view homeopathy as an alternative, and hence "non-mainstream," form of medicine, but, in fact, until relatively recently homeopathy occupied a central place in American healthcare. In Washington, D.C., only one memorial is dedicated to a physician—the founder of homeopathy, Dr. Samuel Hahnemann. In Hahnemann's time, in the late-seventeenth and early-eighteenth centuries, patients often suffered as much from their treatments as from their illnesses: Standard medical practices included bloodletting, leaching, and mercury poisoning. Early in his medical career, Hahnemann rejected these injurious therapies and shifted his focus to finding a different method of healing. He called his eventual discovery homeopathy.

News of his system spread, and by the early 1800s, homeopathy had arrived in America. Its popularity in the U.S. grew considerably after doctors used homeopathic remedies with great success during the cholera epidemic of 1849. In addition, many people were not only seeing homeopathic doctors, but relying on homeopathic remedies to treat common mild ailments at home. By 1900, there were over a hundred homeopathic hospitals in the U.S. alone. Conventional doctors defended their turf, however. The American Medical Association, or AMA, began in direct response to the popularity and success of homeopathy, and effectively forced this once very mainstream medical practice to the sidelines of U.S. healthcare. Likewise, this same contentious history was also played out between MDs against osteopathic physicians in the 1950s.

For children, homeopathy and other forms of holistic medicine can prove to be safer and more reliable therapies than standard courses of antibiotics or over-the-counter medications. Children's bodies grow and change at an incredibly rapid pace, and part of their healthy development is the fine-tuning of their immune system. Mild acute illnesses like colds and earaches are normal and healthy parts of growing up, and natural remedies allow you to treat the discomfort without interrupting the immune response. For non-serious ailments like these, homeopathic remedies are also safe and easy for parents to administer, saving a trip to the doctor's office and a course of antibiotics. One Friday, for example, my son's preschool called me to let me know that he was sick and needed to be picked up. When I arrived, he was sitting in his teacher's lap, crying and clutching a red and painful-looking ear. I anticipated we would be spending the weekend nursing an earache, so at home I decided to give him *Belladonna,* Mullein-Garlic ear drops, and an onion poultice, and he went to bed early. The next day, to my surprise, he was in good spirits and had no further complaints about his ear.

Stories like this are common in my practice, and demonstrate the effectiveness of homeopathic remedies for children. These substances counteract symptoms, but they do not interfere with a young body's natural inclination to heal itself. Allowing the body to work through all the stages of healing is important at any age, but particularly for children, who are developing the immune systems that will keep them healthy through the rest of their lives. Moreover, the homeopathic approach is child-friendly. Most children love the sweet taste of the remedies.

Herbal Medicine

For centuries, cultures across the world have recognized the healing properties of herbs, and have passed this knowledge through the generations so that it remains a vital force in holistic healing today. Herbal medicine is also known as botanical medicine or phytomedicine, and some of its better known remedies include echinacea, goldenseal, and St. John's wort.

Although they are considered safer than standard prescriptions, herbal preparations can still interact with medications, so always check with an herbalist if you have questions about the safety of using a treatment in conjunction with other prescriptions. On the whole, though, herbal medicine works as a wonderful complement to other treatments and can boost your child's immune system. In Part V, you will find several commonly used herbs to treat conditions for children. Children are more cooperative when herbs are either pleasant tasting or pleasantly concealed; liquid extracts from tinctures or glycerites and teas and infusions from dried herbs are suitable for children.

Gemmotherapy

Gemmotherapy refers to remedies made from the buds or shoots of young plants, distinguishing it from herbal remedies, which are typically made from adult plants. In a sense, gemmotherapy can be considered concentrated embryonic plant stem cells. For example, all the vital substances necessary to sustain a sapling so that it may grow into a might giant oak lies in the bud. While use of human stem cells is controversial, the use of plant stem cells is considered by the FDA as a supplement for ingestion and is not as regulated.

Plant bud therapy (gemma means bud in Latin) began in Belgium in the 1950s, and was clinically tested and introduced twenty years later by a French doctor, Max Tetau, who also gave it its name. Because of its ability to aid in eliminating and draining toxins from the body, gemmotherapy is known as the "chimneysweep" for cells, cleansing them of toxins accumulated from food, air, and water, as well as medications and stress.

The body naturally eliminates toxins and waste products through a number of systems, including the digestive organs (liver, gall bladder, intestines, stomach, and pancreas), the kidneys (urinary tract), the lungs (respiration), and the skin (sweating). The heart, blood vessels, nervous system, and endocrine system (hormones) also help promote optimal cell function. While the body has these natural ways to cleanse itself, sometimes it needs a little help in elimination. This is where gemmotherapy can be useful, since gemmotherapy remedies stimulate the function of bodily tissues and promote elimination. There are over fifty "gemmos" which target different organ systems and their functions. *Briar Rose* is a wonderful gemmo for children, especially during the winter months.

Parents have a powerful, safe, and inexpensive means to support their children's health with gemmotherapy. In our practice, we have often found that children taking gemmotherapies experience less severe sicknesses compared to children who did not take gemmotherapies. This also means that when they come in for an acute illness, we have more time to try other homeopathics and other prescription medications before resorting to strong antibiotics or steroids.

Bach Flower Essences

Developed by the British physician Edward Bach, Bach Flower Essences consist of thirty-eight flower essences that work to gently restore various negative emotional states. Bach Flowers are prepared from wild flowers infused in spring water and are considered safe and natural. The most well known, Rescue Remedy, is a combination of five flower essences meant to be calming for emergency situations. They are preserved in 27% brandy.

Aromatherapy

Scent is a profoundly memory-based sense. Beginning from birth, the sense of smell triggers bonding between a mother and child, and for the rest of one's life, a familiar smell can trigger memories and emotional states that are astonishingly vivid. Aromatherapy makes use of our strong scent memory, utilizing fragrant essential oils extracted and concentrated from aromatic plants and flowers to promote restoration and healing. The chemistry of each essential oil distinguishes its color, potency, and fragrance.

Aromatherapy can be employed externally for children through liquid drops (used in the bath and in creams), sprays, vaporizers, radiators, and in healing applications such as compresses, and is recommended for its calming, antiseptic, and anti-bacterial properties and ability to treat aches, pains, fevers, and diaper rash. Our children's skin, mucous membranes, and sense of smell are more sensitive than adults', so when using essential oils, administer fewer drops rather than more.

If you are not familiar with essential oils, it is best to use commercial and natural aromatherapy preparations designed for children and specified for the bath, diaper care, or for calming purposes. Essential oils can be irritating to your child's sensitive skin and most are not appropriate for babies or children. Straight essential oils should not be used for babies six months and younger, since from birth to six months their skin and mucous membranes of the nose are especially delicate. Best to keep it simple!

If you are buying individual bottles of essential oils, they should be packaged in a dark glass bottle and stored in a cool, dry place. Check our resource section for reputable companies that guarantee pesticide-free blends and avoid oils not specifically prepared for children and babies.

Note from Dr. Hoang: At this time, I do not recommend the use of any aromatherapy for infants and young children. Any substance that has a nice fragrance has in its chemical structure an "aromatic" ring which very easily crosses the blood brain barrier. The brains of infants and children are still developing and any possible interference in the brain's chemistry and physiology is a risk.

Naturopathy

Naturopathy is a discipline that employs a variety of natural modalities to treat and prevent illness and strengthen a patient's overall constitution. Most naturopaths (N.D.s) have extensive training in accredited four-year schools in a collection of therapies that include nutrition, herbal medicine, vitamins, supplements, physiotherapy, hydrotherapy, and naturopathic manipulations. Some also have additional training in homeopathy, Oriental medicine and acupuncture, Ayurvedic medicine, midwifery, and other modalities. N.D.s work both as primary care providers and as specialists, and children respond well to the versatile approaches offered by naturopathic medicine.

Chiropractic

Chiropractic care was developed in America by D.D. Palmer in 1895 and centers on the treatment of the spine and its alignment through a hands-on, manipulative approach. According to the chiropractic theory, misalignment of the spine can lead to irritation of the nerves and may provoke health conditions. While many adults make use of chiropractic care for back, neck, and related strains, few realize it is also safe and helpful for babies and children. Many babies experience stress on the spine during birth and throughout the first year as their backs grow and their spines change in curvature. The common bumps and falls of the toddler years may also contribute to spinal and cranial misalignment. Some chiropractors specialize in pediatrics, sports injuries, and rehabilitation, using additional modalities such as heat and ice therapy, ultrasound, exercises, and rehabilitation therapy. Many of my patients take their newborns and children for gentle chiropractic prevention and treatment of the spine.

Osteopathy

Osteopathic medicine was founded in 1892 by Andrew Taylor Still, M.D. Considered on equal footing with medical doctors, doctors of osteopathy (D.O.) share unrestricted medical licenses and the ability to perform surgery and prescribe medications. The difference is that osteopaths are given additional training in Osteopathic Manipulative Technique (OMT), used for preventing, diagnosing, and treating conditions and injuries. OMT is a gentle hands-on soft tissue technique that can be used for birth trauma, colic, ear infections, muscular skeletal injuries and more. Many osteopaths are trained in specialties like obstetrics and gynecology or family practice, and can be a wonderful additional to a birth team. When our son was just days old, our osteopath treated him preventatively, as birth is considered by many specialists stressful on a newborn's body. I often recommend osteopaths to parents-to-be. Developed by Andrew Taylor Still over one hundred years ago, osteopathic principles and soft tissue manipulative technique focus on improving range of motion, correcting the structure of the musculo-skeletal system, revitalizing tissues, and increasing the movement of bodily fluids. Today, D.O.s use a wide variety of hands-on techniques including myofascial release, Cranial-Sacral therapy, lymphatic work, and soft tissue manipulation.

Craniosacral Therapy

Craniosacral Therapy, a gentle, light touch technique developed by osteopathic physician Dr. John Upledger, D.O., focuses on the craniosacral system, which consists of the structures and membranes surrounding the brain and spinal cord, including the cerebrospinal fluid. It may also act as a preventive therapy for scoliosis, hyperactivity, learning disabilities, and dental problems. Many practitioners have studied and used Craniosacral Therapy and you can find specialists among medical doctors, dentists, osteopaths, chiropractors, naturopaths, physical therapists, massage therapists, and professional bodyworkers.

Anthroposophical Medicine

Anthroposophical medicine is based on the teachings of the Austrian philosopher, Rudolf Steiner (1861-1925) who developed a philosophy that encompasses a specific educational approach, natural medicine, and spiritual philosophy. Steiner's most visible contribution is the Waldorf Schools, attended by children throughout the world and staffed by highly trained teachers (see Chapter 7). The medicinal path incorporates homeopathy, naturopathy, and some allopathic principles, which provide the foundation for anthroposophically inspired remedies, homecare compresses, and poultices (see Chapter 9), as well as art therapy, music therapy, and movement therapy (eurhythmy). The information in this book from the Wellness Nurses is inspired from anthroposophical principles.

Acupuncture and Chinese Medicine

The holistic traditions of Chinese medicine and acupuncture span over 2,500 years, predating modern medicine by millennia. Both are based on the theory of chi, the vital energy which courses through channels in the body. Obstructions to chi or imbalances in energy result in discomfort and disease, and the aim of Chinese medicine and acupuncture is to restore the flow of chi through the body. Practiced extensively in China in rural communities and major hospitals, these disciplines make use of acupuncture (needle treatment), acupressure, cupping, moxibustion (warmed herbs), and Chinese herbal medicine to help relieve a wide variety of acute and chronic conditions. Diagnosis is made after an extensive interview that includes an evaluation and treatment of one's chi energy flow in the body based on pulse, tongue diagnosis, and other factors. In the United States, acupuncture is perhaps the most widely practiced therapy from this tradition. Children can benefit from acupuncture, though it may be difficult to get a young child to cooperate with the use of needles. Some acupuncturists use electric stimulation devices to connect directly to the needle. I do not recommend electric stimulation by electroacupuncture or TENS (transcutaneous electrical nerve stimulation) devices. There are a few lone voices in the medical community expressing concern regarding long-term health consequences of direct application of an EMF generator to the body and there is increasing scientific evidence of the harm of EMFs and health consequences of electropollution of our home and sleep environment. Thus, we should be more wary if it is applied on and into our body. Acupressure, which Acupressure, which does not use needles, is better suited to younger children, as is Chinese herbal medicine—although the taste of Chinese herbs can take some getting used to!

Ayurvedic Medicine

Ayurveda is based on the traditional medicine and ancient therapies of India, and includes use of nutrition, herbs, cleansings, massage, yoga, and astrology. Similar to many other healing practices, Ayurveda recognizes that therapies should address each person individually. Ayurvedic healing takes account of a person's body type, which is based on three basic energies—Vata, Pitta, and Kapha—in varying degrees. Recommendations for optimal health, including daily habits and nutrition, are developed according to these body types.

Whichever complementary course you employ, try that system first for yourself before applying it to your children. Whichever system works for you, you should see sustained improvements in your constitution and your health, decreasing need for medicines, and fewer and less frequent flare ups of a chronic condition. These metrics are part and parcel of a successful integration of conventional and alternative approaches.

PART II

Stages and Ages

When the voices of children are heard on the green
And laughing is heard on the hill
My heart is at rest within my breast
And everything else is still

ALTHOUGH CHILDREN ARE UNIQUE IN THEIR physical, mental, and emotional makeup, they develop in predictable ways and follow general developmental stages. These stages are not a precise roadmap for your child's growth, but they do offer you and your doctor a picture of what to expect at specific ages, more or less. Especially for first-time parents, tracking an infant's development can be an unanticipated source of stress: Doctors, friends, and family are all measuring a baby's progress, leaving the parents often feeling as though infancy were a test a child could either pass or fail. What is most important, however, is not that your baby reaches developmental stages earlier than other infants, but that she progresses according to her own rate and timeline, and is encouraged to explore the world at her own pace. Babies rarely mirror the monthly charts exactly, and if your child has not reached a developmental stage at the expected time, it is not a sign of inadequacy on your part or hers: Your baby is simply progressing according to her internal timeline, rather than one set by the medical establishment.

This part will outline major developmental stages from birth through early adolescence, offering an overview of the physical, mental, and emotional milestones you can expect from your growing child. These years are tremendously exciting, characterized by rapid transformation as your child emerges as a unique individual—curious, engaged, and active. Keep in mind that your child's individuality also means that she will progress at different rates in different areas—she may be physically fearless and socially shy; slow to talk but quick to learn sentences; small at birth or large. Your child's development is a process to celebrate, not agonize over, and both you and your baby will benefit from experiencing learning and growth on your own terms, rather than those of your parents, friends, or the "experts."

chapter 4

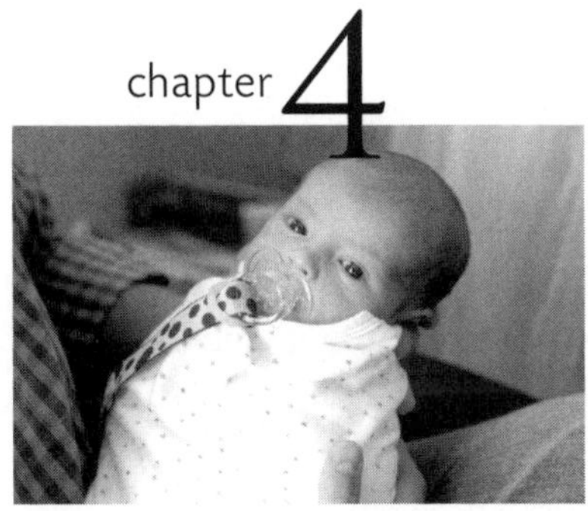

Newborns (Birth to One Month)

It takes a whole village to raise a child.

–African proverb

BIRTH MARKS THE FIRST of so many beginnings for your infant. Each week and even days will bring new discoveries, as your baby encounters its world and develops its personality. When my boys were infants, I tended to focus less on the actual stages of development and more on the enjoyment I took from my day-to-day interactions breastfeeding them, playing with them, and watching them grow. Comparisons to other children are inevitable, though, especially if you are around parents with babies of similar age. Try to avoid becoming emotionally charged; infant development is a process, not a competition. You will always meet another parent whose baby is ahead on skills, sleeps longer, and grows faster than your baby. Early or late development in these areas is no indication of a child's later aptitude, health, or emotional well-being. In fact, being too "results-oriented" about infant development can lead to unhappiness for both you and your baby.

Throughout infancy, your practitioner will help you monitor your baby's developmental progress in three areas to ensure that he or she falls within the guidelines for normal growth.

- Physical indicators of development include movement, muscle strength, and coordination. From fine motor skills (precise hand and finger coordination) to gross motor skills (use of larger muscles in the body, trunk, arms, and neck), your baby's control over her body increases rapidly throughout infancy.
- Mental-cognitive and communicative skills become more apparent as a baby matures. An expanding range of expressions, gestures, and vocalizations indicates an infant's increasingly complex awareness and response to the surrounding world.
- Social and emotional development are also crucial processes throughout infancy. How your baby feels will be communicated through a broadening array of facial expressions, body language, socialization, and vocalizations.

Developmental Milestones

Babies' birth weights can vary by several pounds, and the average weight for term babies is approximately 7 lbs (3.2 kg.). At birth, she may lose as much as 10% of her initial weight by shedding fluid that she does not need. After approximately two weeks, however, she will have regained this weight and will continue to put on ounces rapidly from this point forward. For the first six months of your baby's life, she will gain approximately 0.5 oz (14.2 g) to 1 oz (28.4g) every day.

At birth, your baby's heart will beat at a rate nearly twice that of yours (130 beats a minute compared to your 72), and she breathes nearly three times faster than you do (50 to 60 breaths a minute compared to an adult's 18). Babies' head circumference begins at approximately 32 to 37 cm at birth and increases to 48 cm by two years.

During the first month, your baby will sleep most of the time. She often lies curled up in a fetal position, and her muscles twitch on occasion. Her hands remain in a tight fist and will not hold objects. Her head needs to be supported, though she can lift it slightly for moments at a time. Her sucking and swallowing skills will be progressing smoothly. She is beginning to make eye contact and focus on your face. In fact, she can focus on objects 10 inches away.

Her communication will mostly be cries and grunts to let you know that she is hungry, needs a change, feels tired, or needs comfort. She will have begun to smile, laugh, and coo. During the first month as she begins to know you, she will start trusting her caregivers. She will respond to loud noises and bright lights, and turn toward recognizable voices, like yours. She enjoys your attention as well as skin-to-skin contact.

As a newborn, most of your baby's behavior is reflexive and instinctive—emotional and intellectual responses to her environment will develop later. Beginning at birth and in subsequent office visits, your practitioner will be testing your baby's neurological development. Most of these reflexes probably originate from primitive survival behaviors; they appear at birth and last for varying time periods.

- **Palmar grasping reflex:** If an adult places a finger on your baby's open palm, your baby will tightly grasp the adult finger. Grasp strength should be equal with both hands. This reflex is at its strongest in first two months, and lasts up to six months.
- **Moro reflex** refers to your baby's startle response upon hearing a loud noise or feeling suddenly that she may fall. Momentarily, the baby's arms and legs will open outward, back arched, and then the limbs will return to the chest. This reflex lasts four to six months.
- **Babinski reflex** occurs when the sole of the foot is rubbed from the heel upwards along the little toe side. A newborn's big toe will bend back and toes will splay outwards. It lasts six months to two years.
- **Righting reflex** is elicited when you place a baby on her stomach. In an effort to ensure breathing, she will lift her head and turn to one side.
- **Tongue-thrust (gag) reflex** occurs when an object (other than a breast or bottle) is placed in the back of baby's throat. Automatically, the tongue will push the object out of the mouth. The tongue-thrust reflex is important when introducing solids later on, as it prevents choking. The gag reflex is lifelong.
- **Rooting reflex** is important for breastfeeding: when baby's cheeks or lips are stroked by finger or nipple, she will move her head to that side and open her mouth to breastfeed. This reflex lasts three to four months.
- **Walking or stepping reflex:** When a baby is held upright with her feet touching a table or other surface, she will move her legs as if trying to walk. The reflex lasts approximately two months.
- **Tonic neck reflex** (fencer's position) is elicited when a baby is placed on her back. She will move into a fencing-like position with the head

pointed to one side. The limbs on that side will be straight out and the opposite limbs will be bent. It lasts for six months.

You may also notice soft spots on your baby's head called the fontanelles. In order for your baby to pass through the narrow birth canal, her head bones have to be soft and pliable. As the bones of the head grow, the soft spots eventually come together and close. The diamond-shaped anterior fontanelle in the front of the head closes sometime between four and eighteen months, while the posterior fontanelle, which is smaller is size and triangle shaped, closes earlier at two months. At birth and at early doctor visits, it is routine to check the fontanelles. If the fontanelle is too sunken or concave, it may be a sign of dehydration, whereas bulging in the fontanelles can indicate an infection like meningitis.

Forty-Day Period

The first month is characterized by intense intimacy between you and your baby, and will build the foundation for a strong bond throughout her infancy, childhood, and beyond. At this stage, she is dependent on you for everything—food, shelter, frequent changing, warmth, and love—and by meeting these needs you establish crucial trust and stability early in her life. This first month is part of the forty-day period in which it is recommended that mother and baby spend time together breastfeeding, resting, and bonding.

When I was a child, our neighbor Connie spent several weeks resting around the house following the birth of her children. I was perplexed, since that kind of extended recuperation seemed old-fashioned. It wasn't until my own pregnancy that I learned about the age-old custom of the forty days, which I ended up adopting just like our neighbor and millions of women around the world. If there are other children in the family, this period will encompass family adjustments to the new member. It is said that baby and mom should stay within nine feet of each other during this period. Although it is customary in our culture for friends and family to inundate you with social visits, resist these visitation rights and the obligation to entertain for several weeks. After all, what's the rush? You will always have the opportunity to introduce your baby to the world, but these first weeks together are irretrievable.

The forty-day period can also help ease the transition into parenthood, which can be fraught with overwhelming and often conflicting emotions. During this time, it is important to protect your baby from too much stimulation and to allow mother and family to rest. A good rule of thumb is to sleep when your baby sleeps. Ideally, have friends or caregivers take care of all other activities, such as food preparation, errands, household chores, and helping with other children. In my own experience, giving my baby and me a concentrated period of time together restored my energy, which I needed as I knew I would be going to work soon after. In fact, I have found that women who deny themselves this special period of rest and attachment can end up fatigued for several years. Do the best you can, ask for help when you need it, and be careful not to overdo it!

Doulas

Having support during one of the most momentous experiences of your life is vital. In the past, women were surrounded by other women—a midwife, a mother, and women of the village. Nowadays, fathers are playing a more active role in the birth experience and, along with family and friends, can offer great support during childbirth and in the postpartum period. However, many eager friends and family members may not have the experience to deal with issues during birth, breastfeeding, and the postpartum period. At my first birth, my mother had never seen a birth before, and had never breastfed. She was able to give me support, but not much guidance.

Fortunately for mothers-to-be, professionals are available to offer support during and in the postpartum period. In my mother's generation, women hired a baby nurse to come and help in the first few days and weeks following birth. Today, more parents in my office practice work with doulas, who are trained to support a mother during labor and first days and weeks following labor. *Doula* is a Greek word that refers to the main female servant in a household. Research shows that women who labor with a doula at their sides have lower rates of cesarean sections and forceps deliveries, fewer requests for epidurals, and shorter labors. Doulas are trained professionals in the birth process and postpartum period. Although they do not actually deliver babies, their nurturing presence can enable a woman to smoothly transition into motherhood. Depending on the agreement between the doula and the family, doulas can stay by the woman to make her experience more comfortable, whether it be through massage, reassurance, physical comfort measures, or even assisting with meals and other family members.

Tests and Procedures Following Birth

When I was expecting my first baby, I was led to believe that the greatest hurdle I would face was childbirth itself. After that initial obstacle, the hard work was over and my "bundle of joy" and I could live, I hoped, happily ever after. It was true that childbirth proved a profound experience, accompanied by feelings of indescribable elation as well as weakness and exhaustion. Like most mothers, I was simply glad that labor was finished so that I could hold my baby, but I found, as all parents do, that even the first moments of my child's life brought a number of challenges and decisions. Whether you are delivering in the hospital, at a birth center, or at home, you will be faced with procedures, conditions, and decisions that may seem like distractions from the vital work of meeting your baby. They are important nonetheless, so you will want to avoid surprises as much as possible by informing yourself before birth what these initial tests and decisions will entail. From my experiences as a mother and a doctor, I have found the homeopathic and natural parenting suggestions to be enormously helpful. In this section we will summarize the basic procedures of the first week.

Apgar Score

At the moment you give birth, your midwife or doctor will evaluate your baby using a scale called the Apgar Score. The Apgar scoring system was devised by Virginia Apgar, a doctor and former director of the March of Dimes. It assesses a newborn based on five criteria, each of which is assigned a point value of either zero, one, or two. The numbers are tallied for an overall assessment of an infant's health. Scores are taken one to five minutes following birth.

I am often asked the extent to which the score determines a baby's future. Most babies do not score a perfect 10. The Apgar test is designed for the medical assessment of your newborn baby by your healthcare provider. I encourage you to focus on your baby and bonding, not on the score. When I was giving birth, I remember my midwife telling me, "Okay, Lauren, take out your baby." I do not recall what his Apgar scores were; what I remember instead is my son's strong, warm body and smooth skin as I lifted him into this world.

	0	1	2
HEART RATE	Absent	Less than 100	Over 100
BREATHING	Absent	Slow, irregular	Strong, crying
MUSCLE TONE	Limp, weak	Flexes arms/legs	Active, strong
SKIN COLOR	Blue, pale	Arms/legs blue, body pink	Pink
RESPONSIVENESS	Absent	Grimace	Lusty cry, protest, cough, sneeze

Scores:

7 to 10	Normal
4 to 6	Baby may need suctioning of airways or use of oxygen
Below 4	Requires more medical intervention and observation

Eye Drops for Newborns

After your baby is born, practitioners routinely give newborns a course of antibiotic eye drops, used preventatively for the rare occasions in which a newborn's eyes can become infected during birth. Eye infection in newborns, or *Ophthalmia neonatorum*, can be contracted from an infected mother's birth canal. It occurs in 30% of babies whose mothers have gonorrhea or chlamydia, both sexually transmitted diseases (STD). In those cases the infections cause an inflammation of the eyelid and cornea which appear within two or three days after birth. Gonorrhea has been known to cause blindness, conjunctivitis, and other infections.

Erythromycin ointment is the current standard medicine, replacing silver nitrate, which was common in past years. While the antibiotic ointment is considered harmless by the medical profession, it can cause a baby's eyes to become red or swollen, as well as lead occasionally to infection with the characteristic "goopy eyes." In addition, the ointment can blur baby's vision, which can hamper bonding between parents and baby.

Current research suggests that the routine use of antibiotics to prevent eye infections in newborns may not be necessary. A study by the National Eye Institute concluded that no eye treatment was reasonable for women who tested negative for sexually transmitted diseases while pregnant. If you are planning on using the eye drops, keep in mind that they can be delayed an hour or more in most medical settings, allowing you uninterrupted time to bond with your newborn. Be sure to discuss this with your health practitioner ahead of time.

Vitamin K

Newborns are also routinely given vitamin K at the time of birth. Vitamin K is important for blood clotting, and is produced by normal intestinal bacteria. Since the 1960s, vitamin K has been administered for preventive measures, based on the rationale that newborns normally have low levels of this vitamin until they are able to manufacture it on their own.

Researchers believe that vitamin K deficiency can lead to spontaneous bleeding, known as Hemmorhagic Disease of Newborns (HDN), which occurs in approximately 1 in 10,000 babies. Early HDN occurs in the first 24 hours, classic HDN is from day 1 to day 7, and late HDN from 2 to 12 weeks of life. Early HDN has been linked to mothers who took such medications as anticonvulsants, anticoagulants, or antibiotics during pregnancy. HDN is seen most frequently in preterm infants, low birth weight infants, babies who suffered traumatic deliveries or had surgery following birth (including circumcision), and breastfed babies.

Traditionally, vitamin K has been given as a shot. In the conventional medical community, the general consensus is that that the vitamin K shot has no risks and ensures that any baby who has a predisposition to HDN will be protected. However, controversies have begun to emerge regarding the vitamin K shot. In the early 1990s, several medical papers investigated a link between the vitamin K injections and childhood leukemia. It had been suggested that vitamin K or one of the constituents (which contain synthetic petrochemicals) may increase the risk of childhood cancer. But these studies have been inconclusive.

Although it seems incompatible with the laws of nature that healthy babies would require supplementation at birth, in reviewing the information, it would be sensible to consider giving your newborn vitamin K. As an alternative to the shot, which can be painful and may have other side effects, most of my patients who opt for vitamin K use the oral form. Although most pediatricians administer one dose of oral vitamin K, some clinicians advocate giving breastfed infants three doses of oral vitamin K during the following intervals: first week, between weeks two and three, and at 28 days. Baby formula is supplemented with vitamin K.

Mothers who are breastfeeding may want to eat more foods high in vitamin K, such as dark green vegetables, during pregnancy and while nursing, as research has shown that this boosts the levels of vitamin K in breastmilk. Although breastmilk is low in vitamin K, baby's first milk, colostrum, and mother's hind milk contains higher concentrations of the vitamin. To receive the benefits of vitamin K in breastmilk, mothers are encouraged to nurse unrestrictedly, especially in the first few days following birth, as well as to allow baby to nurse and finish one breast before nursing on the other (in order to receive hind milk).

Neonatal Screen Blood Test

Several blood tests will be completed shortly after your baby is born. At birth, umbilical cord blood is taken to check for baby's blood type and Rh factor. Later, within the first week, the neonatal screen blood test checks for several groups of diseases that are not apparent at birth. In California, they include cystic fibrosis, endocrine disorders, metabolic disorders, hemoglobin disorders, and severe combined immunodeficiency disorder. Several of the specific disorders common in tests in most states are: phenylketonuria (PKU), hypothyroidism, and galactosemia. Different states may have different types of disease groups on their screen. Check with your state health department or ask your obstetrician. Although many of my patients prefer to forego the vitamin K and eye prophylaxis, the comprehensive newborn screen is a state mandated blood test.

Phenylketonuria (PKU) is a genetic disease in which an infant lacks the enzyme phenylalanine, necessary for metabolizing essential proteins in the body. PKU occurs in approximately 1 in 15,000 newborns. A baby born with PKU appears normal for the first few months, but if the condition is left untreated, he or she can become mentally retarded by one year of age. PKU affects all ethnic groups, although it is most common in families of Northern European ancestry. Currently, there is no cure for PKU, though the condition can be managed with a specific diet. Through nutritional management, these children are now able to lead normal lives.

Although rare, hypothyroidism is the most common of the three infantile illnesses that are part of the test. Caused by a low functioning thyroid gland, hypothyroidism (which occurs in 1 in 5000 infants) can lead to mental retardation if left undetected and treated. Symptoms of hypothyroidism in infants can include poor feeding, low muscle tone, a puffy face, swollen tongue, poor growth, constipation, and lethargy. Babies born with congenital hypothyroidism are treated with thyroid hormone.

A rare disorder occurring in approximately one in sixty thousand infants, galactosemia is a familial disease caused by an enzyme deficiency. Early detection is essential to prevent progression to mental retardation, cirrhosis, and growth failure. Symptoms include poor feeding, fatigue, edema (swelling), enlarged liver, and cataracts. Like PKU, galactosemia is treatable by a specific diet.

The newborn screen blood test is done after birth. The baby's heel is pricked and a few drops of blood are taken and sent to the laboratory. It is recommended that the test be performed when baby is older than 24 hours and less than seven days old. As women are often leaving the hospital earlier than 24 hours, some babies are tested too early, leading to potentially inaccurate results. If your baby was tested too early, it is recommended that she be tested again at two to three weeks of age. Since the blood test is uncomfortable for your newborn, have the test done once in the recommended time period. (Hint: Prior to the needle prick, you can prepare baby's heel with warm compresses or hand massage to increase blood flow to the area.) I gave my baby *Ledum palustre* which is excellent for healing puncture wounds, as this test required several heel pricks. (See the *Injuries* entry in Part IV.)

Umbilical Cord Care

At birth your baby will be born with her umbilical cord, which varies in length, attached to the placenta. While in utero, she was nourished through the blood which circulated from placenta to baby via the cord. Ideally, the cord should be cut after all the blood has drained from the placenta and received by baby. This can take as long as ten minutes, and most doctors will not wait the time allotted for most believe this is an unnecessary practice. When baby's umbilical cord is cut, your doctor or midwife will place a clamp around the cord stump. Within several days to three weeks, the stump dries up, heals, and falls off. Most practitioners recommend cleaning the stump with alcohol. However, research shows that no specific treatment is necessary. During this time, though, it is important to keep the area clean and dry.

Avoid submersing your baby in a tub of water. Instead, sponge bathe her as needed and place her diaper turned down below the navel. Clean the cord at least four times a day or as directed by your pediatrician. I used the following protocol with both of my sons and their stumps healed quickly: Apply *Calendula* tincture with a cotton swab to the stump at least four times a day. Use goldenseal powder around the stump following the *Calendula*. You can apply the goldenseal by opening a capsule and sprinkling the powder on the area.

Allow the cord to come off on its own, as bleeding can occur if the cord is pulled off. On rare occasions, the umbilical cord becomes infected and starts to bleed. Signs of infection include redness, tenderness, or foul-smelling yellow drainage around the cord. If you notice any complications, call your doctor immediately.

Circumcision

Circumcision is a surgical procedure that removes the foreskin on the penis. The foreskin, in males, protects the glans penis and the urinary tract. As part of the immune system, the foreskin produces antibacterial and antiviral proteins to protect against infection. Sexually, it is rich in nerve endings and as sensitive as the fingertip, with a greater concentration of nerve receptors than any other part of the penis.

Circumcision is performed in both the Jewish and Muslim traditions. For Jews, circumcision is a sacred pact between Abraham and God that is to be performed on the eighth day after birth. Muslims circumcise later in childhood. In the United States, circumcision became popular in the late nineteenth century to discourage masturbation; by the mid twentieth century, nearly 90% of American boys were circumcised. The United States has the highest rate of circumcision in the world for non-religious reasons, while globally 10 to 15% of men are circumcised.

In 1989, a report concluded that circumcision reduces the risks of urinary tract infections, cervical cancer in women, and sexually transmitted diseases. Many doctors have since dismissed these findings and, currently, the American Academy of Pediatrics recognizes no medical benefits in circumcision. Circumcision prevents neither cancer of the penis, nor cervical cancer in sexual partners, nor sexually transmitted diseases. As a result of these conclusions, fewer boys are being circumcised. Since the late 1960s, circumcision has steadily decreased to 60% presently.

Circumcision is the most common surgical procedure in the United States, and, up until recently, it was also the only operation in which the patient was not given anesthesia. The American Academy of Pediatrics now recommends that boys undergoing circumcision be given a local anesthetic to prevent pain and psychological trauma from the surgery. In the Jewish circumcision ceremony (called a *bris*), a trained *mohel* uses a wine-soaked cloth or local analgesic cream for the ceremony.

During circumcision, a local anesthetic is injected into the base of the penis. The baby is placed on a restraining board with hands and feet securely strapped. Using a medical instrument, the foreskin is mechanically separated from the head of the penis, then placed in a metal clamp while it is being cut. The procedure is painful and your baby will cry. Some parents prefer to not be present at this moment; however, I strongly encourage parents to be there and offer comfort. Anatomically, circumcision can remove as much as 80% of a male's penile skin, including veins, arteries, and nerves. The surgical complication rate is one in 500 and, occasionally, scar tissue may cause the penis to appear disfigured.

It is not uncommon for mothers and fathers to disagree about whether or not to circumcise. Although there is no medical need to circumcise, many parents feel very strongly about having their babies circumcised for religious or cultural reasons. Often, fathers want their sons to look similar to them. My response is, "By the time your son will look like you, he will be a teenager, and he won't want to compare!" Neither of my sons are circumcised. When my son was in second grade, he commented that he looked different than some of his friends and I explained to him that the other boy was circumcised. My brief description of the procedure satisfied his curiosity and he never asked about it again.

If you do decide to circumcise, there are several remedies that can relieve pain and speed healing after the procedure, which are listed in the *Surgery* entry in Part IV. While many herbs and medications should not be used at the time of a surgery, there are no contraindications to using homeopathic medicines after surgeries, including circumcision procedures.

If you decide not to circumcise, you may need to educate your practitioner and family members on how to take care of the foreskin. Many pediatricians and grandparents grew up in an era when circumcision was standard, and it is common for them to not be familiar with care of the foreskin.

Adequate bathing is sufficient for most boys. If you ever notice any unusual redness, pain, or discharge, call your healthcare provider immediately. In addition, the foreskin should not be retracted. According to pediatrician Dr. Paul Fleiss, "A child's foreskin, like his eyelids, is self-cleansing. For the same reason it is inadvisable to lift the eyelids and wash the eyeballs, it is inadvisable to retract a child's foreskin and wash the glans." In babies, the foreskin opens enough to allow for urination. When he becomes older he will begin to retract it himself. Up until puberty, there is no particular age when the foreskin retracts. By puberty, the penis will have developed, and the foreskin will retract.

Jaundice

Jaundice is not uncommon in newborns and is caused by an accumulation of bilirubin in the body. Normally, bilirubin is produced from the breakdown of red blood cells and then excreted by the liver. Infants are born with an abundance of red blood cells, but their livers are still immature, which can cause the yellow pigment in bilirubin to amass in the skin and eyes, giving them a yellow hue. If your baby is just slightly yellow, that is considered normal and should clear up within two weeks. If the yellowish tinge persists or if she is also unusually sleepy or lacks interest in nursing, which can lead to dehydration, you should contact your practitioner, who can give her a heel prick blood test to determine her bilirubin level. Excessively high levels of bilirubin can lead to deafness, cerebral palsy, or brain damage. These abnormally high bilirubin levels can occur if baby is born prematurely or stressed after a difficult birth, if the mother is diabetic, or if the mother and infant have incompatible blood types.

Babies who are breastfed also tend to have higher bilirubin levels than those who are formula-fed. For pediatricians who are not well educated in breastfeeding, the higher bilirubin in breastfed babies can sometimes cause unnecessary concern and they may recommend that a mother temporarily discontinue breastfeeding and give babies bottles of formula in hopes of reducing bilirubin levels. This method, however, has been proven ineffective and may even increase a baby's jaundice. Mothers instead should continue breastfeeding, since nursing promotes bilirubin excretion in the stools. Furthermore, research has concluded that a slight elevation in bilirubin may actually help prevent bacterial infections in newborns, as well as functioning as an antioxidant in the brain.

If your baby is at risk for jaundice, you can try *Arnica montana* as a preventive measure. Numerous other homeopathic medicines, which are covered in the *Jaundice* entry in Part IV, can be used in conjunction with allopathic therapies to treat jaundice. The most common allopathic treatment is light therapy (also referred to as bili lights, or phototherapy). Phototherapy helps break down bilirubin in baby's skin. Phototherapy has been traditionally done in the hospital over the course of one to two days, where the baby is placed naked under lights specifically designed to counteract bilirubin. The treatment can also be done at home using a fiber-optic blanket or band that wraps around the baby. The latter takes longer than the conventional hospital treatment and is more commonly recommended for babies with less severe cases of jaundice. Adverse effects of phototherapy include burns (similar to sunburn), skin rash, loose stools, temperature problems, damage to the retina (if the eyes are not properly protected), and dehydration.

Take the following actions with your newborn to prevent jaundice from becoming a problem:

- Check your baby for any changes in coloring. It is best to observe in natural daylight. Gently press your finger on the tip of your baby's nose or her forehead. If the skin looks pale when pressing, there is no jaundice (this can be done on babies of all skin colors), while a yellow hue indicates jaundice. If this is the case, don't panic! Call your doctor to discuss a course of action to take, if any.
- Breastfeed more frequently. For slightly elevated levels, frequent nursing is helpful in flushing out the bilirubin.
- Sunbathe your baby. Both of my sons were slightly yellow during their first week, so as a precaution, I let them "bask" in the natural daylight. If the weather is cloudy or cold, a blue incandescent light or "grow light" may be used. Place your baby in only a diaper on a blanket next to a closed window in direct light. "Sunbathe" for approximately fifteen minutes, three times a day. Avoid allowing baby to become chilled (through exposure to drafts), overheated, or sunburned and cover her eyes.

Diapers: Disposable versus Cloth

Disposable diapers: the blessing and curse of modern parenthood. In our convenience-oriented culture, disposable diapers are almost universally viewed as an improvement over the cloth diaper of the past. But unfortunately life offers few short cuts, and we will be paying for the health and environmental consequences of our disposable dependency for generations to come: an estimated one billion trees are used yearly to make them, and thousands of tons of disposable diapers pile in landfills daily. Disposable diapers are not recyclable and pollute the earth and groundwater with raw sewage and chemicals.

Before my firstborn, I diligently ordered a supply of cloth diapers from the diaper service. As a staunch believer in cotton diapers, I was proud that my son wasn't in disposables, though we did supplement with them on day outings, while traveling, and occasionally at night. In general, though, we found cloth diapers convenient and easy to use on a day-to-day basis, and rarely found ourselves tempted toward disposables.

Disposable Diapers

The disposable diaper is made of an absorbent cotton-like material produced from wood, which is sandwiched between an outer waterproof plastic layer and an inner liner. The diaper also contains fragrance, dyes, toxic chemicals, and plastic. Disposables can absorb nearly 100 times their weight in water due to the chemical sodium polyacrylate—the same chemical removed from tampons after it was linked to toxic shock syndrome and allergic reactions, and shown to be lethal to animals. Dioxin, a chemical used in the manufacturing process, can cause cancer, liver damage, skin conditions, and birth defects; while diapers do not explicitly contain dioxin, they may still carry residual amounts. Diapers can also be pulled apart and present a choking hazard.

With its super absorbent qualities, the disposable diaper gives the impression of being dry, but it is not magic. The first time I used a disposable diaper, I was confused because it felt dry inside. In fact, a dry-feeling diaper is not the same as a dry diaper. Disposables do not reduce the presence of bacteria from the urine, which is irritating to a baby's bottom and produces ammonia. They also prevent the skin from breathing, trapping the ammonia close to the skin and leading to more diaper rashes. When you evaluate the risks of disposable diapers, it makes sense to use them sparingly because they will be wrapped around your child's genitals for several years.

With all the concern about the environmental impact and health risks of disposable diapers, some companies have attempted to produce a "better" more eco-friendly disposable alternative. When my boys were in diapers, I chose to use these when I wanted to use the disposables. These brands are currently advertising themselves as:

- Chlorine free
- Unbleached
- Gel free

- Natural blend cotton
- Softer feeling
- Hypoallergenic
- No dyes or perfumes
- Latex- and TBT-free (tributyl tin, or TBT, is harmful to the immune and hormonal systems)

Cloth Diapers

Buying and cleaning your own diapers is cost effective, environmentally safe, and nontoxic to your baby. While cotton diapers will always require more effort than disposables, today's options now come in several different styles meant to make diapering easier: flat, fitted, and all-in-ones. The flat diaper is the simple old fashioned cotton square that can be folded to fit around baby's bottom. It is secured by ties, fasteners or pins. These diapers are the most economical and never go to waste. You can also use them as burp cloths, blankies, and, after your child is out of diapers, dish towels and cleaning cloths.

Pre-folded diapers are similar to a flat diaper except that they contain an extra layer of cloth down the center. Contoured diapers are form fitting and are held in place with a diaper cover. Fitted diapers are contoured, with elastic around the waist and leg area. The all-in-ones contain a waterproof outer layer, which makes them the most similar in convenience to a disposable diaper as they does not require an outer diaper cover. The all-in-one is one-stop-shopping. The flat and fitted diapers require that baby wear a diaper cover.

What about the extra work? My patients who are cloth diaper devotees find the few extra loads of laundry simple. "You easily get used to it." Long gone, too, are the days of diaper pins. Although sometimes we clipped the diapers together, the velcro diaper covers held the diapers in place.

Diaper covers for cloth diapers range from inexpensive plastic covers to polyester, nylon, water-resistant wool, and fleece covers. Some mothers add liners and inserts to the cloth diaper for extra absorbency, allowing for longer periods between diaper changes, especially at night or during naps. There are excellent quality diapers made from organic cotton and hemp. Hemp is a natural fiber that is grown without pesticides, It is naturally absorbent, more durable and has antimicrobial properties. This means there is less chance of diaper rash.

Cloth diapers encourage children to toilet train at younger ages since the diaper feels uncomfortable and wet to the skin following urination. Currently, with the ease of disposables, parents also have less incentive to begin toilet training, meaning children will often stay in diapers longer than they have to. My European mother-in-law, on the other hand, toilet trained all her five boys before they were one year old, mainly because it would mean fewer diapers for her to wash. This helps makes cloth diapers more cost-effective than disposables in the long run. Although cloth diapers are more expensive at first, you can save up to $1600 over a 30-month period.

With me working full time and my husband in school, we did not want to spend our free time doing diapers. Fortunately, we were able to use a convenient diaper service that provided the diapers. As our baby grew, the diaper company accommodated us with larger and larger diapers. The procedure was simple: a soiled diaper was placed in a bin and would be picked up by the service on specific days. None of the dunking, washing, or drying of my mother's day. If you are concerned about the risks of disposables but reluctant to give up the convenience, give a diaper service a try. For more information on diaper services in your area and where to find good quality cloth diapers, see the Resources and Further Readings section.

Diaper Changing

It's something of a cliché to tease new parents about the number of hours they will spend changing diapers. While initially awkward and complicated, however, diaper changing will quickly become a habit. To prevent rashes and other change-related hazards, keep in mind the following common sense measures:

- Use an appropriate surface for you and for the baby, usually a flat, preferably firm surface, at a comfortable level for you. To prevent any accidents of falling off a changing table, rolling off a sofa, or scooting off a bed, it is advised to change your baby on a changing pad placed on the floor. There is zero risk of injury done this way.
- Avoid any place that baby could easily roll off or fall.
- Always keep one hand on your baby.
- Avoid allowing baby to put containers, lotions, or diapers in her mouth. In fact, keep all of them out of her reach, as some of the ingredients are toxic. Keep baby busy while you are changing with other interesting child-friendly objects.

The best wipes for baby, the environment, and your pocket book are the homemade versions. Reusable wipes are available as well. Many commercial brands of wipes are filled with irritants and toxins, including alcohol, dioxin, chlorine, and perfumes, and should not be used, especially when your baby has a diaper rash. For babies with sensitive skin, if you must use generic store-bought wipes, use a sensitive skin version and pull them all out into a bucket of water, double rinse the wipes, and put them back in the container.

To make homemade diaper wipes:

- Use a soft cotton cloth (such as the 100% cotton squares sold for makeup removal) or washcloth mixed with water and soap. We kept a spray bottle full of soapy water by the changing table.
- Store dry cloth wipes nearby.
- For outings, place damp cloths premixed with water and soap in a container or plastic bag, or bring a container of soapy water with a supply of cloths. After use, place the wipe in a separate plastic bag.

Diaper Creams and Baby Powders

While we rightly think of our skin as a barrier protecting us from our environment, it is in fact quite permeable, allowing moisture, nutrients, and toxins to pass in and out of the body. The body takes in more chemicals through the skin and lungs than from the food we eat. Because your baby's skin surface area (relative to her body weight) is higher than an adult's, she is particularly vulnerable to her environment. One of the first steps that you can take to avoid harmful contaminants is to evaluate the creams that you rub on your baby's body and bottom.

Diaper creams are meant to be barrier creams, protecting and soothing a baby's bottom from the irritants in urine, feces, and disposable diapers. Typically, I recommend that parents use creams only if needed. If baby's bottom is fine, no need for a cream—less is more! If your baby does need a cream, avoid standard commercial preparations that contain mineral oil, petroleum jelly, lanolin (unless pure or organic), and other chemicals, which can block the release of toxins and cause dry skin or acne. Instead, choose natural healthier versions. Look for the following ingredients.

Lanolin: Used for ages, lanolin is the natural oil found on the wool of sheep (it is also known as wool fat or grease). A natural emollient, it makes skin soft, and is also acquired without having to kill an animal. On the downside, lanolin can be contaminated if the sheep has been exposed to chemicals. Therefore, be careful to look for the pure (ultrapure) variety.

Zinc oxide: It provides a protective barrier on baby's bottom and is safe to use.

***Calendula*:** An excellent healing agent for the skin made from marigold. Effective for treating diaper rash, *Calendula* has natural antibacterial properties and is soothing and antiseptic.

Grapefruit Seed Extract (GSE) made from the seeds and the pulp of a grapefruit works against microorganisms and has bactericidal, antiviral, fungicidal, and antiparasitic properties. It is excellent to prevent and treat diaper rash. In a spray bottle, dilute 5 to10 drops of GSE in one ounce of water, and use as needed on baby's bottom. It can be applied at the same dilution with a cotton swab for thrush in baby's mouth and mother's nipples.

Baby powders are supposed to make baby's skin soft and absorb moisture, reducing irritation and chafing. But as with creams, if a baby's bottom looks good, I do not recommend using anything routinely. If there are instances where you will be using both a cream and powder, apply the powder first.

Talcum powder (talc) should not be used on babies at all, as its inhalation can harm their lungs, causing cough, vomiting, pneumonia, and potentially even cancer. Talc can also contain traces of toxins like arsenic or asbestos. I am amazed that Johnson's Baby Powder still contains talc and fragrance even as the label carries the warning, "Keep powder away from child's face to avoid inhalation, which can cause breathing problems." This is sometimes easier said than done. As of October 2016, three lawsuits against Johnson & Johnson ended with jury verdicts totaling $127 million. Victims were women who claimed daily use of their talcum powder caused their ovarian cancer. Bottom line: avoid altogether any product with talc.

Instead, use cornstarch on a baby's bottom or purchase herbal non-talc powders made with cornstarch, herbs, and essential oils.

Swaddling

When we tell our children to "sleep tight," we are wishing them a sound and secure night, wrapped tightly in sleep's protective cocoon. For this reason, the term also reminds me of the ancient art of swaddling, which binds a baby closely in cloth for the first several months of their life. For nine months, your baby has been tightly enveloped within you, so it is hardly surprising that she will respond well to close surroundings: the feeling of being tightly wrapped is familiar territory for her. Around the world, mothers have recreated this womb-like feeling by keeping baby swaddled or worn in slings for months following birth, and veterans in the art of swaddling claim babies are more content and calmer when they are wrapped in this protective state.

Swaddling can be especially helpful for fussy babies with flailing arms and legs since the wrapped position prevents them from triggering the Moro (startle) reflex, which can upset them even more. It can also encourage a baby to sleep for longer stretches and can help him focus when breastfeeding. For half the day baby can be swaddled, with the duration extending from several months to a year depending on your infant's comfort level. According to pediatrician Harvey Karp who wrote *The Happiest Baby on the Block,* babies are born "too early"—not properly equipped for exposure to the world—and therefore need to live in an imitation womb for at least their first three months of life, which he refers to as the fourth trimester. The paradigm he has developed closely mimics the essence of being in the womb and revolves around the "five S's": swaddling, side or stomach position, shhhh-ing sound (reminiscent of the sound of blood flow in the uterus), a swinging motion, and sucking.

To swaddle your baby:

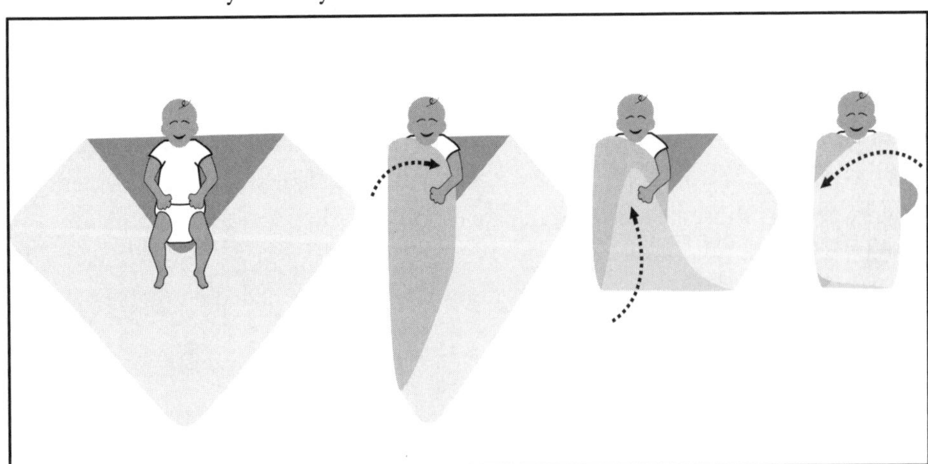

- Place a blanket flat on a level surface
- Fold one of the corners down (6 inches/15 cm)
- Place baby on her back, neck along the fold
- Place her arms by her side
- Lift the left corner of the blanket over her right arm and chest, and tuck it behind her back on the left side
- Then lift the bottom corner over her feet and body and place over chest
- Lift the right corner and wrap it over baby's left arm, and chest and tuck it as far as you can around her back on her right side
- Both arms should be wrapped (though there are variations in which the arms are free)
- Always keep baby's head and face exposed

Babywearing and Carrying

The use of handmade devices to carry a baby is as old as parenting itself. In many cultures, babies are strapped onto parents, allowing parents to keep their baby safe and warm while they work, cook, or walk. Similar to the concept of swaddling, wearing and carrying your baby in a sling simulates the feeling of being nestled in the womb and replicates the natural motions experienced for nine months in utero. Many childcare experts talk about the eighteen-month gestational period—nine months in the womb and nine months without—and the swaddling and carrying of your baby is effective in providing just this kind of extended womb experience. Baby carrying offers benefits to parents and infants alike: studies have shown that infants who are frequently carried cry and fuss 43% less than babies who are kept in a stroller or crib.

In cultures that practice natural child-rearing, most mothers or caregivers carry babies for months before their little feet literally touch the ground. Many parents here, on the other hand, worry that wearing their baby consistently will be an impediment. Often, however, quite the opposite proves true. Newborns worn in a sling are often quiet and unobtrusive company. When Étienne was six weeks old, we were at a friend's party in a restaurant and I was wearing Étienne in the sling. One of the guests exclaimed that she did not realize there was a baby in there until she saw a little hand emerge.

Upright Baby Carriers

Not all carriers are created equal. Nowadays, I see more parents "wearing" their baby; however, many are using upright baby carriers, or harness. You may be surprised to learn upright carriers can be harmful to your baby's spine, leading to back problems. Your baby is born with two normal curves: middle back and base. (The adult spine has four normal curves: neck (cervical spine), middle back (thoracic spine), lower back (lumbar spine), and base (sacrum). In the popular upright carrier, in which your baby is harnessed with her legs dangling from either side, her body weight is being held in her pelvis at the base of the spine.

As with baby walkers and jumpers, the upright infant carrier places your baby is a position where the spine bears all of her weight, a posture your baby is not physically ready to handle. This can influence her back development, and according to chiropractor Rochelle L. Casses, may cause spondylolisthesis (a painful back condition in which the vertebra of the lower back slips out of place). In addition, it places baby's legs in a bowlegged position, and can hinder circulation. The upright vertical carrier can also lead to a whiplash type of injury in the neck if used before a baby has proper head control. Moreover, the front carriers do not allow for a baby to change position. Given the risk of lower back conditions, I strongly urge you to avoid the upright infant carriers, as well as baby walkers and jumpers that place the weight on the base of the spine.

The Sling

My preference for carrying a baby is a sling, used by families for centuries, allows baby to be held in many different positions (worn front or back of the parent, and baby can be facing out or in) and makes it easy to take her in and out with minimal disturbance, especially if sleeping. The baby is comfortably confined in a horizontal or inclined position, and as she matures (around five months), will be ready to begin sitting up in the sling, preferably in a cross-legged position, which helps disperse the weight throughout the legs. The sling can be used up to toddler age.

For infants, the sling is recommended for its versatility and ability to accommodate your infant in a position that is natural for her. Babies who are carried are more involved in the family life, as they are right there in the middle of all the action. Carrying a baby also promotes breastfeeding and bonding.

Just be careful when wearing your baby in a sling. Try to avoid walking through narrow places. Do not drink hot beverages when wearing your baby.

The Backpack

From the time our babies were older and sitting up, we ventured out on hikes with them in tow in the backpack. I even used it around the house, as I found it a comfortable way to keep my sons close while I did other things. The backpack, constructed with a metal frame for support, is different than an infant carrier. Before you use it, your baby needs to have adequate head control and should be able to sit up unsupported. Typically, you can begin using a backpack when your baby is approximately six months old and can continue until she is about four years old (or when she is around 40 to 45 lbs). Our backpack lasted through both of our children. Limitations to the backpack include a lack of eye contact with your child and the fact that your child will only be able to sit in one position.

Backpacks come in all shapes, sizes, and prices, and many can accommodate different toddler weights. Be sure to try it on for comfort before you buy one, if possible with your child in it. My husband is nearly a foot taller than I, but we managed to find a frame that was equally comfortable for both of us. I preferred one with padded straps at the shoulder and waist. Features to look for include:

- **Ease in placing your child in the backpack:** In our model, the backpack could stand upright on a firm surface while I placed my son in myself, without the help of another adult.
- **Comfort for your baby:** She should be able to sit comfortably, her whole bottom supported, with a foot rest for added support and ample arm and leg room. Consider the high-backed padded seat.
- **Good visibility for baby:** She should be able to see to the front and sides.

Bonding and Attachment Parenting

As a child, my mother used to tell me that before I was born I was a twinkle in her eye. To a young one, this made perfect sense. Pregnant women communicate with their babies through a myriad of ways, including song and talk, physical massage and movement, and spiritually through prayer and meditation. Emerging research now validates what mothers have innately known; namely, that the bonding relationship with a baby begins before birth.

This bonding is not restricted to the mother, but also includes fathers and partners. Babies in utero react to their environment: they experience, perceive, and feel emotion in response to those around them. While many parents sense intuitively that their baby communicates with them, conventional medicine has yet to fully explore this deep prenatal connection. As a medical doctor, I was trained to think about bonding in more technical terms, inquiring generally about pregnancy, labor, and delivery. As a holistic doctor, however, I was also encouraged to ask in detail about relationships, emotional states, and any stresses during pregnancy. My own experience as a parent and those of many of my patients make clear that bonding is a process not an event; it starts before your baby is born and continues for the rest of your years together.

The hub of the natural parenting approach begins with bonding, incorporating a wide array of practices meant to foster physical and emotional connectedness. Perhaps the most well known proponents of bonding are the pediatrician William Sears and his wife, Martha, who coined the term *attachment parenting* to encompass the techniques that promote closeness between babies and parents. Their seven attachment tools are:

1. birth bonding
2. breastfeeding
3. babywearing
4. bedding close to baby
5. responding to baby's cry
6. avoiding rigid approaches to baby-rearing
7. balancing one's own needs

The Sears' suggestions are versatile and can be applicable to newborns or can be adapted to a child adopted at one year old. An example of adaptation would be to hold a bottle-fed baby in your arms as you would a breastfed baby.

In the past, fathers and their feelings were often afforded only minimal consideration in the birth and bonding process. Fortunately, attitudes and assumptions are changing, and the father or partner's role is recognized to have a major impact on pregnancy, birth, and bonding. Fathers are playing a larger participatory role in parenting than in previous generations, and the conventional wisdom on bonding now includes a number of ways for fathers and partners to contribute. This includes bottle feeding with breast milk, carrying, and babywearing.

Between mother and infant, the bonding process usually occurs effortlessly in a loving environment, assisted by the intense biological affiliation experienced in the hours, days, and weeks following birth. Sometimes, however, obstacles can interfere. Separation of the mother and baby following a difficult birth, treatment in the neonatal intensive care unit, or postpartum depression all prevent close contact between a mother and child in the crucial period of time following birth. According to researchers, the two hours after birth offer a window of opportunity to enhance the relationship between mother and baby. This sensitive period, called a quiet-alert state, is characterized by a heightened alertness between mother and infant and presents a higher chance of breastfeeding success since the sucking reflex is also strong. Studies show that infants respond to a mother's voice immediately following birth, and that high levels of endorphins are released in both mothers and infants following delivery. Dr. Michel Odent suggests that these natural opiates may foster bonding.

Because these hours can be so important to bonding, you will want to consider this time period when you are preparing your plan for a hospital birth. If you are planning on giving your baby the vitamin K shot or newborn eye drops, consider delaying this for several hours following birth to allow your child to focus on you. Keep in mind, too, that newborns are often sleepy following this period and may not be interested in nursing the first day. This does not mean that you have lost critical bonding time; simply that it will happen later, when your baby is ready to nurse. Despite the research on early bonding, many families achieve strong lifetime bonds even if they are not able to be together right after birth. What is important is that you continue bonding with and nurturing your child for the months and years to come.

SUMMARY

DEVELOPMENTAL MILESTONES

The developmental milestones give you a general overview of child development. However, each child is unique and will go through these stages according to her own physical, mental, and emotional makeup.

Physical: May lose up to 10% of initial weight but will regain it by the first two weeks. Sleeps most of the time. Hands are tight fisted. Head needs support. Sucking skills mature.

Mental: Begins eye contact. Focuses on objects 10 inches away.

Social: Communicates with cries and grunts. Early smiles and coos. Responds to noise, lights, and your voice. Enjoys skin-to-skin contact.

FORTY-DAY PERIOD

For the first forty days, it is recommended that mother and baby spend time together at home to allow time to breastfeed, rest, and bond.

DOULAS

Doulas are trained professionals in the birth process and postpartum period who can help a woman transition smoothly into motherhood.

TESTS AND PROCEDURES FOLLOWING BIRTH

Apgar Score. Evaluates your newborn's wellbeing at one minute and five minutes of life.

Eye Drops. Commonly given to newborns to prevent the eyes becoming infected in the event that mothers have gonorrhea or chlamydia. Currently, many mothers who test negative for these diseases, are waiving the eye drops. If you choose to have the eye drops, delay the procedure for several hours to allow special time for bonding with your baby.

Vitamin K. Vitamin K is recommended by doctors to prevent bleeding but some studies have suggested a controversial link between vitamin K injection and childhood leukemia. Oral vitamin K, given in three doses, offers the benefits without the side effects of the shot. Also, pregnant women and nursing mothers may want to eat more foods high in vitamin K.

Newborn Screen Blood Test. This test is done to rule out rare diseases that can be treated successfully if diagnosed early. An accurate blood test should be done when baby is older than 24 hours and younger than seven days old.

Umbilical Cord Care. The umbilical cord should be clamped after all the blood from the placenta has emptied. It can take up to several weeks for the cord stump to heal. Keep the area clean, and use *Calendula* and goldenseal.

Circumcision. Circumcision is a procedure that removes the foreskin on the penis, originally performed on boys in the Jewish and Muslim traditions. The American Academy of Pediatrics recognizes no medical benefits in circumcision.

JAUNDICE

A slight amount of yellow tinge to the skin from bilirubin is considered normal and should clear up within two weeks. Frequent breastfeeding, sunbathing, and remedies are helpful in flushing out the bilirubin. If it persists or your baby is overly sleepy or does not want to nurse, contact your practitioner regarding treatment options.

DIAPERS: DISPOSABLE VERSUS CLOTH

Cotton diapers have the following benefits over disposables:

- **Health:** Fewer skin reactions and diaper rashes, less likelihood of asthma.
- **Cost effectiveness:** You can save up to $1600 over a 30-month period.
- **Environment:** Cotton diapers and covers can be reused as rags.

In addition to diapers and wraps, you will need diaper wipes and creams:

- The best baby wipes are made from cotton cloth. Minimize the commercial brands, which may irritate diaper rash.
- Use creams only if needed.
- Avoid standard commercial creams that contain mineral oil, petroleum jelly, lanolin (unless pure or organic), and other chemicals. Instead, choose natural healthier topical versions that contain ultrapure lanolin, zinc oxide, *Calendula,* and grapefruit seed extract.
- Use powder, such as corn starch, sparingly, and avoid any preparation made with talc (talcum powder).

SWADDLING

Many claim that swaddled babies are calmer and sleep for longer stretches when they are wrapped. Babies can be swaddled for half the day beginning at birth. Continue for several months to a year depending on your baby.

BABYWEARING AND CARRYING

Babies who are carried rather than placed in a stroller are known to have less periods of fussiness. My preference is to use the old fashioned sling in which baby can be carried in many different positions. Upright baby carriers, baby walkers, and jumpers can be harmful to baby's spine. Another type of carrier, the infant backpack, is suitable for infants older than six months old.

BONDING AND ATTACHMENT PARENTING

Attachment parenting tools suggested by pediatrician William Sears include birth bonding, breastfeeding, babywearing, bedding close to baby, responding to baby's cry, avoiding rigid approaches to baby-rearing, and balancing one's own needs.

chapter 5

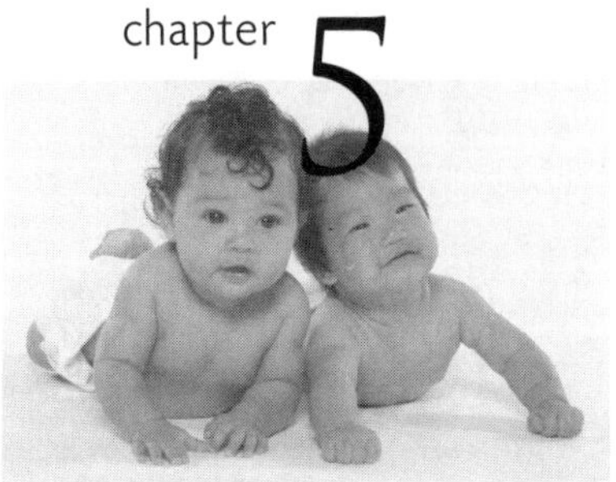

Infants (One Month to One Year)

> You are the bows from which your children as living arrows are sent forth.
>
> –*Kahlil Gibran*

INITIALLY, YOUR BABY WILL RESPOND from instinct and reflex, but as she gets older, her cognitive and mental skills begin to unfold. She will think about her actions before performing them, and her communication will be more specific and discernible—first with cries, and later on with motions, expressions, sounds, and words.

Developmental Milestones

During her first year, your baby's birth weight will usually double by four to five months of age and will triple by nine months to one year old. At two years of age, her weight will be double the weight at five months. Her height will increase by ten inches (25.4 cm) by her first birthday.

By two months, your baby will begin to emerge from her cocoon. Physically, her tight-fisted, flexed body is starting to relax, and she twitches less. She can lift her head 45 degrees, but it remains unsteady. Colic-like symptoms with gas, digestive upset, cramps, and fussiness are common. The quality of her cry differentiates between different needs, whether she wants a diaper change, is hungry, or feels tired. As she is becoming more interested in the world around her, she enjoys visual stimulation such as looking at mobiles, and black and white patterns. She will start to smile and become more interactive with the world around her. At this stage, she is beginning to show interest in you, studies your face, and makes more eye-to-eye contact. She also begins to make cooing sounds—music to a parent's ear.

By three months, your baby will be able to stretch out her body and open and close her hands. She will clutch and shake a rattle longer than before, and plays with her hands, pulls hair, and swipes at hanging mobile objects. When you hold her and allow her to stand on your lap or on a hard surface, her legs will be stronger and push off. When placed on her stomach, she can hold her head higher than her bottom. When held in a sitting position, she is able to hold her head upright. Often her fingers, hands, and fists will be in her mouth, an early sign of teething (although her teeth probably won't come in until five or six months). Cognitively, she is learning about cause and effect—i.e., that when she shakes a rattle, it makes a noise. She will also have made a stronger connection with you. Your baby will smile in response to your voice and will begin to be more vocal, communicative, and expressive. She knows the differences between parents and strangers, and may cry when you leave the room.

By four months of age, your baby has more control of her body when lying down and may begin to roll over from the tummy to the side or back. It is important to be careful where you place baby at this stage, as she is becoming more mobile. Be sure to protect her from falling. At this stage, she gains more control of her head and is able to lift it up to 90 degrees and scan 180 degrees around her. She is able to stand up with support and can sit with her arms propped up. When using a sling, she is now able to enjoy the forward facing position. She reaches and grabs a toy or object with precision, and will be able to follow moving objects with both of her eyes. Her nighttime sleep may begin to increase to six-hour stretches. Visually, baby will now be more aware of colors. She is more aware, responding to stuffed animals, music, picture books, and games like peekaboo. Be careful at this stage to avoid choking and other hazards, as she will begin to put things in her mouth out of curiosity. She recognizes that persons and things have labels, and learns that sounds change when she changes the shape of her mouth. Socially, she can reciprocate with a smile, and may begin to be timid around strangers. She laughs hard if tickled and is learning social gestures, such as greetings.

By six months, she will turn her head in the direction of sounds, roll over (stomach to back or vice versa), play with both hands, and start to use the pincer grasp. If held in a standing position, she will bear some weight on her legs. She is now beginning to sit without toppling over, and once she is comfortable sitting unsupported, she will soon try lunging forward and, later on, crawling. She begins to get up on all fours, and rock. This is followed by movement in the direction of a favorite toy, including pivoting on the belly to a particular direction and scooting. Usually solid foods are introduced around this time, giving baby the chance to sit in a high chair. She can sip from a cup. At this age, she is also beginning to notice small details, and study and point at objects. She can play with one toy at a time, and may bang them. Her verbal skills are more specific, she begins to find her voice (loud and soft), and begins babbling and repeating vowel-consonant combinations (ma-ma-da-da). Through body language and gesturing, she begins to let you know her wants and desires. She is beginning to respond to her name and imitates facial expressions.

Usually by nine months, baby is sitting, making efforts to begin crawling (if she hasn't mastered it already), or trying to cruise (lifting to stand and holding onto furniture). She is more dexterous and can hold a sippy cup or bottle. By this age, most babies have begun solid foods. Her language has graduated to two syllable sounds and she can understand the meaning of the word "no." She is very curious and wants to explore the world around her. She can stack several large sized blocks. She is beginning to enjoy being praised and point to objects that she wants. She reacts to whispers. She plays games like pat-a-cake. This is also the age where she may show separation anxiety. Also, many pediatricians will now routinely check your baby for anemia between nine and fifteen months old. Anemia may occur in babies who were preterm, are formula-fed, or are given cow's milk after one year of age. Symptoms of anemia range from fussiness, low energy, and pale appearance to delayed growth, swelling of the tongue, loss of appetite, and sores at the corners of the mouth in more severe cases. Between 9 months to 1 year, as part of the well child visit, her doctor will check for anemia and lead exposure with a simple blood test. If she is anemic, she will be prescribed an iron drop. Some parents prefer to begin with dietary changes, as the iron can cause constipation. To increase iron, provide healthy foods rich in iron, use an iron pot while cooking, and increase your child's intake of vitamin C. If the condition persists, consider iron supplements.

By the end of the first year, most babies will have mastered cross-crawling, and many will have begun their first step or can walk alone. Her newborn reflexes begin to fade, and she becomes more precise and specific in her motions. She begins to show hand dominance. Cognitively, she will develop the ability to learn and remember. If you leave for awhile, she will comprehend that you exist, even though she does not see you. This is referred to as object permanence. Throughout the year, her language skills increase almost as much as her weight. Like a little sponge, she absorbs the world around her. She enjoys bouncing to music, singing and looking at books. She may begin to say several words and when upset she can have a temper.

Colic

Colic is a commonly used term to describe fussiness, irritability, and crying in newborns. Although the true definition is uncontrollable colic symptoms lasting longer than three hours a day, three days a week, many parents and practitioners use the term "colicky" more loosely in the first few months. Colic usually occurs from three to six weeks of age but can last up to four months. Although researchers are not sure of the exact cause, most agree that it probably is due to an immature nervous system. Babies are subjected to totally different stimuli (and a lot of it!) following birth compared to the warm protected confines of the womb.

Most physical complaints come from discomfort in the digestive system. Symptoms such as abdominal pain, gas, distention, burping, spitting up, constipation, and diarrhea are characteristic. Treatment is aimed at providing relief, so that everyone can get a good night's sleep. Soothing natural measures include carrying, swaddling, babywearing, breastfeeding, infant massage, and homeopathic medicines. Many nursing mothers will change their diet to avoid aggravating the condition. Often parents will comment that just as the colic phase is leaving, the teething one arrives. See the *Colic* entry in Part IV for remedies.

Crawling

Crawling, which typically starts between six and twelve months, marks a major development for your baby, and a major shift in your life as a parent. Prior to this stage, you were in the "driver's seat" when it came to your baby's mobility, steering and directing her moves from location to location. Now, she is more independent and more eager to explore the world around her, but with her newfound freedom comes a greater chance that she could get "into" things. This is the time when you need to begin baby-proofing the house. Locks and hooks can be placed on low cabinets, and drawers; and plugs placed on electrical outlets.

Once your baby possesses enough strength in her arms, legs, and trunk to allow her to sit, she will begin the steps that lead to crawling. If she is seated on the floor and sees a toy or object not within reaching distance, you will notice that she will first try to grasp for it. If unsuccessful, she will then begin to move towards it, first with a forward motion. It is not uncommon that these first motions often result in her toppling over, as the arms and legs want to move, but the heaviness of baby's bottom keeps her firmly planted. She will then begin to move her bottom in an effort to gain momentum as she starts to move forward. Baby begins to fully crawl on all fours after she is able to negotiate the heaviness of her bottom and tummy between her arms and legs.

The crawl has many variations, but the standard is the cross-crawl, accomplished when the left arm and right leg move forward and touch the ground simultaneously in alternating motion with the opposite limbs. Researchers report that the act of crawling on all fours plays a role in developing the brain's network of neural communications, strengthening connections in the corpus callosum where the left and right hemispheres of the brain join together. This network allows the brain to communicate from one side to another and is responsible for coordinating the use of the eyes, ears, hands, and feet. Crawling is a complex physical task: ideally, 50,000 motions are needed for adequate connection of the left and right sides of the brain.

Some researchers believe if crawling is inadequate, learning difficulties such as dyslexia may result. Practitioners have made use of the cognitive and physical benefits of crawling for older children as well, incorporating its motions to help improve learning skills, physical coordination, and focus; the most famous of these systems is known as *Brain Gym,* developed by Dr. Paul Dennison. For your infant, crawling marks a crucial step in linking the body, the mind, and the will, as she learns to assess her environment and move freely within it.

Some parents report that their child simply did not crawl, and instead went from sitting to cruising and walking—and many have no problems. I have found you cannot make a child crawl if she is not inclined to do so. Parents also report that their baby wants to stand all the time. I would discourage you from helping your child to crawl, stand, or walk earlier than they are naturally prepared to. Standing and walking early causes stress loading of the growth plates in the long bones and sometimes the legs are bowed just above the ankle where there is a growth plate. Normal ages to walk vary widely, and will sometimes depend on whether a child has an older sibling she is trying to "catch up with." My older son, for instance, walked at thirteen months, while my younger son began at ten and a half months.

Your Baby's Teeth

At the time of birth, your baby's twenty primary teeth are fully in place under the gums. They developed while your baby was in utero, and consist of ten upper maxillary and ten lower mandibular milk teeth. In addition to their function in eating, these baby teeth (also known as milk, deciduous, or primary teeth) play an important role in developing jaw proportions, talking, and permanent teeth.

Teething

While the teething timeline differs for each child, most babies follow a typical pattern, with pre-teething often lasting months before the actual appearance of a tooth. Often heralded with drooling, a fist in the mouth, diarrhea, fever, discom-

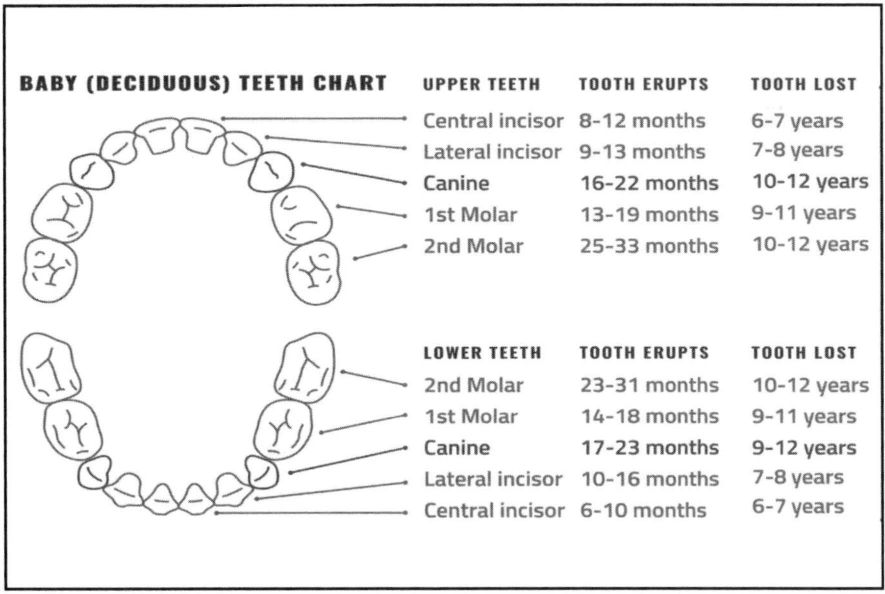

BABY (DECIDUOUS) TEETH CHART

UPPER TEETH	TOOTH ERUPTS	TOOTH LOST
Central incisor	8-12 months	6-7 years
Lateral incisor	9-13 months	7-8 years
Canine	16-22 months	10-12 years
1st Molar	13-19 months	9-11 years
2nd Molar	25-33 months	10-12 years

LOWER TEETH	TOOTH ERUPTS	TOOTH LOST
2nd Molar	23-31 months	10-12 years
1st Molar	14-18 months	9-11 years
Canine	17-23 months	9-12 years
Lateral incisor	10-16 months	7-8 years
Central incisor	6-10 months	6-7 years

fort, fussiness, and difficulty sleeping, teething can be a trying time for baby and parents alike.

At the six-month mark, some babies may have already begun to have teeth, and some not—both instances are normal. By two and a half to three years old, most children will have a full set of milk teeth. When teeth do start to appear, they often do so in groups of four, in upper and lower pairs, with the lower pair frequently showing first in the middle lower jaw. An easy rule of thumb for the teething process is "4 by 4": four new teeth appear approximately every four months. Keep in mind that boys may teethe later than girls. Teething usually begins with the central incisors (lower before the upper), followed by the lateral incisors, first molars (double teeth for chewing), canine (pointed fang-like teeth), and finishes with the second molars.

Brushing the Teeth and Gums

Oral hygiene is in large part a matter of taking preventive measures: brushing teeth and flossing regularly, eating a healthy diet, and visiting the dentist. Unless there is a specific concern, the ideal time for your child's first visit to the dentist is after her primary teeth have come in, usually by two and a half to three years old.

Begin these habits early. Even before the teeth have erupted, you can begin to accustom your baby to the brushing routine by massaging her gums with your finger, a wet washcloth, or gauze. Alternatively, you can use a soft rubber tip that fits on the end of an adult finger. These can help with the discomfort associated with teething and stimulates blood flow in the gums. Once teeth have erupted, continue massaging the gums as well as gentle cleaning of the teeth, by adding an infant size soft bristle brush. Brushing in this early form is more important after your baby has begun to take solids. Drinking water after meals is also helpful.

When my sons were close to two years old, we began "brushing" our teeth together. While I was brushing my teeth, my sons would mimic my behavior; this proved an effective way both to teach them how to brush and to get them excited about doing it by themselves. By three years old, your child can begin to master simple brush strokes by herself. Effective brushing should be done with intention and can take up to two minutes. Apply a pea size amount of toothpaste on the brush; I prefer to use the natural toothpaste brands for children without fluoride, artificial sweeteners and alcohol. The latter dries the gum tissue. Place toothbrush at a 45 degree angle where the teeth and gums meet. With small circular motions, gently brush both gums and teeth. Do this on both the inner and outer surfaces of the teeth. With the toothbrush flat, brush the chewing surfaces of the teeth, as well as the tongue. A toddler's toothbrush should be small for their mouth size with soft bristles, and they should be brushing in the morning and at night before bedtime. Older children and adults should also use soft bristles.

In addition to brushing the teeth, you should also be using dental floss. Flossing cleans between the teeth where a brush is not able to reach, especially those teeth which are in tight contact. It helps prevent cavities and gum disease. Although most children can brush their teeth themselves, in the early years flossing between the teeth requires the skill of a gentle and patient adult. Place toothpaste in the mouth prior to flossing. According to my dental hygienist, flossing without toothpaste is like running the dishwasher without soap. For optimal results, use floss that is wide, flat and waxed for adolescents and adults. Younger children prefer the children's floss with fruity flavors. Cut a piece of dental floss (up to 18 inches in length and less when possible) and gently slide the floss in between the teeth down to the gum line, using both hands. Gently move along the surface of the tooth with the dental floss. Repeat for each tooth. Floss your child's teeth daily. In our home, I find it easier to accomplish this with my children in a reclining position similar to the dentist's chair. Usually by age 12, an adolescent has the dexterity to properly use dental floss and should be encouraged to floss at least first thing in the morning, and after dinner.

Fluoride

A trip to the dentist usually includes a speech on the benefits of fluoride for your children's teeth. For decades, we have heard that fluoride helps fight cavities by strengthening tooth enamel, and in daily life, we receive it from a multitude of sources: in our water and commercial drinks, from fruits and vegetables irrigated with fluoridated water, and from our toothpastes. Fluoride also occurs naturally in vegetables and grains.

A certain amount of fluoride correlates with fewer cavities; however, there exists a narrow range between helpful and harmful levels. Currently, given all our various sources of fluoride, we are ingesting more than safe amounts, making many of us vulnerable to a condition called *fluorisis*. In dental fluorisis, the teeth become mottled, first with white areas and, in more advanced stages, with stains that range from yellow to brown to black. Fluoride meddles with the enamel on the teeth, but it also affects ligaments, muscles, and skin, and is associated with lower IQ levels, arthritis, and cancer. Fluoridated soft water appears to be the most toxic, as it allows more fluoride to be absorbed into the body. Moreover, boiling fluoridated water can increase concentration, making it even more harmful. You can avoid fluoride by using fluoride free toothpaste, drinking filtered water, avoiding fluoridated water (baby formula, sodas and reconstituted juices are often prepared with fluoridated water), and avoiding Teflon-coated pans.

According to many advocates of cleaner water, large corporations were responsible for the propaganda encouraging the use of fluoride for preventing tooth decay. Their motivation could not have been further from public health: they were looking for a means to unload their toxic waste product, sodium fluoride. As a result of their lobbying efforts, many industries now eliminate their waste in our water, legally. New Jersey state assemblyman John V. Kelly's investigation of fluoride in our water in the 1990s revealed that after 50 years, there had not been any clinical trials that demonstrated the effectiveness of ingested fluoride, and it had not been approved by the FDA (Food and Drug Administration), Regarding water fluoridation, Nobel Prize scientist Dr. Arvid Carlsson wrote, "Nations who still practice it should feel ashamed of themselves." Currently many European countries, Egypt, and India no longer allow water to be fluoridated.

Cavities

As a child I never suffered from cavities, so I was surprised when my younger son was diagnosed with several in his primary teeth. Our dentist chose to fill some of the ones with deeper decay. When dentists fill cavities in primary teeth, they take into consideration several factors such as the severity of decay, age of the child, her ability to cooperate, and closeness of the permanent teeth. Unless the primary tooth is within six months of being lost, cavities should be filled, since there is a tendency for cavities to grow and affect the nerve. To avoid cavities, begin with a preventive approach: brush, floss, and visit the dentist regularly. Minimize (or avoid altogether) consumption of sweets and processed foods. Do not allow your baby to sleep with a bottle of milk or juice. According to holistic dentist Joseph Sarkissian, "Do not brush teeth right after drinking sour or acidic drinks [which temporarily deplete the tooth's enamel surface]. Just rinse with water. Nibbling on a piece of hard (non-creamy) cheese (preferably sheep or goat) will re-calcify the child's teeth." In addition, just waiting an hour will allow saliva to remineralize the enamel.

Fillings come in two major varieties: composite and amalgam. The composite filling is made from plastic resin and is the preferable option, while amalgam fillings are made with silver mercury. The mercury in the amalgam fillings is known to be toxic and may release vapors even after it has hardened in the mouth. Pregnant and nursing mothers should also avoid dental work involving amalgam mercury fillings. Mercury toxicity can lead to damage to the brain, kidney and immune system of children. There may also be fatigue, poor memory, psychological disorders including personality changes, irritability, insomnia, and autism.

Introducing Solids

Give her solids and it will help her sleep through the night! Popular wisdom holds that a full stomach will keep a baby satiated and sleepy. When I was growing up, my mom followed doctor's orders and started my siblings and me on solids (rice cereal in the bottle) when we were just a few weeks old. Times have changed! Studies have shown that it is simply not true that full babies are sleepy babies. Nowadays, the American Academy of Pediatrics recommends waiting until at least four months of age, and preferably closer to six months, before beginning solids. Waiting to six months (and sometimes longer) is more suited to your baby's developmental and nutritional needs.

Young babies have young intestines. From four to seven months old, your baby's digestive system will mature in preparation for solid foods, but before this time, the intestine is more vulnerable; beginning babies on solids before their bodies are ready to properly absorb nutrients can lead to allergies. Along with the intestines, infant kidneys are also immature. High protein foods such as cow's milk, if given at too early an age, can negatively affect the kidneys. Not good!

Developmentally, babies are simply not able to ingest solid foods before six months. Have you ever seen a baby "eating"? Especially early on, more food ends up on the face and hands than in the tummy. This is because it takes a certain level of development to coordinate the tongue, mouth, and throat in order to properly swallow solid foods. Up until baby is around four months old, she is developmentally protected from choking by the tongue-thrust reflex that pushes out any object (like a food-filled spoon) placed in the mouth. This strong reflex makes it difficult for a baby to keep food in the mouth. By six months old, this reflex has substantially decreased. Teeth are also a good indicator that your baby may be ready for solids, and most do not begin to appear until at least six months of age.

Also, before four to five months old, baby cannot communicate when she's had enough to eat, which can lead to overfeeding. By six months old, she can lean and move forward to show that she wants to eat, and move back in order to refuse food and give you other signs that imply, "I've had enough!" Ideally, when baby is ready to start solids, she should also be able to sit upright. This developmental milestone typically occurs between five and seven months old.

Most importantly, I encourage you to observe your baby, and take cues from her. She will let you know when she wants to eat what you are eating. Initially, it may begin with a serious stare at your food-filled fork. She will then imitate you. When you open your mouth to eat, so will she. This will be followed by serious motions to grab your food. If baby is ready to eat, she will open her mouth eager for her first bite.

In addition, if your baby is showing signs she is hungry (irritable between meals, wanting to feed more frequently, unsatisfied), and you are not sure if it is time yet, try increasing the frequency of breastfeeding (or formula). If increased feeding does not meet her needs, it may be time to introduce food. Begin slowly and in small amounts—once a day to start. There should be no time pressure as slow and steady is the key to encouraging your child to take solid food. Most importantly, listen to yourself: parents often instinctively know when their child is hungry, and when their child is ready to take the next developmental step.

Feeding your baby is like singing a duet: it takes two. Now that you have determined your baby is ready to begin solids, it is time to make sure that you are ready and prepared. It is not uncommon when you begin feeding for food to end up in every nook and cranny in the feeding area, as well as all over you and your baby. Be practical, situate yourselves in areas that are easily cleaned, and wear clothing that is easily washable.

The Feeding Arena

I take many of my food preparation cues from my husband René, a former chef and athlete from Switzerland. Like his relatives from the old country, his kitchen is his kingdom—I am barely allowed in it. Food meals are prepared freshly, and meant to be pleasing to the eye, palate, and stomach. He stresses that this is as important for a baby as an adult. Not all—or even many—of us have the time or ability to cook like a chef, but we might take some cues from the professionals. Meals do more than make sure we are not hungry: as any chef knows, food preparation is a creative act, a way of expressing oneself and sharing oneself with others.

Mealtime is also a social time for family and friends to come together. Although in Europe lunch is the larger meal, here in America the evening dinner typically constitutes the most important meal of the day. Unfortunately, due to busy schedules, many families no longer have the chance to come together around the table for a family meal. Whether for dinner, lunch, or breakfast, I encourage you to eat together as a family for at least one meal a day. If you begin early, with your baby's first solid food, you can establish rituals that will bring your family together for years to come.

As most children appreciate steadiness, it is helpful to establish at the outset where your baby's feeding area will be. I prefer it to be in the place where the family eats—which I hope is not in the family room in front of the TV. If this is the case for you, as it has been for many couples, it may be time for you and your partner to consider a more traditional eating area, like the kitchen or dining room. If you live in a small space, even setting up a table away from the television will help divide the mealtime from other activities. As you begin to forge healthy eating habits for your baby, you can also do a check-in for yourselves: if you are eating the majority of meals in front of the TV, now marks the perfect time to change the habit.

In the interest of preserving your flooring, you will want to consider also the area in which your baby will be eating. If food would ruin the area (in the case of carpet or rugs), keep it protected with a waterproof covering. If the walls or shelving nearby are worth protecting, do it. Food can end up anywhere. As much as possible, situate your baby's feeding area in a place that is easily cleaned. And don't forget a bib—or a camera. Babies' first experiences with solid food often make for great photographs.

The High Chair

Once you have determined where your family meals take place, it is time to think about the particular needs of your baby. By six months, most babies are able to sit up, and will find this position the easiest and most comfortable in which to eat. Initially, you may have the urge to keep baby in your lap, but this position can often prove awkward. For one, your baby is used to either nursing or taking a bottle from you, and the introduction of food may be confusing from this position.

With your baby sitting on your lap you may also find it more difficult to see her mouth. Consider the high chair when you are ready to introduce solids. The bulky chair will seem like a radical change at the dinner table, but it also marks an important new phase in your baby's development.

High chairs and feeding chairs come in all shapes and sizes, so, before purchasing, you will want to pay attention to adjustable heights, tray size, stability, and how easy they are to clean. If you are buying a new one, consider those with the consumer safety certificates. Hand-me-down chairs have their advantages, but make sure baby is safe: you will want to double check that the baby is not able to slip easily under the tray. The high chair should rest on a stable, level surface, with brakes locked for rolling high chairs. Before using, familiarize yourself with the features of the chairs, including the braking mechanism, adjustments, and straps, and in particular ensure that you are able to easily and quickly remove your baby from the chair in the case of a choking event.

Dishes and Silverware

When my son Étienne was born, our friends gave us a lovely first bowl and plate set in the style of Beatrix Potter. Unfortunately, it was made from china. I decided that this was not suitable for my son's first meal (or perhaps any meal) and, instead, treasure it as a keepsake. In other words, always use non-breakable plates, bowls, and cups.

Use a rubber-tipped infant spoon, small plastic spoon, or your clean finger tip. Avoid using the silver spoon baby gift as it can feel hard on baby's gums, and can also hold too much heat with warm foods or likewise be too cold in baby's mouth.

Digestive Changes

Be prepared for changes in your baby's poop. The consistency, color, and odor, as well as habits, will change. You may even notice fragments of undigested food in baby's stool—not to worry. Binding foods like bananas and rice may be constipating initially. When introducing solids begin with single ingredients and add one at a time. Signs of food intolerance or allergy include spitting up, bloating, gas, skin rash, and extreme bouts of constipation or diarrhea. (See "Food Allergies and Sensitivities" in Chapter 13 for more information about food intolerances and allergies.)

Pacifiers and Thumbsucking

Your baby is equipped with an innate desire to suck. This is most obviously vital in breastfeeding, but the sucking reflex serves a variety of purposes. Sucking at the breast offers feelings of comfort, warmth and love, and also places pressure on the gums, which can be soothing while teething. Sucking that is unrelated to feeding, such as on a pacifier or thumb, is known as non-nutritive sucking.

Considered an essential part of baby paraphernalia, the pacifier is meant to do just what its name implies: pacify your baby when she is agitated or unhappy. It is for precisely this reason that I have always been uncomfortable with pacifiers and chose to not have them around the house when my boys were babies. The pacifier always reminded me of an artificial plastic plug, stopping a baby from expressing what is truly bothering her and distracting parents from the real work of soothing and comforting. I had also heard horror stories from parents whose toddlers would wake screaming in the middle of the night because the pacifier was nowhere to be found.

All too often I see parents use the pacifier as an indirect way to comfort a baby and replace nurturing. In the typical scenario, a baby starts to cry and is immediately given the pacifier to calm her down. Pacifiers often work, but in relying on them, parents forget how much their touch, love, and comfort means to the baby—both in that moment and in the future.

Pacifiers may also cause nipple confusion if used in newborns. Like a bottle nipple, the pacifier requires a different sucking action than a mother's breast and may lead to a baby preferring the bottle and pacifier over the breast. The resulting decrease in milk production makes breastfeeding increasingly difficult for both mother and child. A study found that babies who were given pacifiers by the time they reached six weeks of age showed an earlier rate of weaning. Prolonged pacifier use can also manipulate developing facial bones, leading to crooked upper front teeth, overbites (if used after age two), and an increased likelihood of ear infections.

If you are currently using a pacifier, choose one that is constructed from one piece, made of flexible inert material, has ventilation holes, with an easy to hold handle and a shield that is a minimum of 1.5 inches wide. Avoid attachment cords that could possibly cause strangulation. The pacifier should be large enough that baby cannot swallow it.

One of the best ways I found to pacify my children was to breastfeed them, but if I was too tired or my nipples too sore, especially in the first few weeks, we used other methods of comfort. A clean finger can work for a short period of time, but we found our most effective technique was bodily comfort—being carried in dad's arms or worn in a sling proved immensely soothing to our boys. If your baby still enjoys the comfort of sucking over other forms of pacification, be assured that she will eventually find her thumb. It is a habit that starts early; while still nestled in the uterus, many babies are sucking their thumbs.

According to researchers, sucking causes the brain to release chemicals similar to endorphins, which provide a calming effect. On the downside, thumbsucking, like pacifier use, can lead to orthodontic problems if it continues to three to four years old and beyond. According to studies, statistics show that thumbsuckers were more likely to be bottlefed, weaned on a schedule rather than on demand, and slept separately from their parents.

If your child is already hooked, consider weaning. If you are trying to prevent or cut down on a child's thumbsucking or pacifier use, consider trading the binkie for a blankie. These kinds of gradual substitutions—replacing a comforting thumb or pacifier with another attachment object such as stuffed animal, toy, or special blanket—are among the best methods for reducing non-nutritive sucking. Some parents have success keeping the pacifier out of reach, and eventually "losing" it. Engage your child, so the distraction will take her away from reaching for the pacifier or sucking her thumb.

Cribs, Playpens, and Walkers

Many new parents complain that it is easy to become overwhelmed with all the decision making regarding the latest gadgets, furniture, and baby paraphernalia. From cribs to playpens and walkers, there comes a time, when many realize that most purchases can wait in attempt to keep it simple and focus on breastfeeding, bonding and catching up on sleep.

When purchasing a new crib or obtaining a hand-me-down, you will want to be aware of safety recommendations on cribs. A crib should have a two step lock-release system, and the distance between the mattress and crib slats should be no more than two finger spaces. Older cribs made before 1991 may not meet current safety standards. For information on yours, consult the U.S. Consumer Product Safety Commission at 1-800-638-2772. Do not use a crib if the paint is lead based or if the slats are wider than 2⅜ inches apart. (For more information, see "The Family Bed" in Chapter 11.) Playpens may be useful for short periods of time while a parent or caregiver is unable to fully watch or attend to baby (for instance, while you are on the phone), but they should not replace your attention to your child. When I was pregnant, we were given an old wooden playpen that only ended up collecting dust. We found we were much more inclined to watch our children closely if they played in the same area as us.

If you do use a playpen, play it safe. Use only soft toys and select a playpen that ascribes to high safety standards. As with cribs, these safety guidelines should be advertised by the manufacturer and can be easily researched on the internet or in consumer advocate publications. Avoid wood playpens if the bars are wider than 2⅜ inches (6 cm) lest baby get her arms or legs caught in between them. The newer mesh playpens should have small weave (less than ¼ inch), as the larger holed mesh can catch buttons.

Walkers support a baby's bottom and allow her legs to "stand" and lift off from the floor. Usually baby does not have the body strength or coordination to achieve a standing-like movement on her own, and instead, placed on wheels, she learns to move in a walker before she's ready. This kind of mobility is dangerous, particularly around stairs and places where she can fall. Up to 40% of babies using walkers have suffered injuries. Studies have also shown the use of a walker can interfere with and delay the motor skills important for walking, so I do not recommend them.

Sudden Infant Death Syndrome (SIDS)

Sudden Infant Death Syndrome (SIDS), also known as crib death, is a devastating tragedy for any family. Defined as the unexpected sudden death of babies during sleep, it is the third leading cause of death in infants from one month to one year of age and affects over 2,000 babies a year. The exact cause of SIDS is unknown, but since recommendations were published that babies sleep on their backs or sides (rather than on their stomach), SIDS has decreased over 40%.

SIDS could be due to a variety of different factors. Most cases occur between one and four months of age, during the winter months (and hence during the cold and flu season), and incidence is higher in Native American and African American babies. Risk factors also include sleep position, prematurity, birth defects, metabolic abnormalities, heart rhythms, infection, vaccinations, family history (a sibling who had SIDS), poverty, teen mothers, and maternal tobacco use during pregnancy. Sleeping in a crib also seems to be a risk factor, as the majority of cases occur while the child is sleeping alone. SIDS occurs more often towards the early morning, and boys are more often affected than girls. Most research, however, focuses on the potential relationship between a baby's irregular breathing patterns and the onset of SIDS (see "Your Baby's Sleep Patterns" in Chapter 11). Babies up to six months of age experience periods of apnea (temporary pauses in breathing) that can last up to fifteen seconds. Most babies automatically start breathing on their own, but occasionally the apnea period is abnormally long, and breathing fails to start again.

Babies reported to not be breathing for prolonged periods of time are called near-miss SIDS. Observers of near-miss SIDS report that the infant turns pale, blue, and limp. Usually gentle stimulation like touch will trigger baby to begin breathing on her own, though sometimes a baby requires more drastic measures such as resuscitation. Studies have shown that near-miss SIDS infants wake up less often in the night. According to researchers, SIDS is up to four times higher in cultures, like ours, that promote separate solitary sleep.

The following suggestions may be helpful in lowering the risk of SIDS:

- **Prenatal Care:** Maintain good prenatal care, including avoiding tobacco and other risk factors for premature or low-weight babies. Provide a smoke-free environment after baby is born.
- **Sleeping Positions:** Infants sleep safest on their backs. The side position can be used with the baby's lower arm placed forward to avoid rolling over to stomach. Sleeping on the stomach may get in the way of a baby's normal protective mechanisms of arousal during periods of apnea.
- **Breastfeeding:** Some studies have suggested that SIDS is less common in breastfed infants, possibly because breast milk protects baby from infections that may lead to SIDS.
- **Vaccinations:** Is there a connection between SIDS and vaccinations? According to the Center for Disease Control (CDC), studies show no connection between SIDS and the DTaP vaccine. But a University of Nevada School of Medicine study found more than two-thirds of children who died of SIDS had been vaccinated with DTaP prior to their death. In addition, the National Vaccine Information Center, which was started by families whose children suffered injury or death following vaccination, has tracked other cases of SIDS following the

DTaP vaccine. The first three DTaP shots are given at two, four, and six months of age. This also coincides with most cases of SIDS, which occur between two to four months of age. (For more information on shots, see "The Pros and Cons of Vaccination" in Chapter 14.)

- **Co-sleeping:** Developmental studies revealed that infants' heart rates, breathing, and arousal during sleep are affected by parental sounds, including common sounds during the nighttime such as stirring in one's sleep and breathing. It is suggested that these stimuli aid in a baby's development, and may lower the risk of SIDS in babies. In other words, it may actually be just as important for baby to monitor parents, as it is for parents to monitor babies. When your baby sleeps in the bed with you (also known as co-sleeping), she can do this easily. If you choose to have your baby sleep in another room, consider having a double-way monitor—so that you can monitor her, and she you. (See "The Family Bed" in Chapter 11.)

Working Parents and Caregivers

Like many mothers, I knew soon after my boys were born that I would be going back to work. I was fortunate to have a husband who enjoyed cooking, cleaning, and food shopping for the house, but we still needed extra help in caring for our baby. We wanted to find a nurturing person (or center) who respected the natural parenting approaches that we were beginning to establish: these included use of my breast milk, frequent carrying or wearing, use of cotton diapers, interest in healthy nutrition, and use of natural remedies when needed.

It was also important to me that the caregiver take a class to become CPR (cardiopulmonary resuscitation) certified in the case of choking or another emergency. I highly recommend CPR certification for all caregivers (including parents) working with your children. Ask at your daycare or during interviews with prospective caregivers whether employees are certified or willing to take a class. Schedule one for yourself, your partner, and, if necessary, your caregiver. Classes are also available in Spanish.

Choosing the right person and situation requires a carefully educated decision, so give yourself time to consider several places and people. Parents can find out about caregivers from work, the internet, agencies, and word of mouth. Both of our caregiving situations came from friends I met in my pregnancy yoga class, and I recommend that you ask friends, coworkers, or other trusted individuals for referrals. Most new parents are also constrained by budget. Good child care is not inexpensive, and if you are concerned about affording a nanny or daycare, consider hiring part-time or sharing with another family. Be prepared to interview any prospective caregiver thoroughly.

Daycare and Preschools

Daycare centers and preschools should be licensed by the state, have a low staff-to-child ratio, offer strong and available references, and reflect your priorities as a parent. Consider talking with other parents who enroll children in the program about their experiences and opinions, and trust your gut feeling: If you feel uncomfortable in any way with how the daycare is run, look elsewhere.

Daycares generally come in two varieties: those run in homes by private individuals and those operated commercially in centers. Home daycares are typically run by a mother who established it in order to be able to stay home with her own children. As with any caregiving situation, the quality of the daycare depends on the caregivers, their childcare philosophy, the cleanliness and safety of the environment, and the number of children. Home daycares are often smaller, more informal and flexible than commercial daycare centers. Regulations for home daycare vary throughout the United States. With any type of daycare, it is important to note the staff-to-child ratio. In a small home day care where there may be only one or two adult caregivers, the suggested ratio depends on ages of the children, as infants require more supervision than an independent older toddler. A home daycare should have no more than one 1-year-old, two 2-year-olds, three 3-year-olds, and so on. These guidelines are slightly different compared to a larger formal daycare setting. The American Academy of Pediatrics (AAP) has suggested guidelines for out-of-home child care programs that would allow for a safe, stable, and stimulating environment.

Commercial daycare is not recommended for infants, especially those under one year old. Sometimes, however, a daycare center is the only appropriate option. As with home daycares, be choosy when you are selecting a place: consider staff-baby ratios, the number of children, the activities and environment, and references. The American Academy of Pediatrics recommends that the child-staff ratio be 3:1 for infants up to 12 months old, 4:1 from 13 to 30 months, 7:1 for three-year-olds, and 8:1 for four- to five-year-olds.

Daycares can offer many advantages. Typically they open early and close late to accommodate working parents, and they are often the most affordable option. The other babies and children on the premises allow a child to begin to socialize appropriately for his age. However, this is also daycare's primary disadvantage, since the number of other children means germs are in constant circulation. Children in daycare (and school) pass germs through runny noses, coughing, sneezing, and play, and as a result, infants and children in daycare can be sicklier than those in home care environments.

Home Care

Home care presents the ideal caregiving situation, since your baby stays in her own environment, freeing you and her from the stress of a strange place, multiple caretakers, and numerous other children. The caregiver could be a family member, a hired caretaker who comes to the house, or a combination of the two. A number of families also take part in shared home care, working together to coordinate caregiving across several different homes. One parent might take care of their child and two others one day, alternating with the other parents for the next days. Our first experience with a caregiver occurred as part of a shared home care situation with Suzanne, a friend I met in prenatal yoga class, whose son Alexander is the same age as my son, Étienne. Suzanne had hired two women from Nepal to care for both of our sons. When I went back to work, I would take my son over to her house every day. We recently had a reunion, and both boys are now taller than their original caregivers.

When Étienne was five months old, we hired a nanny to care for him in our home. Fortunately, she stayed with us for years, and though both of our sons are now school age and we no longer need her, she is godmother to our younger son and still part of the family. Our situation is unusual in this regard, but many parents find that a nurturing caregiver becomes an integral part of family life and can play a large role in children's emotional and intellectual development and health.

When we were interviewing prospective nannies, I naturally wanted a caregiver who enjoyed children and was responsible and nurturing. I also wanted someone I implicitly trusted and enjoyed being around. These qualities often take some searching, so if you are looking to hire someone to come into your home, take your time with the interview process. Make a list of your needs, your approach to parenting, and your priorities beforehand. Be thorough in checking references and inquiring into background and experience. This person is about to become a second parent and your thoughtful decision is of utmost importance.

Some parents worry that private caregiving will isolate their children from playmates their own age. It was only after we started working with our nanny that I realized quite the opposite was true, and that my son would soon be meeting other children in the neighborhood. In our area, most nannies are Spanish-speaking. This meant that when she and Étienne went to our local park or took a walk near the house, they encountered the other local children and their nannies. Soon they began to establish a large social gathering of similar-aged children in the area, and on certain days some children would come to our house and vice versa. When my son Quentin was little, we had five to eight children and their nannies over our home every Tuesday for a potluck lunch and afternoon of play. They enjoyed themselves immensely—all sixteen of them.

Family Care

Family care encompasses a variety of situations in which a child is looked after by someone in the immediate or extended family, either in the home or elsewhere. In some families, parents have flexible hours, part-time jobs, or work out of the home, allowing one parent to take care of baby while the other is gone. As often as not, the stay-at-home parent these days is dad, a big change from my parents' generation when fathers were generally less active in childcare. Many families also combine family care with daycare or hired home care as an effective form of budgeting. A baby might be looked after by dad one day, grandma the next, and a nanny the day after that. As you are planning childcare options, think creatively. Often combining strategies allows for a mix of childcare situations that fits both your budget and priorities.

Grandparents and other extended family can be wonderful regular caregivers if they live nearby and are willing. My parents enjoyed babysitting, for instance, but were not able to commit as caregivers. If this is the case, be sure to still take advantage of your parents' wisdom, affection, and experience, since most children benefit from knowing their family's culture, traditions, and heritage and will bask in the warmth of a grandparent's love. I was fortunate growing up with my grandparents nearby, and share many lovely memories with all of them. In general, however, the notion of an extended family has fragmented over the years so that grandparents, aunts, uncles, and cousins often live in different parts of the country, making the traditional practice of shared childrearing increasingly rare.

Keep in mind, though, that family care can have its disadvantages as well. Parents have confided that some grandparents were not willing to follow their instructions—many grandparents enjoy the role of spoiling the child and sometimes allow too much television or sweets. A grandparent's age, too, might make it difficult to "keep up" with the rambunctious energy of a child. As a rule, evaluate a family care situation as you would any other. Does the caregiver meet your requirements for nurturance, safety, childrearing philosophy, and availability? If not, don't be afraid to seek your primary help from another source.

Resource for Infant Educarers (RIE)

The months following the birth of a child can be a heady, exhausting, and, for some women, lonely time, as she is separated from her usual routines and social outlets. Fortunately, numerous mommy-and-me groups have sprung up to provide parenting instruction, physical activities, and social interaction for new parents. Soon after my own kids were born, I joined groups with other moms that I had met in my prenatal yoga class.

One such parenting approach is RIE (pronounced *rye)*, an acronym for Resources for Infant Educarers. RIE is based on the philosophy that "from the day they are born, all infants are cared for with respect and are seen as unique individuals with surprising capacity to participate in relationships." According to one of the founders, educator and infant specialist Magda Gerber, the word *educarer* encompasses an educational approach that espouses, first and foremost, respect for the infant. For example, parents are taught that prior to picking up baby, first tell the infant of the intention and wait for the child to respond. The RIE approach seeks to provide a safe and nurturing environment that encourages the child to become a self-learner with the freedom to explore her world, initiate her will, and become an active social participant. You can read more about RIE in *Your Self-Confident Baby: How to Encourage Your Child's Natural Abilities—From the Very Start,* written by Magda Gerber and Allison Johnson.

SUMMARY

DEVELOPMENTAL MILESTONES

Your baby's birth weight will usually double by four to five months of age, and triple by one year old. Her height will increase by ten inches (25.4 cm) by one year old.

TWO MONTHS

Physical: Tight body and fists relax. Lifts head 45 degrees. Colic-like symptoms are common.

Mental: Cries for different needs. Enjoys visual stimulation (mobiles, black and white patterns).

Social: More eye contact, social smiles, and cooing sounds.

THREE MONTHS

Physical: Stretches out body. Swipes at objects. Rolls back to side. Holds head up. Early teething symptoms.

Mental: Learns cause and effect. Begins vowel sounds.

Social: Responds to your voice. Knows difference between parents and strangers.

FOUR MONTHS

Physical: Rolls over from tummy to side or back. Lifts head 90 degrees. Stands with support. Reaches for objects.

Mental: More aware of colors. Recognizes labels. Mouth changes shapes for different sounds.

Social: Reciprocates smile. Timid around strangers. Gestures for "pick me up."

SIX MONTHS

Physical: Rolls over. Plays with both hands. Uses pincer grasp. Sits unsupported. Solids introduced.

Mental: Notices small details. Uses loud and soft voice. Babbles and repeats, "ma-ma, da-da."

Social: Communicates through gestures. Responds to her name. Imitates facial expressions.

NINE MONTHS

Physical: Comfortably sits. Crawling stage. Holds sippy cup. Stacks several blocks.

Mental: Uses two syllable sounds. Understands meaning of words, "no."

Social: Enjoys praise. Reacts to whispers. May show separation anxiety.

ONE YEAR OLD

Physical: Mastered crawling, or has begun to walk. Shows hand dominance.

Mental: Increased ability to learn and remember. Develops object permanence.

Social: Enjoys music, songs and books. Exhibits a temper when angry.

COLIC

Colic, an extreme irritability that usually occurs from three to six weeks, is probably due to an immature immune system. Treatment is aimed at soothing and providing relief.

CRAWLING

Crawling, which begins between six and twelve months, is a complex physical task which is important for learning skills, coordination, and ability to focus. Now is the time to babyproof your home.

YOUR BABY'S TEETH

By six months of age, some babies may have their first primary teeth while others show signs of teething, which include drooling, fist in the mouth, diarrhea, fever, or fussiness. By two and a half years old, most children will have their full set of teeth—ten on the top and ten on the bottom.

Massage the gums and gently clean the teeth as they come in. By three years old, your child will be able brush her own teeth but flossing must be done by a parent. For toothpaste, use the natural brands for children without fluoride, artificial sweeteners and alcohol.

If your child suffers from decay and requires fillings, composite fillings are preferable over amalgams, which can be a source of mercury toxicity.

INTRODUCING SOLIDS

Although most babies are ready to begin solids by six months old, breastmilk or formula still remains your baby's main source of nutrition. Watch for signs that include staring at your fork, imitating your feeding gestures, and grabbing for food. Begin slowly and in small quantities. Make sure you have a high chair, nonbreakable plates, bowls, cups, rubber-tipped infant spoon, and bib. Change in stools, constipation, diarrhea, spitting up, and gas will not be uncommon.

PACIFIERS AND THUMBSUCKING

Pacifier use and thumbsucking can lead to nipple confusion, increased ear infections, and orthodontic problems. To wean a child from non-nutritive sucking, substitute another attachment object, and keep her busy and distracted.

CRIBS, PLAYPENS, AND WALKERS

Cribs should have a two step lock-release system, and the distance between the mattress and crib slats should be no more than two finger spaces

Wood playpens should have bars narrower than 2⅜ inches. Mesh playpens should have less than ¼ inch weave.

Walkers can cause injury and delay the motor skills important for walking, so I do not recommend them.

SUDDEN INFANT DEATH SYNDROME (SIDS)

Could be due to a variety of different factors. To lower the risk of SIDS:

- Maintain good prenatal care. It's especially important for the mother not to smoke.
- Place infants on their back to sleep.
- Breastfeed.
- Have your baby sleep in your bed.
- If you choose to have your baby sleep in another room, use a two-way baby monitor.

WORKING PARENTS AND CAREGIVERS

Working parents have a number of caregiving choices, including daycare, home care, and family care. Daycare centers, not recommended for infants under one year old, should be licensed by the state; consider staff-baby ratios, the activities offered and safe nurturing environment. Be thorough in checking references for daycare, nannies, or babysitters.

chapter 6

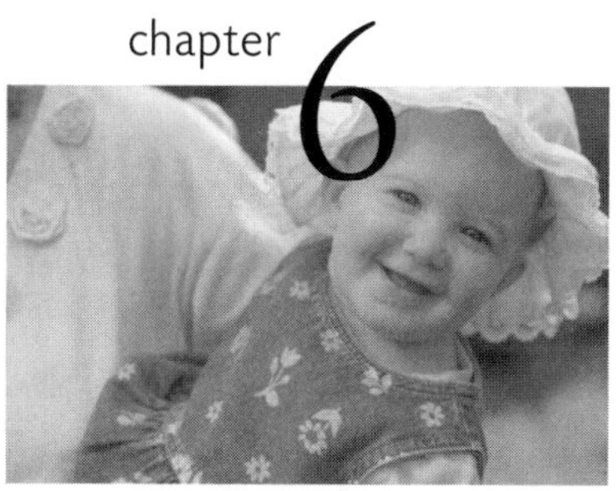

Toddlers (Ages 1 to 4)

Nothing dries sooner than a tear.

–*Benjamin Franklin*

Developmental Milestones

The one-year mark is a special one for parents. In addition to celebrating the anniversary of your baby's birth, you are now leaving her first year, along with all the challenges, rewards, and surprises that accompanied it. As my grandma Janet used to say, "It's amazing how much fuss we make over such a small person!" Your small being is now a toddler, by definition a child who is beginning to walk. Twelve months marks a big leap into toddlerhood; your baby is moving, communicating, and growing in unprecedented ways.

One Year

By one year, your baby will weigh from 17 lbs to 27 lbs and be 27 to 32 inches long. There is a wide variance in physical skills: most babies are able to sit unsupported and are probably crawling, pulling to stand, and may have begun to walk (normal range is from nine to seventeen months, with an average fourteen months). As she becomes more mobile, she begins to lose some of the baby fat around her face and tummy and becomes more muscular and lean with increased activity. She will open her arms to allow you to put clothes on her, and is able to finger feed herself. On a good night, devoid of teething or other complaints, your baby may sleep from 11 to 13 hours a night. By this time, she is taking solids, and may be enjoying up to three meals and two snacks a day.

Cognitively, she is beginning to make specific sounds like ma-ma or da-da and is starting to imitate words. She may even have a few intelligible words in her vocabulary. At this point, she starts to remember experiences—this will manifest by repeating newly learned skills, such as throwing a ball. As toddlers become older, their learning expands to connect words with a certain object; the word "ball" will be associated with the object. She is beginning to make simple yes-no gestures with the head. She will also begin to use objects, such as utensils, properly—many one-year-olds in my office enjoy coming behind my desk and picking up the phone or using the cups in my child's kitchen to "drink" from.

Socially, she is more able to express her preferences, both for familiar people and for toys. A stranger knows where they stand with her, for at one year old she can timid or friendly. She likes to imitate motions, sounds, and people, and is beginning to show an interest in picture books. She laughs at funny pictures or behaviors.

One and a Half Years (18 Months)

By 18 months old, most toddlers have mastered walking without support. She has the dexterity to take off her shoes. At mealtime, she is able to hold a cup herself, drink from it without spilling, and feed herself.

She is able to say or repeat up to 20 words. During playtime, she can sort shapes of blocks. This period can be a rollercoaster ride of emotions for both toddler and parents. Toddlers can be quite obstinate, and persistent in trying to be independent. They insist on their ability to perform certain tasks, and can become extremely frustrated or angry if not able or allowed to. Often these struggles end in fits of tears.

Because of her increased capacity to remember, your toddler may experience separation anxiety, believing when you leave that you will not return. With age comes easier separation; in the interim, this anxiety may be comforted by offering an object such as a blanket or stuffed animal. Toddlerhood also brings an increased sense of possessiveness. When my children had difficulty sharing, I put away any object or toy that my sons would not be willing to share when guests came over.

Two Years

At this age, your child's activity level is extremely high. However, a child's ideas about the world are often illogical and limited by the inability to understand other points of view. Unlike the first year, which boasts huge strides in growth and height, a second-year baby may only grow 3 to 5 inches (7.6 cm to 12.7 cm) in height and add 3 to 5 lbs (1.4kg to 2.3 kg) in weight. At two and a half years old, children are considered one half of their height as an adult. Two-year-olds show tremendous strides in physical ability and coordination. Most can walk and pull toys behind them, go up and down stairs with support, run (usually after your child has been walking well for six months), kick balls, and climb up furniture.

By two years old, your child's vocabulary is rapidly expanding, potentially to as many as 20 to 55 words or more. She has a greater command of her language, may be piecing together three-word sentences, or even be able to say her first and last name. Of all the skills, however, language milestones can be the most variable. If your child is taking longer to talk, it is generally not a cause for concern. They are able to categorize and sort objects by color or by shapes, and some enjoy reading picture books, while others prefer to help around the house. Each child is active with her or his own interests. Your child's social interactions may include parallel play, in which children play beside each other, but not with each other. At this stage, children begin to understand time concepts (later vs. now) and show an increased appreciation for how others feel. Tasks that seem simple and trivial to an adult can be extremely frustrating. So it will help to keep both a sense of compassion and humor as your child asserts her selfhood for the first time. Bouts of frustration can lead to tantrums as your child enters the "terrible twos."

Three Years

By age three, children have all their primary teeth and many children by now are of toilet training age. Gross motor skills, including running and jumping in place, and fine motor skills such as dexterity continue to solidify. She can pedal a tricycle.

Cognitively, three-year-olds are able to recite name, how old they are, and their gender. They understand most conversation and speak in four to five word sentences. Some are beginning to show an interest in the alphabet and counting. They hold a pencil in writing position, and draw with crayons. Imaginative life is rich and varied, and they enjoy playing with puzzles. They tend to experience less separation anxiety and can show affection with playmates. They may have difficulty with a change in the daily schedule.

Four Years

Four-year-olds are now riding a tricycle or bike with training wheels. They can catch balls and throw overhand. They can recognize colors, draw a stick figure with three parts, and use scissors. Their speech is intelligible, and they can recount stories and sing songs. They know basic rules of grammar. As their imaginations and fantasies expand and grow more active, children at this age also begin to acquire fears, like monsters in the closet. A four-year-old has difficulty differentiating between fantasy and reality. They like to play dress up and "mom" and "dad." In general, they are more independent.

Five Years

By age five, they can dress themselves, and physical skills include hopping, swinging and performing somersaults. With greater independence, most can dress and undress unassisted. At mealtime, they are able to use forks and spoons and, in some cases, cut with a knife. Cognitive skills have grown by leaps and bounds. They can recognize many letters, count up to 10, and often know their address and phone number. Language and verbal skills expand rapidly and their speech is understood by most strangers. They are able to write several letters. Drawing skills now include a person with head, body, arms and legs.

Socially, children still enjoy imaginative play but are now distinguishing reality from fantasy. In their activities, five-year-olds still feel at the center of their universe, and parents can help nurture their imaginative play. While recent decades have debunked a number of sex-based assumptions about boys and girls, this is also the age when children begin to play according to gender: boys tend toward more physical activities (e.g., with balls), while girls are more often involved in social types of play.

Babyproofing

As your baby becomes more mobile, you will need to anticipate both her growing curiosity in the world around her and her expanding ability to reach objects and cover distances she hasn't previously been able to. If you have not babyproofed your house already, doing so during the toddler years is crucial. Because every home presents its own opportunities and dangers, you will want to assess its potential hazards as well as the places where children can safely play and explore. In some houses, every room becomes the setting for the toddler playroom. Since we socialize a lot in our home, I preferred to have rooms set aside for kids, saving our living and dining room for my husband and me. While the choice of décor was still child-friendly in these rooms, they were not used on a daily basis for the family.

Babyproofing your home allows everyone to live a little more comfortably, and cuts down on the need to constantly say "no!" Many parents tell me that their child is attracted to handling anything that is not appropriate for her, so be sure to put away any dangerous, irreplaceable, or valuable objects. When our boys were of toddler age, we found it necessary to keep items on tabletops away from the edge (more than twelve inches or thirty centimeters) where they could be easily pulled off. We also babyproofed cupboards and drawers that we did not want our boys to open, and instead offered a drawer and cabinet space set aside especially for them. It contained mostly non-breakable plates, cups, spatulas, and containers that they could use, bang, and play with.

For toddlers, life is a constant adventure. Although their intellectual and cognitive skills are developing at a fast pace, children at this age usually respond more to a fearful parent's scream than a wordy explanation of the risks and dangers of the crossing the street, handling a sharp object, or touching a hot stove. Recently in my office, a mother recounted how, when her rambunctious eighteen-month-old son rushed toward a busy street, she screamed so loudly that the frightened boy ran immediately back to her. While a sudden warning can be effective, in more calm moments children are likely to begin to understand repeated words that connote danger, such as "hot," "pointy, "ouch," and "hurt." One day when my husband was baking in the oven, he taught our toddler about the word "hot." René repeated "hot" and "ouch" as they both touched the warmth of the outside of the oven. The lesson was both safe and effective in teaching our son the meaning of the word.

Babyproofing begins with you. By examining your house carefully for any potential dangers, you can effectively babyproof your environment on your own, though professional enterprises are also available for parents who want an outsider's eye. Hot pans, hot liquids, and knives should not be within a child's reach. As soon as your toddler can stand, make sure objects are more than twelve inches from the edge of a table where she will not be able to get to them. Household cleaners are notoriously toxic, so keep them in a latched cabinet, high above ground level. Because we live in earthquake country, Southern California, all of our upper cabinets are latched to prevent dishes and glasses from falling. In general, though, you will probably find that you will want to keep your baby out of most drawers and cabinets, so make it a rule to keep them latched, too.

Babies have drowned in toilets and even pails of water, so I recommend keeping all toilet lids latched and pails and other containers empty of water. Swimming pools, too, should be adequately enclosed to protect wandering babies.

Keep your medications and vitamins in an upper cupboard. Although homeopathic medicines are safe and nontoxic, it is prudent to keep them out of reach as well. Faucet water in the sink, bath, and shower should be not too hot, and all electrical outlets should be covered. Pay attention as well to cribs, toys, playpens and all other objects that your child will be exposed to regularly.

In all of these environments, your baby or child should ideally not be left unattended. One way to avoid hazardous situations for your toddler is to create places and activities that evoke her curiosity while still being safe. If you see your toddler headed toward a potential problem, quickly redirect her attention to something equally or more interesting.

Tantrums

Tantrums come in all shapes and sizes, just like toddlers. Considered a normal stage in their emotional development, tantrums allow young children an outlet for expression, and more specifically, for expressing their frustration. For some children, stormy moods are a rare occurrence and for others tantrums can manifest several times a day. Heightened levels of frustration can begin as early as one year old, but are more common around age two (hence, "the terrible twos") and into the preschool years.

Many children go through a phase in which they exercise aggressive behavior, including biting, hitting, pulling hair, and kicking. These kinds of physical displays can coincide with temper tantrums or meltdowns, which may have your child kicking and screaming on the floor, often in the most inappropriate public places. Needless to say, this phase is unpleasant for both child and parent.

Tantrums and difficult behavior can stem from a myriad of causes: hunger, fatigue, illness, new environments (daycare, caretaker, or home), over-stimulation, stress in family relationships, natural tendencies, and medications. Tantrums, aggression, and chronic destructive behaviors are often a manifestation of a child who is not feeling good. They may not be sleeping well from poorly controlled eczema, may have had a recent head injury causing headaches and personality changes, or any number of physical complaints. Consider having your child evaluated for a medical condition that may need to be addressed. For abrupt changes following injuries, we often have patients come in for osteopathic treatment and counsel parents that the first thing that must be improved is their sleeping. Depending on the duration of the behavior, the child will need to "catch up" on the lost sleep. We advise parents to let their child rest and sleep, even allowing them to skip a meal to catch up on sleep. The behavioral changes are often evident within a week of catching up on sleep. See Chapter 11 for more information on sleep. Some parents who bring their children to my office with physical complaints like chronic coughs or eczema also reveal in the course of the interview that the child's disposition has been problematic. Often parents are surprised to learn that aggressive behaviors can be linked to other physical symptoms and that homeopathy is able to address biting, head banging, and impulsiveness at the same time that it can relieve other physical ailments like eczema. For practitioners in the holistic field, a child's mental and emotion states are never separate from their physical complaints—we treat the totality of symptoms, rather than focusing on one aspect of health in exclusion to all others.

Many childhood experts agree that tantrums are a natural part of your child's development, and offer a healthy means to clear blockage in her mental and emotional sphere, allowing her to think clearly again. Tantrums, in other words, work something like emotional detoxification. On the other hand, some tantrums will not be relieved until the triggering condition, such as hunger or fatigue, is alleviated. By paying attention to these types of triggers and your child's early warning signs, you may be able to ward off a number of tantrums. Employing a routine nap schedule and providing healthy snacks if meal time is not appropriate are two of the best ways to avoid common tantrum triggers. If tantrums are manifesting as a more chronic behavioral problem and interfering with your child's relationship to peers, self, and family, consider seeing a holistic practitioner in your area.

Disciplining a child's tantrum is never an easy task—it requires patience, firmness, and a clear sense of boundaries for both you and your toddler. All children need boundaries; their limits offer a sense of safety and security, provide a gauge for inappropriate and appropriate behaviors, and protect a child from danger.

Establishing boundaries with your child means also establishing boundaries for yourself, being clear about what is and is not acceptable behavior around you. Avoid, therefore, quelling a baby's tantrum with an adult tantrum. Both of you will expend a lot of unnecessary energy, and you will likely find yourself less able to deal positively with the next episode. It is better to stay calm, and offer a soothing but firm approach. Avoid giving in to her whims and desires, but choose your battles wisely—if your child is inconsolable and you are not in a position to deal at length with her, save your energy. There is little use in reasoning with a screaming, shouting child who will not be able to hear you anyway. Although your child needs to be educated about her actions and their consequences, also realize that at her stage of development she is not able to control her impulses, and that this will soon pass.

On a practical level, it is important that your child is not in danger of hurting herself or anyone else when in the midst of a tantrum. Once the toddler's safety is established, parents have been known to take a number of approaches, including reinforcing appropriate behavior, redirecting or distracting the child with a toy, game, or something of interest to look at, and reassuring her that you are there. It may also help to allow your child to let off the steam, and wait for her to calm down on her own accord. Consider also a timeout approach—one minute for every year of age—including a brief explanation as to why the timeout is necessary. Often parents are able to recognize the early cues leading up to frustration, and can redirect before it escalates by nursing or cuddling a frustrated toddler. As their vocabulary and verbal skills improve, toddlers will be better able to verbalize their feelings as well, making this proactive approach a more viable possibility for parents.

Whichever approach feels most comfortable to you, it is best to be consistent in your responses; as we all know, however, our responses differ depending on the time, location, and occasion. The way you address a tantrum home will be different than if you are in the middle of a birthday party. At home, some parents allow their child the space to express themselves, whereas on the street the child may hurt herself and the tantrum may need to be contained and redirected. During a tantrum parents can do the following:

- **Stay calm:** Avoid losing control yourself—it gives your child the upper hand.
- **Avoid triggers of tantrums:** Make sure your child is getting adequate naps and food.

- **Stagger errands and household chores:** Instead of planning on two hours of errands, consider going on shorter errands with intermittent breaks geared towards your toddler.

Dr. Harvey Karp, author of *The Happiest Toddler on the Block*, claims that toddlers are like uncivilized, primitive cavemen. In order to work well with one, you need to learn her language and communicate at her level. For this very purpose, Karp developed "toddlerese," a language that consists of sounds like grunting and shouting, overstated expressions, and verbalizations that match the child's state of emotion. He groups children 12 to 18 months as chimpanzees, 18 to 24 months as Neanderthals, 24 to 36 as cavekids, and 36 to 48 months as villagers. Initially embarrassing to learn and use, toddlerese, according to a number of parents, can greatly diminish tantrums. If you feel this is not your style, at least it is good to be aware of Karp's different stages of toddler hood.

Toilet Training

When my mother was young, it was the style to have a baby toilet trained by age one, a goal that seems ambitious by today's standards. Currently, our culture typically follows the child-led toilet training method, which relies on the child's own desire to use the toilet. When our boys were toddlers, we kept a potty for them around to encourage them; I was never one to force them to use it, and as a result we rarely had an accident. I have, however, witnessed parents and children forcing the issue too early, only to result in disappointment for all involved. For all children, though, accidents do happen and learning to cope with them when they do is one of the keys to successful toilet training.

In general, girls tend to toilet train earlier than boys. Many parents begin by allowing a child to walk around the house naked, so that he or she makes the connection between the urge to use the toilet and the consequences of doing so. Toddlers show readiness to use the toilet from as early as eighteen months to over three years old, with an average age of two and a half years. You will know your child is ready when she is uncomfortable in a soiled diaper, interested in the potty, and wanting to wear big-child underwear. She is aware of bodily functions, expresses an interest in simple dressing and learning to use the potty, and will be able to stay dry for one to two hours. Often a parent will sense when their child needs to use the toilet by body language, posture, and expression, and can help her use the toilet properly.

By encouraging proper use of the toilet rather than discouraging mistakes, you can set yourself up for success. Avoid toilet training during times of stress, like a move, travel, birth of a new sibling, family problems, or illness. Cloth diapers generally prompt toilet training earlier than disposable diapers because urine is not absorbed and therefore more readily felt as soon as your child has urinated. According to some, cloth diapers can speed up the toilet training process by five months to a year earlier. Although I prefer to let the child toilet train at his or her own pace, summertime may be a better time of the year for the mere fact that children wear less clothing in the summer and can hang out in training pants around the house. Toddlers generally train with bowel control first in the night, then in the day, after which they acquire bladder control in the day, and last at night.

Daycare and Preschool Germs

As we discussed in the previous chapter, daycare or preschool is a reality for many working parents of infants or toddlers. Once your child enters a daycare or preschool setting, whether it be at someone's home or a commercial venue, she will be in regular contact with other children—learning valuable social skills, making friends, and, unfortunately, coming down with their illnesses. Without a doubt, your child will get sick more often in daycare than if she were at home, particularly if the facility supervises a number of children or has a low staff-to-child ratio. While home care may be ideal for preventing illness, it is rarely practical for parents. Fortunately, there are measures you can take to lessen the frequency of your child's illnesses and ensure her safety and health. If your child is continuously sick, however, consider enrolling her in a daycare with fewer children, which will reduce her exposure to germs.

The daycare or preschool will have protocols for sick children that usually encompass the following conditions. Not all illnesses will keep your child home from daycare, but do be aware of the symptoms of common daycare conditions and treat your child accordingly. For more information on specific illnesses and symptoms, see Part IV.

- Diarrheal illnesses can be contagious and daycare centers have been known to foster outbreaks. Infectious diarrhea is not to be confused with the diarrhea that accompanies teething: it can be frequent, explosive, and tinged with blood or mucous, and can occur in conjunction with nausea, vomiting, and fever. If your child has contracted infectious diarrhea, he or she should be at home with preventive measures against dehydration.

- Pinkeye, recognizable by a telltale bloodshot and goopy eye, usually requires your child to be quarantined until you pick her up. Pinkeye is often confused with a "cold" in the eye, which manifests as simple drainage from the eye without it being bloodshot. The latter can be a result of a cold, sinus infection, or allergy.
- Colds, coughs, and fever are not considered as menacing as diarrheal illnesses and may not result in your child being sent home. In my son's preschool, I saw lots of children with runny noses and coughs, especially during the cold and flu season. But if your child is not feeling well and running a fever, keep her at home.
- Allergies can be confused with colds, as both will present with similar symptoms: a runny nose (usually clear in the case of allergies), sneezing, itchy eyes and nose, and even wheezing. (Wheezing can be dangerous and should be treated by your practitioner). Unlike colds, allergies are not contagious and your child can attend daycare.
- Vomiting and the accompanying nausea will leave your child feeling weak and uncomfortable: this is always a good reason to keep him or her home.
- You may receive a notice from your school or program that a child has head lice and to watch your own child closely. These parasites are commonplace where numerous children are in close contact. They are contagious and if your child has contracted them, you will need to treat her before she can return back.
- Chickenpox is a highly contagious viral infection, and will quickly make the rounds in a daycare, preschool, or elementary school classroom. Both of my boys contracted chickenpox while in elementary school, and they each stayed at home for about a week.
- Impetigo, a bacterial infection, appears often on the face as a crusty golden-colored rash. It is contagious and your child will need to be treated before returning back to daycare.
- Caused by a fungus, ringworm is not considered as contagious as impetigo or chickenpox and is not a cause for dismissal from daycare.

While many parents do not have options other than the commercial daycare setting, certain common sense measures can help boost a child's immune system and ward off a number of the illnesses that frequently circulate.

- At home, make sure your child is eating a healthy diet low in sugar and dairy and high in organic fruits, vegetables, and whole grains. At many standard venues, however, this diet is not always an option. Be aware that you can and should give caretakers specific dietary instructions and even healthy foods to ensure that your baby is receiving adequate immune-boosting nutrition.
- If you are still breastfeeding, keep breastfeeding and pumping while your child is in daycare. Mother's milk is full of nutrients and living organisms that help strengthen your baby.
- Use herbs and remedies as needed for strengthening, preventing, and treating conditions that arise.
- Minimizing the use of medications and antibiotics to cases in which they are absolutely necessary. Ultimately, they weaken and suppress your child's natural immune responses.
- Make arrangements ahead of time, in the likely event that your child will eventually get sick. Know who will pick her up and where she will go.
- Frequent hand-washing is considered effective in stopping the spread of bugs. Traditional washing, including soap, warm water, and a vigorous hand rub followed by rinsing and drying, is considered preferable to the antimicrobial soaps, which can increase antibody resistance. Caregivers should wash their hands after changing diapers, wiping a runny nose, and before handling food, while children should wash their hands before eating, after using the toilet, and after outdoor play.
- Your home and daycare should be clean and dry. Bugs tend to germinate in warm, moist, unkempt areas.
- When you are selecting a daycare, interview the caregivers extensively regarding their illness prevention measures, dietary plans, hygiene and cleanliness, and safety procedures. (For more information on daycare see "Working Parents and Caregivers" in Chapter 4.)

Learning Disabilities

The numbers of children diagnosed with learning and behavioral disorders have vastly increased in recent decades. Most research has been inconclusive as to the causes, however many of the families in my office practice are convinced the blame lies with the vaccines. While more generally, factors such as environment, poor nutrition, pollutants, antibiotics, and changes in family life have all fallen under suspicion as possible causes.

Learning disorders are known to affect 30% of children in the United States, according to the Scripps Howard News Service. Affecting more boys than girls, national trends mirror poorer academic achievements amongst boys, according to the United States Department of Education. As a result, there has been an increase in dropout rates in boys. A learning disability may affect a child's ability to speak (including speech delays), write, read, and calculate in math. In addition, the child's performance may include difficulty with organizing and integrating the subjects being learned. Children with learning disabilities may also be diagnosed with attention deficit disorder, hyperactivity, developmental delays, dyslexia, auditory processing disorder, visual disability, Asperger's syndrome, or autism.

Attention Deficit Hyperactivity Disorder (ADHD) is also known as Attention Deficit Disorder (ADD) or Hyperactivity. The behavioral symptoms of ADHD are grouped under three main categories: inattention, hyperactivity and impulsivity. These traits may manifest in such difficulties as organization, procrastination, restlessness (body and mind), and impulsivity. Compared to a child who is normally rambunctious or spirited, children with ADHD consistently have difficulty controlling their behavior which can affect school, family life, and relationships.

A child with dyslexia may have difficulty with mathematics, reading, writing or spelling. Specifically there may be confusion with right side versus left, writing letters and numbers backwards, as well as hardships with organizational skills. Dyslexia is known to run in families and can affect children of any intellectual capability. Often these children excel in other areas such as the arts or sports and have learned to compensate and become successful in their careers and lives.

Auditory Processing Disorder (APD) refers to a condition in which a child is not able to readily discern the subtle differences between sounds in words. Words such as "lead" may be understood as "letter." In APD a child has difficulty processing in the brain what is heard despite having normal hearing tests. In school this may affect the ability to listen to instructions, understand the class material, and follow multiple-step directions. This often results in behavioral difficulties and poor academic performance.

Some children with vision problems have been diagnosed with a learning disability. Visual tracking problems are complex and can be due to problems in the visual pathways, including convergence and visual processing. Like APD, the vision tests may be normal. Visual tracking problems are diagnosed by a specialist in developmental optometry. According to the American Optometric Association over 90% of children who have reading problems have vision problems. Often the child has been diagnosed with a learning disability, which may include attention deficit disorder. Signs to look for include wandering eye, squinting, clumsiness, and confusion between right and left. The child has difficulty with reading, spelling, and may confuse or reverse numbers and letters. Because of this, the child can easily become frustrated, disorganized, and may be unable to sit still. Once diagnosed, the child is treated with a multidisciplinary approach including vision therapy.

Autism Spectrum Disorder, including Asperger's syndrome, has also increased by epidemic proportions in the last thirty years. Autistic symptoms vary, however it usually is characterized by a child's withdrawal from people and surroundings. Many parents report that their baby or child was fine and either suddenly or gradually began to withdraw from parents and their environment and regress in their developmental skills physically, mentally, and emotionally.

Often, these children have special needs at school. For many, these difficulties become obstacles which prevent them from realizing their full potential. The current conventional approach involves parents, teachers and health professionals to include long-term plans and goals that are specific to the needs of the child. Treatments may employ different therapies (occupational, physical, behavioral), counseling, educational methods, and various medications. Some parents are beginning to include natural treatments such as dietary changes, vitamin supplementation, homeopathy, Chinese medicine, chiropractic, naturopathy, and osteopathy.

Birth Order

Occasionally I will hear one of my parents describe their second child as the "typical middle child" or their firstborn as a "classic oldest child." What do these designations mean? Many of us are familiar with the theory of birth order and its guiding influences on one's behavior in the family and in life beyond. Birth order is not destiny—it is only one of countless factors that shape personality—but research confirms that being an oldest, middle, youngest, or only child impacts self-image, familial behaviors, and future goals. Theories of birth order tell us less about individuals, however, than about trends, and help us identify the particular challenges and opportunities presented to siblings depending on when they were born. Parents should attempt to help each child to see herself as an individual and avoid comparisons with siblings or others. Birth order reminds us that our children are different, possessing their own strengths as well as weaknesses, and should be encouraged to blossom into their full possibilities and unique potential.

The oldest, middle, baby, and only child comprise the four categories of birth order. With families that number more than three siblings, the order begins anew with the fourth child.

Firstborns are the responsible ones—they are known to be dependable, duty-oriented, mature, dictatorial, nurturing, perfectionist, high-achieving, and independent. My grandfather, the eldest of fourteen children, was the first to come to America and begin a life, eventually bringing the family over from Europe, one by one. Older children often bear the brunt of their first-time parents' anxieties and over-protectiveness, making them both cautious by nature and highly ambitious. It is not uncommon for many goal-oriented adults to be the eldest child of the family. Academically, firstborns tend to score higher on standardized tests and in school, though this does not mean they are more intelligent than their siblings—they simply care more deeply about those kind of measurements. Older siblings can also be prone to jealousy. My mother reports that I became jealous at three years old when my sister was born. The first child in my family, I was accustomed to being the center of everyone's attention and wasn't pleased to have to share it with someone else.

The middle child comes from a family of three children and has the difficult role of being born after the oldest and before the youngest baby. For younger siblings, the first child may be a hard act to follow and, to them, life can seem unjust. In my practice, I commonly hear that the middle child lacked attention compared to her two siblings, sometimes leading her to become the problem child. But because middle children often fall between the attention-seekers in the family, they can also be more independent and show particular strengths in playing the role of the go-between or mediator. They learn to adapt, and because they experience less pressure compared to their elder sibling, they are known to be more at ease.

The youngest child tends to be the most babied. Often parents who were strict disciplinarians with the elder siblings have mellowed out by the time the baby has come around and are more lax, tending to give the youngest more freedom than her older siblings. As the baby of the family, the youngest may feel that no one takes her seriously, but she is also demanding of attention and known to get her own way. Youngest children often follow creative pursuits and enjoy being center of attention.

Only children are like little adults from an early age—as the recipient of their parents' energies, both positive and negative, they enjoy and expect to be the focus of attention. They can be independent, but because they have not had to experience the joys and pains of sibling rivalry, they are not known to share as easily and can be self-centered, used to getting their own way.

SUMMARY

DEVELOPMENTAL MILESTONES

ONE YEAR

Physical: Weight varies from 17 to 27 lbs, 27 to 32 inches in length. Walking age ranges from 9 to 17 months (average 14 months). Sleeps from 11 to 13 hours a night.
Mental: Connects words with object ("ball"). Makes simple yes-no gestures. Uses common household objects properly.
Social: Expresses preference for people and toys. Timid or friendly.

ONE AND A HALF YEARS (18 MONTHS)

Physical: Masters walking without support. Holds a cup and feeds herself
Mental: Says up to 10 to 20 words. Sorts shapes.
Social: Easily frustrated. Separation anxiety. Difficulty sharing toys.

TWO YEARS

Physical: Growth slows. Weight gain 3-5 lbs (1.4 kg to 2.3 kg.). Height increases 3-5 inches (7.6 cm to 12.5cm). Walks and pulls toys, kicks balls, climbs on furniture.
Mental: Says name and 3 word sentences. Categorizes and sorts objects. Helps around house. Understands concept of time (now and later).
Social: Parallel play. Sensitive to other's feelings. Tantrums and "terrible twos."

THREE YEARS

Physical: Primary teeth in place. Toilet training. Improvement in fine and gross motor skills (running, jumping, pedaling).

Mental: Recites name, age and gender. Imaginary play. Holds pencil and uses crayons.
Social: Enjoys puzzles. Less separation anxiety. Shows compassion and affection.

FOUR YEARS
Physical: Uses scissors. Rides tricycle, bike. Catches balls.
Mental: Recognizes colors. Draws stick figures (three parts). Intelligible speech. Recounts stories.
Social: Difficulty distinguishing between fantasy and reality. Fears monsters. Plays dress-up.

FIVE YEARS
Physical: Dresses self. Does somersaults and hops. Uses silverware at mealtime.
Mental: Recognizes and writes letters. Counts to 10. Learns address and phone number. Draws person with head, body, arms and legs.
Social: Imaginative play. Distinguishes reality from fantasy. Plays according to gender.

BABYPROOFING

Babyproof your home to create places and activities for your children out of harm's way. Designate child-friendly areas and rooms that are safe for your child. Do not leave her unattended.
Dangerous and Irreplaceable Items: Place dangerous items and valuable objects out of the reach of your child.
Electrical Outlets: Cover all electrical outlets in and out of the home that are not being used.
Toxic Cleaners, Chemicals, and Medications: Keep in latched locked areas. When possible, use nontoxic substances.
Desks, Tables, and Countertops: Keep items more than 12 inches (30 cm) away from edges.
Cupboards, Drawers, and Cabinets: Use child-proof latches.
Toilets and Pails: Latch all toilets. Keep all containers and pails empty of water.
Swimming Pools, Ponds, and Fountains: Keep covered or empty.
Water Temperature: Adjust your water heater's thermostat to avoid burns from overly hot water.
Cribs, Toys, and Playpens: Avoid small pieces that could break off and become choking hazards.

TANTRUMS

Tantrums are more common around age two and into the preschool years. Tantrums can be triggered from hunger, fatigue, illness, new environments, over-stimulation, stress in family relationships, and medications. Tantrums are a natural part of child development. During a tantrum, do the following:

- Stay calm. Make sure that your child is not in danger of hurting herself or anyone else.
- Avoid triggers of tantrums. Make sure your child is getting adequate naps and food.
- Reinforce appropriate behavior.
- Redirect or distract your child.
- Wait for your child to calm down.
- Consider a timeout approach – one minute for every year of age.
- Stagger errands and household chores.

TOILET TRAINING

Toilet training can be accomplished before one year of age; however, most parents usually follow a child-led toilet training around two and a half years. Girls tend to toilet train earlier than boys. Keep a potty around for your toddler early on.

DAYCARE AND PRESCHOOL GERMS

Common contagious conditions in daycares include stomach upset, diarrhea, pink eye, colds, coughs, lice, chickenpox, and skin infections. To lessen the frequency of your child's illnesses:

- Encourage a healthy diet.
- Keep breastfeeding and pumping while your child is in daycare.
- Use herbs and remedies as needed.
- Minimize the use of medications and antibiotics.
- Wash your hands, and your toddler's, frequently.

LEARNING DISABILITIES

The numbers of children diagnosed with learning and behavioral disorders, including attention deficit disorder, developmental delays, hearing or vision problems, and autism, have vastly increased in recent decades. Often times, these children have special needs at school.

BIRTH ORDER

Birth order is one of numerous factors that can contribute to shaping your child's personality. Firstborns are considered the responsible, perfectionist, high achiever. The middle child tends to be more independent and play the role of the mediator. The baby usually has the most freedom and enjoys following creative pursuits and being the center of attention. Only children can be adult-like and independent.

chapter 7

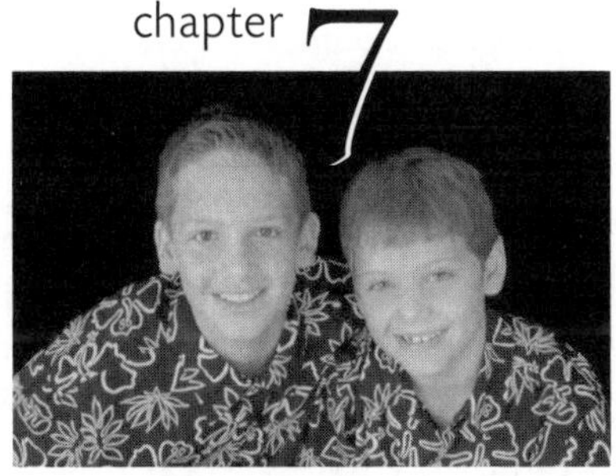

Children (Ages 5 to 10)

Children and fooles cannot lye.

Developmental Milestones

Your child is now in school, and these years will be defined by broadening intellectual horizons, more complex social relationships, and greater physical and emotional independence. School also brings new stressors for children, in the form of increased intellectual demands and social pressures, and busier schedules. They may have to negotiate new responsibilities like homework and soccer, contend with friendships and teasing, and experience grading and academic competition for the first time.

Physically, your child may gain seven pounds a year (3.18 kg.) and grow 2.5 inches (6.35 cm). As she gains strength and coordination, she will also be able to understand the rules and dynamics of team sports and more organized kinds of play. In team sports, the emphasis should be on learning to enjoy the physical exercise and learning to be a team player, rather than on winning or losing. Many children in this age group participate in activities such as team soccer, basketball, and softball, while others prefer independent physical activities such as swimming, tennis, or dance. In both cases, children at this age are able to control their bodies and exert themselves physically in unprecedented ways.

Schools vary, of course, in their academic emphases and educational philosophy but in general, each school year, math skills, vocabulary, and grammar become more complex, and so, too, does your child's ability to reason, think critically, and analyze the world around her. The maturation of your child's thinking skills also means that moments of imagination and fantasy life begin to fade. Cognitively, the egocentric thinking of the preschool years is beginning to change. Though thinking is still concrete, your child will begin to integrate symbols and concepts and consider questions more abstractly. Vocabulary will grow to approximately 14,000 words, and by age 10, children will begin to understand the concept of metaphors and the varied meanings of words. In our home, we play a lot of games: chess, checkers, backgammon, cards, board games, and more. In addition to being enjoyable ways to spend time together, these games have served to build cognitive skills such as memory, counting, and strategy.

Growing Pains

I can recall countless nights when my son Quentin would wake up with an ache in the leg. After a brief massage, a drink of water, and a kiss on the forehead, he was back to sleep and fine the next morning. Commonly known as *growing pains,* or benign limb pain of childhood, these aches are known to affect up to forty percent of children. Growing pains usually occur at two peaks—from three to six years old and then from eight to fourteen. Often growing pains are dismissed by standard medicine, citing a lack of research that correlates the pain to growth. Some doctors believe that they are caused by rapid growth, while others attribute growing pains to the general aches and pain from activity during the day.

Whatever the cause (I am inclined to believe they come from growth), children usually experience growing pains from time to time, and often toward the end of the day and at night in bed. By the next day, the child is back to normal play and activity. There is no residual pain or limp. Growing pains occur in the muscle over a generalized area: the pain is felt in the leg, typically the calf or shin, and sometimes in the thigh, foot, or behind the knee. Pain is not experienced in the joints. They can be worse in the cold and damp weather, and are usually relieved with massage, stretching, and sometimes heat. Growing pains are more common in children who are active in sports and other physical activities.

Although growing pains are considered a mild condition, seek medical attention if your child is consistently limping or has swelling, redness, or a tender arm, leg, or particular joint.

Bedwetting, Sleepwalking, and Nightmares

By around three years old, most children stay dry at night during sleep and are sleeping through the night. As they adjust to new schedules, developmental changes, and environmental stresses, however, many children are prone to conditions that disrupt their sleep, including growing pains, bedwetting, sleepwalking, talking in their sleep, nightmares, and night terrors. Poor eating habits, daytime stresses, and sleeping arrangement can also impact sleep. Make sure your child is not ingesting too many refined foods, particularly those high in sugar and caffeine, and talk frequently with your child about their daily activities—if she has had a frightening, distressing, or exciting experience, discussing it with you may prevent it from keeping her up at night.

Bedwetting

Almost every child will experience at least one episode of bedwetting after the age of five. Enuresis, the medical term for unintentional nighttime bedwetting in children older than age five, is usually not caused by any physical conditions. Bedwetting most often occurs in children who are deep sleepers, and, as a result, not aware of the urge to urinate; many do not even realize they have urinated in bed until the morning. Rarely is bedwetting due to a small bladder.

Bedwetting manifests in different fashions. Some children have never had a dry night, and others were once dry and for some reason begin to wet the bed during sleep. The latter may result from emotional upheavals, including moving, a new sibling, family problems, a new school, and so on. Other causes of bedwetting can include constipation, urinary tract infections (bladder infection), snoring (due to large tonsils and adenoids), food sensitivities (particularly excessive candy and sugar), and Attention Deficit Hyperactivity Disorder (ADHD). Bedwetting occurs more commonly in boys than girls, and family history can also play a role. If both parents wet the bed, their child has a 75% chance also. If one parent did, the likelihood falls to 40%.

Bedwetting can be aggravating for both child and family, interfering socially with activities like sleepovers and frustrating parents who have to face the morning with a wet bed and covers. As a child gets older, bedwetting engenders feelings of embarrassment and shame, and parents will need to be careful not to exacerbate these emotions by blaming or ridiculing their son or daughter. Your child is not wetting the bed intentionally and she should not be punished for it.

To prevent bedwetting:

- See your practitioner to rule out any medical conditions such as bladder or kidney illness.
- Keep a one-week diary, looking for triggers such as foods, events, and emotional upsets.
- Encourage your child to urinate before bedtime.
- Wake your child when you go to bed, as most bedwetting occurs in the first part of the night.
- Moisture-sensitive devices which vibrate if urine touches it are prescribed by some physicians (though they are not one of my favorite approaches).
- See a homeopath or other holistic practitioner. Homeopathy offers a wide array of remedies depending on your child's triggers and personality. *Equisetum*, *Causticum* and *Kreosotum* are examples of the hundreds of possible remedies that can be used for bedwetting. *Equisetum* is indicated when bedwetting occurs without any cause except habit. *Causticum* is used for bedwetting during the first part of sleep, and when worse in the winter. Similar to *Causticum, Kreosotum* is indicated for children who wet the bed early in the night. These children are difficult to rouse during sleep, and report that they dream they are urinating.

Nightmares and Night Terrors

Nightmares are also a major cause of interrupted sleep for children and nearly every young person has awakened frightened from a bad dream. Many nightmares happen in the latter half of the night and can be caused by the events of the day (both pleasant and stressful), overtiredness, medications, relationship issues (among family or peers, and at school), or a new environment. Nightmares are more frequent in girls than boys.

While our first impulse may be to reassure the child that "it's not real," this tendency also dismisses his or her feelings. For your child, the dream appears quite real, and nightmares can easily be confused with reality. Most children respond best with comfort and reassurance. When my boys awaken from a bad dream, we usually snuggle down together the rest of the night. To help prevent nightmares, avoid exposing your child to frightening experiences and media—scary stories, television shows, and movies can all contribute to bad dreams and a bad night's sleep.

Night terrors are not the same as nightmares. In a night terror, a child suddenly sits up in bed screaming, with the eyes wide open. The child is typically inconsolable. Although the child appears awake, she does not remember the event the next day. Night terrors occur during a deeper quiet sleep cycle (nonREM), and although frightening for parents, are not remembered by the child the next day. Night terrors are more common in boys between the ages of three to five years old and commonly occur in the first few hours after falling asleep. Night terrors are thought to be due to an immature central nervous system, and may be triggered by stress, heavy meals before bed, medications, and fevers.

Night terrors, along with sleepwalking, sleeptalking, and bedwettinig are a group of sleep disorders known as "parasomnias." Similar to night terrors, a child who sleepwalks (somnambulism) appears to be awake as he or she walks through the house. In actuality, the child is asleep and can hurt him or herself. Sleepwalking is more common in boys between 6 and 12 years old. Sleepwalking and night terrors are hereditary. Talking in the sleep can range from brief utterances to whole conversations. Like night terrors, it may be linked to fever, heavy meals before bed, and stress.

In my office, children with recurrent nightmares and terrors can be treated with a constitutional homeopathic remedy. One such remedy is *Calcarea carbonica* which is used for a child who has fearful dreams, and wakes up screaming after midnight. She sees horrible faces in the dark and cannot be calmed.

You might also try hanging a dreamcatcher. According to Native American Indian tradition, grandmothers wove dreamcatchers for their grandchildren, placing them above the sleep area to protect the child from bad dreams. Dreams of the spiritual world pass through the dream catcher, with good dreams going through the center and the bad ones catching in the outer webbing until they disappear with the morning sun.

Conventional pediatric medicine sees nightmares and night terrors as "normal" and most approaches are to watch and wait until the child outgrows this phase. However, sleep is necessary for resting the body from the day's activities and rebooting the brain for the next day. Without a full night's rest, we are sluggish the next day. So, nightmares and night terrors should be considered sleep disorders.

Sleep disorders in infants and children over an extended period of time may lead to behavioral issues. These children do not know that they do not feel good, nor feel rested. Some of them may even be having headaches, but they just don't have the words to describe the sensations in their head. In osteopathy, we find that if a child has always been a poor sleeper, it is often because they had a long and difficult birth. For a child who has never had sleep problems, the sudden appearance of nightmares or terrors can be traced back, one to two months prior, to a head injury. A good osteopathic treatment will result in improved sleep the same night. After sustained nights of restful sleep, parents usually see a calmer, happier, and more relaxed child by the end of a week.

Teething in Older Children

According to Kathy Arnos, author of *The Complete Teething Guide*, "Many people are unaware that our children's emotional and physical problems are often related to the teething process. Most equate 'teething' with infancy, when it actually lasts through young adulthood [through the eruption of the wisdom teeth]." Just as teething can affect infants, it can also affect older children, from emotional and mental changes to a weakening of the immune system.

Loss of baby teeth begins between five and seven years old and ends at approximately 14 years old. Children in this age group will lose and replace four primary teeth a year. The first tooth to fall out is generally the central incisor (bottom middle lower jaw), usually at the same time and on the same side that the six-year-old molar is coming in. The molars come behind the baby teeth, but do not replace them. The most intense teething ages (corresponding to the eruption of the molars) are at approximately age two, six, and 12. These are times in a child's life when he or she can be affected physically, mentally and emotionally by the teething process, a fact we generally overlook in children age six and older. Symptoms of teething in older children may include physical discomfort along with moodiness and behavioral problems. Many of these complaints are not traditionally associated with teething in older children. Holistic practitioners treat these conditions by strengthening a child's constitution.

Adult teeth are also called permanent or secondary teeth and usually come in the same order as the baby teeth. They differ in appearance to primary teeth, being rougher and more yellow. By age 16, your child will have fourteen top and fourteen bottom teeth, not including the wisdom teeth. Wisdom teeth, also known as the third molars, are the last teeth to come in. So-called because they erupt by late teens or early 20's, or the "age of wisdom," wisdom teeth may need to be removed if they are crowding the other molars.

Childhood Obesity and Exercise

According to the American Obesity Association, 15% of children in the United States are obese, an increase of over fifty percent in children ages 6 to 11 since the 1960s. Overweight adolescents grow up to become obese adults 70% of the time, and it is now estimated that half of American adults are clinically obese. Obesity in children is more marked in African American communities. This alarming rise in obesity has been blamed upon a number of societal causes, including our more sedentary lifestyle, high rates of television viewing, and the prevalence of fast food and junk food. Children generally consume more calories in front of a television, video game, or computer than they expend, and the food they eat is usually of poor nutritional value—sweets, sodas, chips. Obesity brings with it a host of attendant health problems: diabetes, heart disease, high blood pressure, and higher incidence of some cancers.

We must also consider that some children are by nature born more fleshy than others. Known by the ancients as the "venusian" planetary body type, the full figure, pear shaped curvaceous body was celebrated in art by such painters as Peter Paul Rubens in the 17th century. According to philosopher, Rodney Collin, "Plumpness is connected with fertility, or at least with the rate of survival of offspring." Currently being "large" is not considered attractive as it had been in other eras. Because of this, many overweight children have to endure the endless teasing and mocking that leads to low self esteem and depression. Both health professionals and parents need to consider that each child is an individual and optimal weight standards can vary greatly amongst children.

Practitioners use an objective measurement to calculate the extra weight in a child or adult, called the body mass index (BMI). This is based on the relation of weight and height in comparison to gender and age and is calculated by dividing the weight in kilograms by height in meters squared. A child is considered obese when the BMI is in the 85th percentile relative to charts from the Centers of Disease Control and Prevention (CDC). Pediatricians in America are beginning to take obesity seriously, educating parents and sending children to nutritionists who work with them on establishing healthier lifestyles. Psychosocial factors and counseling also form a key component of this therapy, addressing the ways television, food, and other "escapes" are symptomatic of deeper issues in parent and child relationships. By addressing the emotional as well as physical foundations of childhood obesity, pediatricians and other practitioners concerned with children's health are rethinking both the causes and solutions of the problem.

Whether one is small, tall, or round, all children are encouraged to establish healthy life habits, including physical activity. Every body requires a certain amount of motion to keep it strong, flexible, and healthy. In addition to improving physical health, it has been shown to be helpful with learning skills and emotional wellbeing. Researchers are even considering exercise as a replacement for Ritalin in the treatment of ADHD. A recent study conducted at the State University of New York at Buffalo found a significant improvement in behavior, including a reduction in oppositional attitudes, among children who exercised for forty minutes five days a week.

All children vary in their bodily profiles. Some are fidgety and restless all day long, even during sleep, while others are slower to move and appreciate sedentary activities. As different as these children are, their interests, including exercise and physical activity, will be different as well. In my practice, I encourage my patients to participate in activities that they enjoy because there is a greater chance of continuity. The same holds true for children, who may enjoy an activity they normally wouldn't precisely because they do not see it as "exercise." Dr. Edward Laskowski of the Mayo Clinic suggests to parents to "promote activity, not exercise. Children don't have to be in sports or take dance classes to be active." Encouraging children to participate in physical activity helps sets the stage for maintaining health and optimal weight, through adolescence and through adulthood.

Activities might include playing outdoors, school games on the playground, organized team sports, or playing with friends and family. Although many children are enrolled in organized team sports like softball, basketball, and soccer, competitive sports may not be of interest for every child. If your child shies away from competitive team sports, consider exercise traditions from different cultures, many of which are now becoming mainstream even for children—martial arts, tai chi, and yoga are all wonderful forms of exercise for a child's body, mind, and spirit.

Or encourage more everyday activities like walking the dog or gardening. Gardening is one of my favorite interactive, physical family activities because it also teaches children vital lessons about ecology, communal responsibility, and environmental sustainability. Our city sponsors a smart gardening program that helps families get started on their own growing projects, including providing information on composting and recycling and the bins as well. If your city does not have a similar program, of if you lack the yard space, try looking into community gardens, which will allow you and your child a space to tend to and a community to garden with.

You are a role model for your child. You want your child to be active? Set the stage and be active yourself. Families can incorporate group-oriented exercise like bike rides, hikes, and walks. My family recently joined the YMCA and I play racquetball with my children or we go for swims. My eldest son is old enough now to use the machines and treadmills, and he pushes me! Your children can also accompany you in your own exercise routines; you can hike with a toddler on your back, take your infant running with you in a stroller, or go to the pool with a young child. And don't forget the classic family games: hula hoop, jump-roping, hop scotch, tag, ball play, and Frisbee also make exercise fun.

As far as the type of exercise and length of time, I advocate the practical approach: a sedentary child should do more than she is now. A "recommended" amount of exercise from the American Heart Association for children two years and older is 30 minutes of enjoyable, moderate-intensity activities daily. In addition, they should perform at least 30 minutes of vigorous physical activities three to four days a week for cardio fitness. This period can be divided into two 15 minute periods or three 10 minute periods or of moderate intensity throughout the day.

Childrearing Approaches and Education

Families committed to natural parenting find that schooling presents a number of opportunities and challenges, from negotiating school lunches to investigating curricula to formulating their own educational philosophies. Many learn to supplement classroom learning with hands-on creative projects, outdoor adventures, and extracurricular social activities, taking a more active role in their child's educational process.

Public and Private School

The vast majority of children in the United States attend some kind of public or private school, most from kindergarten onward. The differences in schools vary greatly, and many parents spend time researching the various options available for their children. Families are finding they have choices and are no longer obliged to attend the neighborhood school. Private schools differ tremendously in educational philosophy, special interest programs, and social status. Often these schools come at a high price, and may be unaffordable to many budgets. In an effort to balance the socioeconomic status of the student body, some private schools offer financial aid and scholarships. Parochial schools, such as Catholic school, offer a traditional approach in private education at an affordable price. In the public school setting, many districts have special programs for different developmental levels or have magnet schools for special interests. Some of these programs use a point system for eligibility.

Learning does not stop once your child leaves the classroom, though, and I encourage parents to integrate educational opportunities into home life that both complement the teacher's curriculum and add to it. At the same time, watch out for overscheduling your child: involvement in too many after-school activities does not benefit her emotional wellbeing or yours. Some of our urgency to make sure our kids are in sports, taking dance, learning a foreign language, or practicing an instrument stems from a competitiveness that has more to do with the parents than the children. With some public schools and many private schools restricting entry to only the most competitive candidates, a number of parents have responded by fostering "talents" at increasingly early ages. I see parents of two- and three-year-olds encouraging academics or other activities and wonder, what's the rush? We should allow children to do their work, which is play. The rest will follow at the appropriate age.

While we often assume that school starts when a child reaches a certain chronological age—five years old is typical for kindergarten—learning is more accurately a developmental process and your child's readiness to begin school will vary according to his or her intellectual, mental, and emotional maturation. The term *kindergarten readiness* refers to the developmental milestones necessary for a child to excel in a school environment, and they may not all fall into place at five years old. Boys, for instance, mature at a slower rate than girls—sometimes up to a year-and-a-half in difference—and hence it may make sense to wait another year to enroll him in kindergarten. Since school brings with it a variety of new pressures, both academic and social, I encourage parents to not rush kindergarten enrollment unnecessarily, as your child will tend to succeed when he or she is ready and motivated to learn.

Indicators of kindergarten readiness include:

- **Academics:** Kindergarten will generally introduce your child to writing, numbers, shapes, and colors, and placement in more academic schools may require that he or she has learned these skills in preschool.
- **Dressing:** It is helpful if a child is able to dress herself, as this is a skill needed when using the bathroom.
- **Skills:** Able to color and cut lines with scissors.
- **Attention:** Your child can stay on task or sit in circle time for ten minutes.
- **Social:** Can share with other children.

The following section provides some alternatives to the standard thinking on education, offering suggestions on "natural parenting-friendly" schools as well as ways to promote your own learning agenda in a variety of contexts.

Montessori

Montessori educational programs recognize that children have different educational needs depending on the specific stage of their development. Montessori schools do not segregate children based on age and development, however, but allow them to broadly interact. In any given class, you may find groups of up to twenty-five to thirty children at different age levels within a span of two to three years. A child may stay in the particular class for as long as three years, allowing him or her to feel a part of a stable community. Each child is encouraged to work at her own pace. According to Montessori principles, the older children stimulate the younger ones, as well as act as role models. With an emphasis on child-centric rather than teacher-centric learning, the approach recognizes that it more opportune for a child to learn from another child than an adult teacher. Teachers are certified after extensive education. Most Montessori schools are for children from 3-6 years old. However there are programs that begin in infancy up to school age. There are even a few Montessori high schools.

Waldorf

Waldorf schools are based on the teachings of Rudolf Steiner and comprise the largest group of private independent schools found throughout the world. Learning according to the Waldorf method means educating the whole child's head, heart, and hands with the goal of producing "individuals who are able, in and themselves, to impart meaning to their lives." The same Steiner teacher and child may spend eight years together in elementary school, and, in general, emphasis is placed on cultivating a child's interest in learning rather on grades and performance. Especially in the first years of school, where subjects are presented through the arts, it is common to see a child in a Waldorf school knitting, enjoying fairy tales, or playing the recorder. In the Waldorf school tradition, events such as Halloween and May parades are part of learning as well, designed to appeal to the wonder and imagination of children. Dependence on television, commercial toys, and plastics is discouraged in favor of more self-motivated and creative pursuits. Many Waldorf high school graduates are admitted to top universities. Waldorf schools are available to children from pre-school age up to high school.

Home Schooling

I was very drawn to the notion of home schooling when my children were young, but it proved an unrealistic option in our household, with me working and my husband in school. For many of my patients and other parents nationwide, however, home schooling presents a viable alternative to traditional educational settings. Here in Los Angeles, children who are seriously pursuing acting careers often find it easier to home school so that they can still audition and work. Other parents home school in order to provide a more challenging curriculum, a different social environment, or religious instruction along with the learning basics. In 2001, it was reported that 2 million children are being home schooled, 35% for religious reasons. Curriculum options for home schooling families are as creative or "by the book" as the parent chooses—most prefer to follow their own integrated curriculum; however, a wide variety of course programs are often available privately or provided by the public school system, and many offer contact with a teacher either by phone, online, or in person on a regular basis.

One of the advantages of home schooling is that it can provide a more varied learning experience for children: gardening, cooking, and caring for a relative might all offer opportunities to learn academics and life lessons. Home schooling is frequently perceived as socially isolating, but this need not be the case. Often home-schoolers will connect with other like-minded families to participate in regular meetings including field trips, co-parenting learning, and social gatherings, and many children are involved with scouts, sports, dance, and art classes. With the correct home environment and approach, I have seen children and teens excel in their home studies and enter Ivy League universities. In a *Mothering* magazine article on home schooling, Dr. Lawrence M. Rudner found in a study of 20,000 home-schoolers that "The median scores for home school students are well above their public/private school counterparts in every subject and in every grade, regardless of the presence or absence of formal curriculum use."

SUMMARY

DEVELOPMENTAL MILESTONES

During these school years, your child will experience broadening intellectual horizons, more complex social relationships, and greater physical and emotional independence. With this comes new pressures and stress.

Physical: Weight gain can be as much as 7 lbs a year (3.18 kg). Growth 2.5 inches (6.35 cm) Strength and coordination improve with each year.

Mental: Imaginary life and egocentricity begins to fade. Increased ability to reason and think critically and abstractly.

Social: Stress with increased intellectual demands and social pressures, and busier schedules. Tumultuous relationships. May be impulsive.

GROWING PAINS

Growing pains occur in 40 percent of children in two peak ages from 3 to 6 years old and 8 to 14 years old. Most children find relief with massage, stretching and heat.

BEDWETTING, SLEEPWALKING, AND NIGHTMARES

Bedwetting is usually not caused by a physical condition and is more common in boys. Some causes of bedwetting can include emotional upset, constipation, urinary tract infections, snoring, food sensitivities , and Attention Deficit Hyperactivity Disorder.

Nightmares can be caused by the events of the day, overtiredness, medications, relationship issues, or a new environment. Avoid exposure to frightening stories and media and reassure and comfort your child when nightmares occur.

With a night terror the child is inconsolable and has no recollection the next day. Night terrors are more common in boys, ages 3 to 5 years old.

TEETHING IN OLDER CHILDREN

Teething may affect your older child emotionally and physically. Children will lose and replace four primary teeth a year with permanent or secondary teeth which total fourteen on the top and bottom.

CHILDHOOD OBESITY AND EXERCISE

The rise in childhood obesity has been blamed upon our more sedentary lifestyle, high rates of television viewing, use of video games, and the over consumption of fast food and junk food. Obesity can lead to heart disease, diabetes, high blood pressure, and higher incidence of some cancers. In addition, many overweight children have to endure the endless teasing and mocking that leads to low self esteem and depression. Encourage your children to participate in enjoyable physical activities through adolescence and through adulthood.

CHILDREARING APPROACHES AND EDUCATION

Families committed to natural parenting find that entering the school years presents a number of opportunities and challenges, from negotiating school lunches to investigating curricula and formulating educational philosophies. Private schools vary tremendously in educational philosophy, special interest programs, and social status. In the public school setting, many districts have special programs for different developmental levels or have magnet schools for special interests.

Alternatives to the standard thinking on education include:

Montessori: In a Montessori class, you may find children at different age levels within a span of two to three years. Each child is encouraged to work at her own pace.

Waldorf: The Waldorf method educates the whole child's head, heart, and hands with the goal of producing "individuals who are able, in and themselves, to impart meaning to their lives."

Home Schooling: Curriculum options for home schooling families are as creative or "by the book" as the parent chooses.

chapter 8

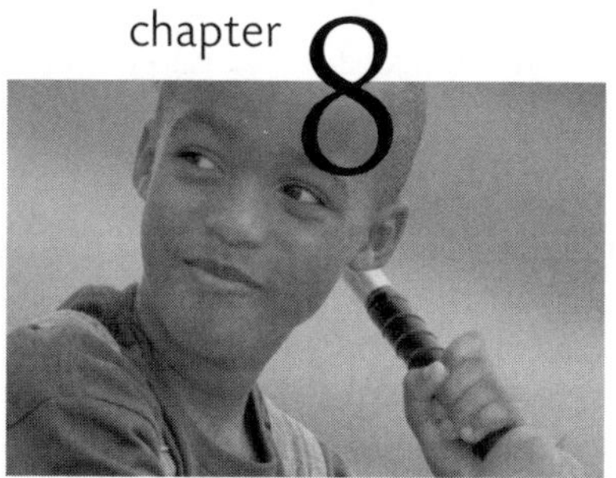

Preteens (Ages 11 to 13)

"If we have virtuous children, we should choose
Their tenderest age good principles to infuse."

—*Phocylides*

Developmental Milestones

Early adolescence begins around the ages of 11 to 14 and is dominated by the onset of puberty, with its seismic shifts in bodily and emotional development. This stage marks your son or daughter's transition from child to young adult and the beginning of his or her sexual development. Many parents anticipate adolescence with no small share of dread, remembering the turmoil of their own teenage years and the often emotional ways they asserted their independence and tested boundaries. Adolescence can indeed be a trying time for both parent and child, but it can also be a rewarding one, as your child "grows up" both literally and figuratively and discovers her potential intellectually and emotionally.

Although adolescent thinking is still predominantly concrete, reasoning will begin to evolve throughout puberty, leading to better comprehension of more symbolic and abstract concepts. According to psychologist Jean Piaget, most children do not have the capability of reasoning as an adult until the age of 15. Many frustrated parents feel this evolution does not come fast enough, although teens' concrete thinking, coupled with their lack of experience and self-control, often hampers their ability to analyze, discern, and make good judgments with an eye toward future consequences. In general, teens are more shortsighted, and may respond better to learning about short-term consequences than long-term. If parents are trying to warn a child about nutrition and junk food, for instance, they may be more successful talking about weight gain and acne than long-term effects like heart disease or cancer.

Emotionally, this time period is fraught with insecurities about esteem, individuality, and identity. This age group tends to put tremendous importance on appearance, and may spend many hours devoted to tending their looks. It doesn't help, however, that puberty is usually heralded by growth spurts, acne, uncomfortable bodily changes, and fluctuating hormonal activity, leading most adolescents to feel out-of-sync with their bodies and awkward both physically and socially. Compassion toward your teen is of utmost importance throughout this period, as the combination of emotional stress and physical change can make many vulnerable to depression, social pressure, and forms of acting out at school and at home.

As children in this age group transition into adolescence, they also become more independent from families and their home. The desire for independence, and a concomitant withdrawal into the bedroom to blast the music, often prompts resentment from alienated family members. Many of these behaviors are considered normal signposts on the path to adulthood and are not necessarily cause for concern. But while your adolescent will be sending you all kinds of signals to stay away, you will need to find ways to stay involved in their lives by starting conversations, inquiring about friends and school, planning parent-child activities, and setting boundaries, curfews, and responsibilities for them. Adolescents need space to explore their own decision-making processes, but too much space may only exacerbate the alienation they already feel. Be prepared to confront your adolescent often about their particular brand of rebellion, and do not hesitate to speak to your practitioner for advice and reassurance.

Puberty in Girls

The onset of puberty in girls varies, with budding of the breasts beginning anywhere from nine to eleven years old and pubic hair appearing six to twelve months later. This is followed by a growth spurt and menstruation, with her first period usually occurring two to two and a half years from the onset of puberty, or around the age of 12 (although it can occur from 10 years old to 16 years old). A girl will usually reach her adult height by 16. With these changes also generally come increased stores of body fat ("filling out"), which in some girls can lead to self-consciousness and body image issues. It is not uncommon that adult women report that their period during adolescence was marked with pain, nausea, and a desire to stay home in bed. Natural remedies can be helpful during this time period (See the *Menstrual Cramps* entry in Part IV).

Early puberty, also known as precocious puberty, is defined as the onset of puberty in girls before eight years old (and in boys before nine years old). It is well documented that sexual development is beginning earlier in children, and is correlated with an increased chance of breast cancer later in life. The incidence is more common in girls than boys and may be more frequent among obese children. Recently, however, studies have also established possible links between the chemicals commonly used in plastic items like microwaveable food storage containers, baby bottles, and teethers to early puberty. These chemicals, phthalates and polybrominated biphenyl (PBB), are so similar to female hormones that they mimic them in the body, potentially leading to early sexual development.

Although the use of plastic is ubiquitous, you can take measures to avoid overexposure by storing your food in unbreakable glass. Minimize plastics, including plastic wrapping and garbage liners, and avoid heating food in plastic containers. If you use a microwave (which is not recommended for many reasons), replace plastic containers with glass.

Puberty in Boys

For boys, the onset of puberty starts between nine and a half to fourteen years old. Similar to girls, the pituitary gland in the brain releases a hormone that activates the male reproductive system. The first change in puberty is marked by the enlargement of the testicles and scrotum. This is followed by growth of the penis within one year. Pubic hair begins to appear between 13 to 14 years old. By 15 years old, the voice changes, pimples begin, and hair appears on the face and under the arms. Facial hair growth in boys usually begins on the upper lip, followed by the cheeks and chin. Nocturnal emissions (wet dreams) are normal and may begin by fourteen years old. Unlike girls, who experience their adolescent growth spurt earlier, a boy may not grow until well into puberty. Girls will therefore remain taller than boys in early adolescence, but once boys start growing, they will continue to do so until age eighteen so that by adulthood, they are taller than the girls. Most boys (60%) experience some growth of breast tissue during puberty, which usually disappears within a year. Puberty for boys can also be filled with emotional changes and mood swings. As for any adolescent, it is important to be able to have close contact with a supportive friend, family member, or other adult.

Menstruation

One of the big milestones in an adolescent girl's life is the onset of her period, which can evoke a myriad of strong feelings ranging from excitement to despair. The onset of a girl's period is known as *menarche* (pronounced meh-nar-kee). During this stage of life, a girl transforms into a young woman, and her body is capable of becoming pregnant.

The onset of puberty is spurred by the release of hormones (follicle-stimulating hormone) from the pituitary gland in the brain. This stimulates the maturation of female reproductive system. At the time of menstruation, one of the ovaries releases an egg (ovum); this is known as ovulation. The ovum travels through the fallopian tubes down into the uterus. Estrogen is secreted by the ovary which causes the build up the inner walls of the uterus with extra tissue and blood. If the egg doesn't become fertilized by a sperm, the lining of the uterus is sloughed off through the vagina. The shedding of the lining which includes, blood, and tissue is known as the menstrual period. A girl's period can last from 3 to 7 days, with a flow that varies from scant to heavy. The common cycle is approximately 28 days, similar to a cycle of the moon. It is not uncommon for a girl's period to begin irregularly and establish a more regular pattern with time. If your daughter's period remains irregular or if cramps are severe and not responding to general home measures, see your practitioner.

In early puberty, it is important that parents (or at least mother) and daughter begin to have an open dialogue about the changes to come. In preparation for this, you will need to have feminine hygiene products (pads or tampons) available. Pads are preferable as they can easily attach to underwear and allow the blood to flow out of the body. Some girls find the pads too bulky, and complain that the blood may contain an odor. Tampons, which are inserted into the vagina, can be more practical for these girls, especially during physical activities. However, they may be difficult to insert and uncomfortable. In addition, tampons carry the risk of Toxic Shock Syndrome. In the 1980s there was an epidemic of Toxic Shock Syndrome, in which women became infected with a toxin producing bacteria following the use of high absorbency tampons. A good rule of thumb when using tampons, change them frequently.

Commercial tampons are made from rayon-cotton blends, both of which are laden with chemicals, and are whitened with chlorine dioxide. Dioxins have been linked to cancer, endometriosis, infertility, skin conditions, and immune system dysfunctions. There have been reports that tampons contain asbestos causing more bleeding, which would increase the sale of tampons. These allegations have not been confirmed and manufacturers deny any use of asbestos in tampons. Instead of commercial tampons try brands made from organic cotton fibers made without any chemicals, pesticides, herbicides and bleaches. When using pads, consider reusable natural ones that are easily washed.

Premenstrual Syndrome (PMS) and Menstrual Cramps

Some girls experience discomfort and pain during menstruation. Painful cramps in the uterus are caused by hormones called prostaglandins, which in turn are stimulated from the hormone progesterone, released by the ovaries after ovulation. Many of the women in my practice report that their period was more painful during the teen years, although this is not always the case.

In addition, many girls will suffer from *premenstrual syndrome* or PMS. PMS is an all-encompassing term used to define many symptoms associated with the week or days just before the period. In addition to cramps, these may include irritability, tearfulness, depression, anxiety, food cravings, headaches, back pain, nausea, bloating, skin breakouts, sleep disturbance, breast tenderness, and more. At least 30 percent of females suffer from PMS and probably every woman at some time in her menstrual history has experienced it in varying degrees. PMS is most often experienced in the second half of the menstrual cycle, known as the luteal phase, which leads to the onset of menstruation. PMS, irregular periods, and painful cramps can be aggravated by hormone imbalance, and stress in the home or at school. As girls get older, the cramps usually diminish. Painful periods and difficulty with PMS can greatly affect an adolescent girl's life and interfere with daily activities such as school, sports, and social life. (See the *Menstrual Cramps and PMS* entry in Part IV for more information on natural treatment of PMS.)

The Birth Control Pill

In standard medicine, painful cramps are treated with non-steroidal anti-inflammatory medicine (NSAID) such as ibuprofen or naproxen. If there is no relief, it is commonplace for a doctor to prescribe the birth control pill to young women with irregular periods or painful cramps.

From my professional viewpoint, I consider the Pill (and variations including the hormonal shots and patches) an unhealthy medication made of synthetic hormones. Furthermore, the Pill contains a combination of the hormones, estrogen and progesterone, which sends a message to the body to prevent ovulating, a natural process in a young woman's body.

The Pill also comes with a list of side effects that include bloating, weight gain, breast tenderness, increased risk to breast cancer, fatal blood clots, stroke, migraine headaches, gall bladder disease, liver tumors, and mood swings. The Pill, which is metabolized in the liver, is known to deplete the body of B vitamins (especially B6 and folic acid), vitamin C, magnesium, and zinc. Use of the Pill is also associated with Candida (yeast) overgrowth in the body. As a method for birth control, the Pill is only one way to avoid unwanted pregnancy. There are other methods which do not have many of the harmful side effects, such as condoms.

At every stage of our children's lives, parents' roles can be influential and important and this applies especially during adolescence. With regards to the changes in puberty, comes the topic of sexuality. Difficult to broach for some parents, the goal is to promote an open dialogue about sexuality so your child feels comfortable to come to you with questions and concerns. The message that many parents, educators and healthcare providers is to encourage abstinence. However, in reality, some teenagers are going to become sexually active even despite their parents protests. Because of this, discussion should include information about preventing pregnancy, AIDS and other sexually transmitted diseases.

Acne

Skin breakouts, or acne, are commonplace during puberty amongst both girls and boys. Emotionally, they can add to adolescent insecurities about appearance. Acne is caused by clogged skin pores from oil (sebum) and dead skin cells. Hormones during puberty are responsible for an increase in oil. Family history may also play a role. Breakouts occur in the form of pimples, cysts, whiteheads, and blackheads and usually occur on the face, as well as on the back and chest. Acne begins to decrease by late teens.

The standard treatment of acne includes washing the face with a mild soap. Scrubbing the face too hard or picking pimples, wearing helmets, moisturizers, medications, and stress may only aggravate the condition. Oily foods and chocolates do not cause acne, according to current popular thought. There are many over-the-counter skin products advertised for acne, containing benzoyl peroxide, which may burn the skin. For severe cases, some doctors may prescribe prescription medications such as antibiotics, or the birth control pill (for girls). Homeopathy and holistic medicine can offer adolescents treatments for acne without the side effects. When washing, use a natural soap product. A good general natural herb taken orally is the gemmotherapy product, Oriental Plane Tree. (See *Acne* entry in Part IV.)

Competitive Sports

For many adolescents, interest in physical activity begins to dwindle and gives way to a more sedentary lifestyle. Physical education programs are unfortunately among the first cut during school financial crises, and nationwide, children are increasingly deprived of exercise during school hours, even as the problem of adolescent sedentariness grows. But physical activity does more than improve cardiovascular and muscular strength; it is essential to fostering a broader sense of health that includes emotional wellness, good nutrition, and improved relationships. Regular exercise has been shown to improve motor skills and coordination, but also just importantly to help alleviate depression and improve brain function, which can boost learning and academics.

The adolescents who remain active in sports, dance and other activities can be quite serious, dedicated and ambitious in their endeavors. This can also make them prone to injuries and pain. A common cause of knee pain is Osgood-Schlatter disease. Osgood-Schlatter disease (OS) affects children from eight to sixteen years old and is the most common cause of knee pain in adolescents in the year after a rapid growth spurt. Children with OS complain of pain and swelling just below the knee cap, caused when the thigh muscle pulls on the patellar tendon. It is more common in boys and among kids participating in soccer, baseball, basketball, track, and other sports. OS affects adolescents intermittently and can last several years, usually healing on its own. Treatment of OS calls for avoiding strenuous exercise, including deep knee bending. For painful areas, rest, ice, compression, and elevation (R.I.C.E) is recommended. Additional standard treatments include leg braces and anti-inflammatory medication.

Sever's Disease is experienced as a pain at the back of the heel and is caused by inflammation where the Achilles tendon attaches to the heel bone (known as calcaneal apophysitis). Because it is painful to walk on the heel, children will be inclined to toe walk. Sever's affects children in a similar age range to OS (nine to fourteen). Standard treatment includes heel pads, R.I.C.E., and ibuprofen. Consider holistic treatments for both Osgood-Schlatter and Sever's if the condition persists.

Some student athletes are using performance-enhancing drugs and supplements to improve performance and increase muscle mass. These drugs are more commonly used in the fields of weight lifting, cycling, swimming, track and field, and others. Known for their serious side effects, many preteens and teens overlook the long term consequences in exchange for short term results. One popular supplement, creatine, is available over-the-counter. Side effects include nausea, diarrhea, muscle cramps, while higher doses may cause more severe heart, kidney and liver damage.

Anabolic steroids, which gained notoriety in Olympic athletes, are now illegal to use and are a controlled substance. Many parents are unaware that their children resort to drugs for sports. Signs of steroid use include mood swings, angry outbursts, aggressiveness, acne outbreaks, and trembling, Steroids can affect an adolescent's sexual development, stunt growth and damage vital organs.

Ephedra, which acts in the body as an amphetamine, has also been used to enhance performance. In December 2003, ephedra was banned because of side effects that include strokes, heart attacks and convulsions. Ephedra and anabolic steroids can be addictive. As adolescents begin to claim their autonomy, it is evermore important that parents maintain an open dialogue with their children about school, sports and relationships.

Eating Disorders

Preteen and teens are barraged with unrealistic body images that are defined by "the thinner, the better." This, coupled with an abundance of food, have been suggested as causes that lead to eating disorders. For the past several decades, the number of adolescents diagnosed with eating disorders, such anorexia nervosa or bulimia, has grown. According to the American Academy of Child and Adolescent Psychiatry, as many as 1 in 10 young women suffer from an eating disorder in the United States. Boys can also be affected, especially if they are involved in sports that include weight classes, like wrestling or boxing.

Girls with anorexia nervosa stop eating out of fear of becoming fat, even when they are underweight. Symptoms of anorexia nervosa begin with difficulty sleeping and fidgetiness. As the weight decreases with loss of body fat, the period ceases and soft hair grows on the face, back and extremities for warmth. If starvation continues, the vital signs slow, the organs become affected, and this could eventually lead to death. Possible causes include difficulty accepting the physical changes of puberty, stress following parents' divorce or death, or increasing pressure with school work and activities. Commonly anorectic girls are high achievers, have a strong sense of responsibility, and present an outward image of perfection despite having low self-esteem.

Bulimia is defined as binge eating followed by purging with self- induced vomiting. Often there is concurrent use of laxatives and diuretics. Bulimics spend a lot of time in the bathroom, secretive about their activities. Consequences can include electrolyte imbalance, irritations in the back of the throat, dehydration, constipation, anemia, and digestive complications. Psychologically, girls with bulimia may feel loss of self control, guilt and helplessness.

Eating disorders are complex diseases caused by multiple factors that greatly affect the children and their families. Standard treatment for both anorexia and bulimia includes specialized therapy (individual and family), nutritional counseling, medication (i.e. anti-depressants) and sometimes inpatient treatment programs and hospitalization. Outcomes are more positive with early treatment. In my own office practice, I have found homeopathy to be invaluable in aiding the healing process.

Junk Food

When my eldest son started school, I was shocked to see how junk food permeated the classroom, playground, and other children's lunch boxes. Nowadays, vending machines selling candy and soft drinks are fixtures in many elementary and high schools. An in-school television program throughout the United States, carries ads for junk food such as Hostess Twinkies, Mountain Dew, and M&M's. With financial restrictions and cutbacks a reality at many schools, the vending machines have become a money-maker for the schools. Approximately 20% of schools have fast-food outlets on campus.

I realized I couldn't completely shield our children from new tastes. Although we avoid processed food and junk in our own kitchen, I have come to terms with the fact that having sweets at a friend's home or at a restaurant aren't always avoidable. Ultimately, raising children to make healthy choices in nutrition begins with a strong foundation in the home—with parents as the role model. This doesn't mean that you have to have begun healthy eating patterns since your child was a newborn. In my own household, I grew up on bologna and cheese sandwiches with white bread. When I was 11 years old, my stepfather came into our lives and introduced us to the concept of healthier eating. My mother stopped buying processed meats, cereals and snacks. Because our entire family switched to eating more whole grain breads, fresh fruit and vegetables, we all easily accepted it.

Most of us recognize junk food: candy, cookies, sodas, chips, and French fries are all high in fats, sugars, salt, and chemical additives, and low in nutritional value. Some junk foods, though, are less obvious than others, leading us to mistake "junky" snacks for healthy ones. For instance, many white foods, including white bread, white rice, and baked goods made with white flour, are low in nutrients and high in calories. Other popular, healthy-seeming snacks include goldfish crackers, many cereals, and the convenient juice box. Reading the nutritional labels on these products reveals just how much sugar and additives they contain—and how little actual nutritional content.

Fruit juice is a prime example of a snack that seems healthier than it is. The largest consumers of juice are children, indicating how many parents substitute fruit juices for sodas on the one hand, and water on the other. Like soda, however, juice has a high sugar content, which can lead to tooth decay, childhood obesity, and diarrhea. The sweetness in juice acts in the body like any other kind of sugar, affecting insulin levels, suppressing the immune system, and stimulating allergies. Unless the drink is 100% fruit juice, it is a flavored drink or cocktail and full of corn syrup. Even if a juice is 100%, it lacks the crucial fiber of whole fruit. With the exception of nursing infants, one should not take in more calories from liquids than solids.

To reduce your child's consumption of junk food, the easiest thing to do is not to have it around the house. This will help you, too! Honestly, I have very little willpower. If I am at a party and there is a bowl of chips or goldfish, I will happily snack on them. Just like the ad says, "EVERYONE LOVES GOLDFISH® CRACKERS!" So I just don't buy them. Instead, have healthy snacks ready to go for a hungry child or adult.

Screen Time: Television and Video Games

According to a study by Johns Hopkins researchers, a high school graduate will have spent up to 18,000 hours watching television compared to 12,000 hours in school, averaging approximately 30 hours a week in front of the TV. The thought of children spending this many hours in front of a television is abhorrent to me, as I would rather see them enjoying themselves out of doors, playing together, or working creatively or imaginatively. As much as I tried to avoid my children becoming part of the television generation, I realized I could not completely avoid it. I knew that my plan of minimizing television was marred forever when my neighbor, who worked for Disney, kindly left us 25 brand-new tapes of the best of Disney at our doorstep. But like many parents, I also learned that there are some intelligent and interesting television programs that I could monitor, as well as movies and DVDs to choose from. If necessary, there are technologies that allow parents more control over television channels and internet access.

As my children entered school, television video games became a bone of contention. My children would complain, "We are the only family in Los Angeles that doesn't have one!" Although they do promote hand-eye coordination, my husband and I long ago agreed that any toy, like a video game, known to cause seizures in susceptible children is not one we wanted in the house. Rapidly flashing and flickering lights can cause seizures in susceptible people, particularly people who are sensitive to light. The Epilepsy Foundation has made recommendations to avoid and prevent these rare occurrences. In general while watching television, video games, and computer screens, keep the room well lit, reduce the screen's brightness, avoid sitting close to the screen, do not watch while tired or for prolonged time periods.

I do, on the other hand, allow them a Game-Boy, saving me from complete insensitivity, according to my sons. Not that a hand-held gadget is necessarily any better. In this instance and others, I have found that decision-making around television and video games is a process of limits and compromise. While I couldn't allow my sons to watch and play whatever they wanted, I also knew that forbidding all exposure would only strengthen the allure. Plus, it can handicap them socially! By setting firm boundaries about how long and in what setting they could play or watch, I let them join friends while not sacrificing family time, homework, and other kinds of activities.

The American Academy of Pediatrics suggests that children younger than two years old avoid television viewing altogether, as it takes time away from direct interactions with others and can affect their brain development. For older children and adolescents, TV and video games expose them to vast array of violent and sexual images, in addition to discouraging physical activity. While many people downplay the impact of violent and sexually explicit material on children's emotional and psychological health, in 1996, the American Medical Association published the *Physician's Guide to Media Violence*, in which they listed the potential adverse consequences of excess media exposure. Among these were:

- Increased violent behavior
- Higher rates of obesity
- Decreased physical activity and fitness
- Increased cholesterol levels
- Excess sodium intake
- Repetitive strain injury (from video and computer games)
- Insomnia
- Photic seizures in vulnerable individuals
- Impaired school performance
- Increased use of tobacco and alcohol
- Increased sexual activity
- Decreased attention span
- Decreased family communication
- Excess consumer focus, resulting in feelings of envy and entitlement

So what can you as a parent do to help prevent and reduce the adverse effects of television and video games?

- Know the shows your child is watching. The younger the child, the more impressionable. Even some "benign" shows may be too potent right before bedtime.
- Avoid using the media as a babysitter. Teach children about other forms of entertainment, such as playing outside, reading, or doing crafts.

- Limit television watching (no more than two hours a day of quality shows after homework is done). Some parents limit TV altogether during the school week.
- Avoid eating meals in front of the TV. This interferes with social interaction.
- Keep the TV and computer in a common area and not in the child's bedroom. Our family computer is in our bedroom, as I like to know what my sons are viewing and who they are IMing (instant messaging).

Advertising and Your Child

From television to billboards to the Internet and movies, children are inundated with consumerism—they will absorb as many as 40,000 advertisements in a single year. Product placement and brand-name clothing are not lost on kids; quite the contrary, children are incredibly sensitive to the trappings of consumerism and strongly influenced by "must-have" items, be they a new game, a food product, or a toy.

Children make such avid consumers in part because they are so sensitive to advertising methods. As psychologist Dale Kunkel notes, "While older children and adults understand the inherent bias of advertising, younger children do not, and therefore tend to interpret commercial claims and appeals as accurate and truthful information." While watching television, for instance, young children are often not able to distinguish between a television show and a commercial, believing the ad is part of the program. In older children, advertising can work more subtly to influence lifestyle choices. Much of the controversy around tobacco advertising stems from just this concern that the cigarette manufacturers are marketing an image of smoking implicitly appealing to adolescents looking to be "cool." It is for these reasons that the American Psychological Association (APA) is calling for restrictions in advertising directed at the youth market, particularly children younger than eight years old.

Advertisers take advantage of the fact that in the marketplace, little ones are big consumers. In a family, children carry considerable weight in how money is spent, with older children spending money on junk food, video games, music, and clothing, and younger children exerting considerable pressure on their parents to buy the latest toys and snacks. While I was at the museum with my son, Quentin, he wanted to buy a magic wiggly worm prominently displayed in the museum store and advertised with a video presentation. To my seven-year-old, the presentation looked persuasive, and he immediately wanted to get it. However, when the clerk pulled the magical worm out of his pocket and showed him how it actually worked, my son was no longer interested.

Quentin learned a vital lesson about advertising that day; namely, that an ad is meant to introduce you to the product without giving you all the information about it. Since advertisers "show off" the product using special camera angles and lighting, the picture does not tell the whole story, and may even be misleading and deceptive. Childcare experts in advertising recommend that parents discuss with their children what a product is really like, aside from advertising gimmicks, before purchasing. Say, for instance, that your child sees an ad for a cheerleading baton; it features an adolescent girl performing fancy maneuvers and tricks, and your daughter eagerly wants to get the same baton. The APA recommends you go to the store to see how a product works before buying it and that you also ask your child several practical questions to help distinguish fantasy from reality, such as:

"How much practice do you think she had before she could do that?"

"If you bought the baton, do you think you would be able to perform as well as she does?"

"Would you be willing to put in the time to learn to be able to do it as well as she does?"

Screen Time: The Internet and Cell Phones

The 21st century has opened up an entirely new aspect of media in our culture, known as the Internet, or the World Wide Web. Useful for learning, pleasure and communication, it can be a wonderful tool and often children are more computer savvy than their parents. However, parents need to monitor its use as they would any activity. Because of the vast exposure on the Internet, parents need to make sure that the material their children are viewing is appropriate, and that their children are safe in the realm of communication.

Children are repeatedly taught to not talk to strangers, and the Internet is no exception. According to Ruben Rodriguez, director of the National Center for Missing and Exploited Children's CyberTipLine (NCMEC), adults in chat rooms may solicit underage children for sexual reasons. A vulnerable child may think the other person is another child, or may not be able to discern when an adult is lying. In order to protect our children from both physical and emotional harm, it is important that parents speak to their children about internet safety and appropriate websites.

In addition to meeting strangers on the internet, children can land on adult websites or receive sexually explicit spam emails. There are filters on the Internet as well as programs that allow you to block sites that are devoted to sex, crimes and other unsuitable material. If your child uses email, become knowledgeable about mail options that have the capability to block senders, apply junk email filters, and safe lists. In our home, we keep the family computer in a common area which allows me to be aware of who they are instant messaging. As with television and video games, consider monitoring the time your child spends at the computer.

More children are walking around with cell phones in their pockets. Many parents like the sense of security that they can easily be in contact with their children, day or night. However, with additional features like text messaging, camera, video, music, and Internet usage built into smartphones today, the same rules of caution apply to cell phone use for children as on the Internet. Teach your child not to give your phone number to someone you don't know or don't trust, not to reply to text messages from unknown people, and to block numbers from people with whom you don't want to receive calls. In addition, speaking on the cell phone can distract people from safely doing other activities such as crossing the street and driving a car.

Some parents are also concerned about a possible link between mobile phone use and cancer, as some phones emit high levels of radiofrequency (RF) energy. To reduce the risk of radiofrequency energy exposure, it is best to limit the amount of conversation time. In addition, the use of text messaging, speaker phone, and any device such as a headset that allows your child to use the phone without keeping it too close to the head would be preferable. Like any other aspect of life, use your parental wisdom to teach your child about common sense regarding these gadgets. This is also a good opportunity to teach your child about responsibility; our older son has learned to keep track of his phone (so that it is not lost or stolen) and not to run up huge bills by talking for too long.

The Wired World

We live in an increasingly wired world and are constantly surrounded by technology. Technology is part of our daily life, from which there is little escape. Electropollution or electrosmog are new terms to describe the phenomena of electromagnetic fields generated by various sources in the course of our daily lives. Increasingly, research has shown how EMFs affect human health.

From the time we wake up in the morning, we have the digital alarm clock generating a field next to our head. Perhaps we went to bed with our smartphone, checking the latest news, weather, sports update, or email and placed our phone on the nightstand. Maybe some of us watched a little cable television or have a satellite dish beam our favorite shows. Regardless of the specific choice of companies delivering our entertainment, there most likely is a Wi-Fi router running all night in our household. When we go to work one of the first things we do is log on to a computer and check our email. For our kids, perhaps our infant slept next to an infant monitor. As we are preparing for the day and packing the kids' lunches and snacks, we may have the television on to check the news and weather. When we drop the kids off to school on our way into work, we look up at the skyline and see celltowers in the distance in every direction. Those of us with longer commutes may see a cell tower disguised as a pine tree or palm tree. When the kids are in school, perhaps their new school has bad wiring or, even worse, new wiring for powerful wi-fi connections or may have smart meters that remotely transmit data on power usage. Our elementary school aged children likely take their computer classes on a weekly basis and have homework which requires some computer usage. After dinner, some of us relax by watching television or playing video games. When it is time to put our young children to bed, we turn on a nightlight to comfort their fear of the dark. We then go to bed and settle ourselves through the same routine. And the cycle of EMF exposure continues again.

According to www.internetlivestats.com, in 2016 the US is the third most populous country in the world (behind China and India) and internet access was at a high of 88.5% of households. This rate is up from Pew Research's 2014 finding of 73% of households in the US. Pew Research also finds that in 2015, 68% of the US had a smart phone and in 2014, 50% of the US had a tablet or E-reader. How can families take advantage of modern conveniences, while still protecting our health and raising our children optimally? There are several simple, practical safety measures that can be we can put in place to minimize our children's exposure to the EMFs around us.

The electronic devices we use that make our modern life so convenient have three sources of EMF radiation that we can easily protect against to minimize our and our children's exposure. Most of our devices are wireless. When they connect and transmit data it can only happen when the antenna is on. On a smartphone, those of us who are electrosensitive can feel the buzz, and some of us get a headache when we put the phone to our ears. This wireless connectivity EMF field can cause headaches and sleep disorders, alter the blood-brain barrier, alter DNA, and increase cancer risk. Several simple rules with smartphone use include: 1) always use the speaker or, for privacy use ear buds but never put the phone directly in contact with the body when in use; 2) Never carry your phone directly on the body when not in use; 3) at night, leave your phone outside of the bedroom.

The second problematic source on our devices is the back of the device where the circuits heat up. But the danger is not so much in the heat, rather what coincides with that heat. That electrical activity generates an EMF field that can disrupt our cellular activity. For most larger devices like tablets and computers people can feel an unusual sensation when the device is placed on the lap. Most laptops EMF fields (up to 3 Gauss) can be measured up to 3 inches below the laptop. Nowadays, laptops are more frequently called personal computers; perhaps the industry is quietly acknowledging the risks by quietly changing its name. A simple rule to reduce exposure would be to always put the laptop/personal computer or tablet on a hard surface and not directly on the lap.

The third area where an electronic device causes harm to human health is the screen. All electronic devices emit a blue light, even the newer energy efficient LEDs (light emitting diode). A 2015 Harvard Health Newsletter warns of the dangers of blue light. Blue light disrupts the body's production of melatonin which is responsible for our day/night cycles. There is preliminary evidence that links disturbed sleep cycles to depression, diabetes, obesity, and cardiovascular effects. Several simple rules and changes of habit can improve the overall health of the family: 1) always turn the brightness level down on the television, computers, and tablets; 2) never allow digital device usage 2 hours before bedtime; 3) if your child needs to use a computer for homework, there are blue light screen filters that can be fitted over the device; 4) always have ambient room lighting on, preferably from good old-fashioned incandescent bulbs, while devices are on in the room.

These simple changes in habit will result in profound improvements in sleep and health for you and your family. This is what I do for my family and this is how I counsel families in my offices. For our family, the two most dramatic changes in our two childrens' (born 17 months apart) behavior occurred the day after I decided to reduce their exposure. The first was when I decided to turn off our wireless router. In general, routers are automatically set to a medium to high signal. Pulling up to our driveway, our devices pick up the wi-fi and readily connect. So even if your child's bedroom is clear across the house, far away from the router, very likely the whole family's sleep is disturbed if it is on all night. The next morning after unplugging the router, our whole family slept in 1 hour later. When the children awoke, they sat at their seats in their own world, not bothering each other; just from a better night's sleep, there was less fighting! My husband is so convinced, that if we forget, he will be the one to get up, plod across the house and turn off the router. The second most dramatic event I noticed occurred shortly after reading the 2015 Harvard Newsletter wherein Stephen Lockley, a sleep researcher, stated that the equivalent of two night lights was enough to disrupt sleep. All children, at some phase, have a fear of the dark. Part of the nighttime routine in putting our children to bed consists of turning on a nightlight. Inspired by Dr. Lockley, one evening, I snuck into my childrens' room and turned off their beautiful nightlight. After a week of consistently pulling out the router and the nightlight, my husband remarked surprisingly, that there seemed to be fewer fights. It is now a nightly routine in our household. Calmer and happier children that fight less is evidence of children that are getting quality sleep.

There is increasing scientific evidence that children are more sensitive to EMF than adults. In the school environment, it is up to parents to enquire as to the situation in their school districts. Parents need to be informed and active in participating and informing other parents and school officials of the dangers of EMF. In France, Italy, Spain, Australia, and Israel wi-fi is banned in elementary schools; all computer lines are hard wired. In a few countries, it is illegal to give a smartphone to a child under two or for businesses to sell phones targeted to children under seven. Other countries are starting to recognize the dangers of EMF to human health and are taking action to protect the most at-risk population. Here in the US, we can start to change that and protect ourselves and our children.

Digital Addiction

As of 2008, internet addiction became recognized as a mental health disorder. Increasingly, experts are recognizing that screen time can be as addictive as drugs and require rehabilitation, both outpatient and inpatient. Recognizing the health effects in children from technology exposure in terms of obesity, sleep, and social and family relationships, the American Academy of Pediatrics came out with recommendations in a policy statement in October 2016. Children under 2 years of age should have no exposure to digital media. Children over 2 years should have no more than 1 hour per day of digital media exposure.

Once children have been exposed, the changes in their sleep and later behavior are slow and insidious. Parents don't even realize what has already taken place. Once the behaviors of tantrums, clinginess, and fighting take place, it is time for an intervention. The first and easiest thing to do for younger children and even teens is to have family time out at the beach or park. From then the next step is withdrawing of digital devices; it is never easy to remove the electronic devices once home. It usually takes about two weeks of resistance: for younger children, this takes the form of more tantrums and crying and whining; in the older kids there is anger, resentment, bargaining, and eventual acceptance. These withdrawal behaviors are why Dr. Peter Whybrow, psychiatrist and director of neuroscience at UCLA, calls electronic devices "digital heroin."

In our family, I experienced these behaviors to a lesser degree with my children. On the weekends when visiting their grandpa, they wake up expecting their tablets. One weekend I decided that we were going to be free of all electronic devices. There was such initial resistance with the whining and crying but once they realized that I was determined, they gave up and the best thing happened: they started playing with each other, using their imagination and pretending. They engaged in lots of laughing and giggling. Three weekends later, their father stated, "You girls were so well behaved, I think you should be rewarded with the tablets." I had successfully weaned them and now one of us had weakened and the temptation was returned. It took a serious discussion but we are now at a good balance of some limited electronic device time.

Across countries, cultures, and governments agreement is consistent with the AAP policy statement that children under two should have no exposure to any electronic device. Infants and toddlers may become over stimulated and parents are unsuspecting. In the office, I see more infants and toddlers that are described by their parents as "very active." When I specifically ask about electronic devices and parents admit to using the smartphone, tablet, or television for distracting their child, I do several things to prove that their child is overstimulated and not born "hyperactive." Often overstimulated infants get fussy and whiny unless the parent holding them rocks them and picks up the pace to match their overstimulated states. In other words, the hyper child is not happy unless the parent becomes hyper and, in effect, they are training the parents too to become hyperactive and thus continue the cycle. In the span of 20 minutes, I prove this to parents and can easily "wind down" an overstimulated young child. Parents can do this at home. First, keep lighting at home mostly warm incandescent or halogen set at dim (or better, turn off lights and flood the home with natural sunlight). Instead of speaking at a normal pace, speech, tone, and volume should be slowed down and lowered even slower than normal speech. Within minutes, the child will visibly slow down. With infants, using the hands and fingers in slow motions will settle them down. For toddlers, opening a board book and reading very slowly will often be enough to slow them down. The secret is engagement with the child and slowing all sensations: visual, auditory, and pace of play. Also, make sure that the home EMF environment is reduced, if not completely eliminated.

SUMMARY

DEVELOPMENTAL MILESTONES

Physical: Puberty begins around the ages of eleven to fourteen. Beginning of sexual development, including budding of breasts and menstruation in girls and enlargement of testicles and penis, voice changes, and hair growth for boys.

Mental: Reasoning continues to evolve. Better comprehension of more symbolic and abstract concepts.

Social: Tremendous importance on appearance, due to emotional insecurities about esteem, individuality, and identity. Fluctuating hormones lead most to feel awkward both physically and socially. Become more independent.

MENSTRUATION

During menstruation, pads or tampons can be used. Commercial tampons contain harmful chemicals; use organic natural cotton brands. Pads are preferable; natural pads, which are reusable, are available.

Some girls experience premenstrual syndrome or menstrual cramps. Holistic medicine can treat abnormal periods and monthly discomfort.

ACNE

Acne is caused by clogged skin pores from oil and dead skin cells. Holistic medicine can treat acne without side effects.

COMPETITIVE SPORTS

Some student athletes use performance-enhancing drugs and supplements. Such drugs as creatine, anabolic steroids, and ephedra are known for their serious side effects.

EATING DISORDERS

Eating disorders, such as anorexia nervosa and bulimia, affect as many as ten percent of young women. Girls with anorexia stop eating out of fear of becoming fat. Bulimia is defined as binge eating followed by purging with self- induced vomiting, and can include use of laxatives and diuretics. Standard treatment includes specialized therapy (individual and family), nutritional counseling, medication (i.e. anti-depressants) and sometimes inpatient treatment programs and hospitalization.

JUNK FOOD

Junk food is all around our children. Healthy eating begins in the home, in your own kitchen, with you as the role model. One of the easiest ways to avoid indulging in junk food is to not have it around in the house.

TELEVISION AND VIDEO GAMES

TV and video games can lead to violent behavior, poor school performance, decreased family communication, and decreased physical activity. Know the shows your child is watching, limit television watching, avoid eating meals in front of the TV, and keep the TV and computer in a common area and not in the child's bedroom.

THE INTERNET AND CELL PHONES

The Internet and cell phones are useful for learning, pleasure and communication but it is important to monitor the computer use as you would with any activity. Use Internet filters and teach children not to give their email address nor phone number to strangers.

PART III

Natural Parenting Basics

When I approach a child
He inspires in me two sentiments:
Tenderness for what he is,
And respect for what he may become.

MANY PARENTS ARE INTERESTED IN USING natural remedies for childcare, yet do not know where or how to start. This section will guide you on the practical aspects of how to use remedies, whether commercially bought or prepared from your kitchen. Parents have commented to me that since learning about these remedies they feel more empowered and confident in treating their children's basic illnesses and offering relief. Even before I learned about homeopathy and natural medicine, I had little use for medications because I often found the side effects more bothersome than my symptoms. My husband would complain to me that our medicine cabinet was bare, except for a bottle of aspirin. Now it is full of a variety of remedies for all types of ailments. It is comforting to have a selection to choose from when I am looking for a remedy in the middle of the night to treat a cough, cold or fever. In fact, I never "leave home without it." I keep homeopathic *Arnica* 30C in my purse at all times in case of any accidents, bumps or bruises. On trips, I bring a traveling medical chest of commonly used remedies specifically chosen for the type of voyage. When I travel to Mexico, for instance, I make sure to take remedies in case of traveler's diarrhea, while on a ski trip we keep take along remedies in case of bumps, bruises, and sprains. If this is unfamiliar territory for you, keep this book handy too!

chapter 9

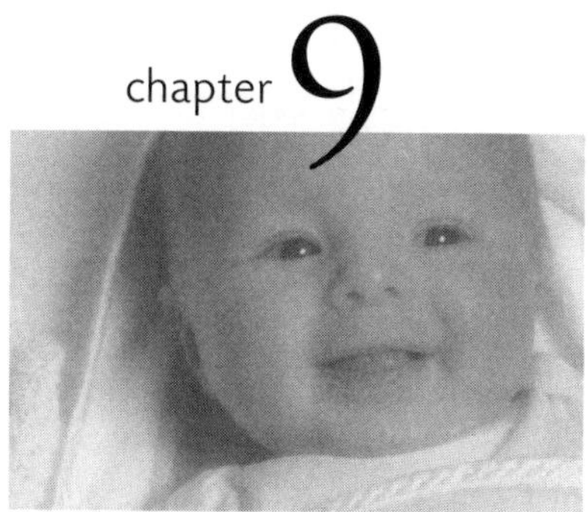

Applying Natural Remedies

Take care of the sense and the sounds will take care of themselves.

—*Alice's Adventures in Wonderland* by Lewis Carroll

The ABCs of Case-Taking

The natural treatments described in this book are for basic, self-limiting conditions that do not require a medical diagnosis (see Part IV). These are minor illnesses with few symptoms. The natural treatment of severe illnesses and chronic diseases like eczema, chronic allergies, attention deficit disorder, recurrent ear infections, and asthma requires the expertise of a professional.

Homeopathy and other forms of natural medicine expand your options for treating common ailments at home. In order to prescribe the correct treatment for your child, however, you will need to begin to think a bit like a homeopath, going through the "case-taking" process that will lead you to choose a course of action or remedy, be it a home treatment, medication, or visit to the doctor.

Your Child's Chart

To find the correct course of treatment, first requires compiling a detailed history of a patient, which in this case is your baby or child. When treating your children for mild, self-limiting illnesses at home, I recommend you keep a journal, similar to the file your doctor has at the office. Having a *home chart* for your child allows you to keep track of your observations and prescriptions over the years. In medical school, we were taught a simple note-taking method that most doctors still use in their practice known by the acronym, *S.O.A.P* (subjective, objective, assessment, plan). The soap note allows you to process your observations in an organized manner, and enables you to construct your home journal so that it keeps track of the same basic information.

Subjective

Under this heading you will write down the history of your child's complaint. As a *parent practitioner*, you will want to make accurate observations about your child's condition, paying particular attention to the signs and symptoms that present themselves spontaneously and unprompted. Just as you do in your practitioner's office, you will have to interpret for your child, especially if she is an infant. In young children, leading questions such as "Does your ear hurt?" can often illicit a yes reply just to placate, so be sure to base your assessment on other factors as well, framing your questions so that the child does not necessarily know the "right" answer.

A sign includes anything you perceive and may include, for instance, a runny nose, redness of the cheeks, or a cough. Symptoms are subjective sensations experienced by your child, such as stomachache, headache, or nausea. Use the following questions to organize the subjective section of your journal.

Who? Keep separate records for each child and include her age. Date each entry.
What? List the main complaints. Begin with the most important ones first.
Why? If you can pinpoint it, write down the cause.
How? Indicate how this illness affects your child mentally, emotionally and physically. Include details particular to complaints, such as:

- season (i.e., spring)
- weather (i.e, damp)
- time of day or night (i.e., 4 to 8 P.M.)
- temperature (i.e., chilliness)
- company (i.e., desires be alone, clingy)
- appetite (i.e., food cravings or aversions)
- what makes symptoms feel better or worse (i.e. noise, light, touch)

Objective

The objective section of the journal records the signs that you observe in your child. Some of the information under the *subjective* heading will already include many of your observations. Examples include:

- Temperature (including thermometer readings)
- Energy Level (i.e., exhausted or listless)
- Snoring
- Doubled over in pain

Assessment

In this section, you write your opinion. For your home chart, you do not need a formal diagnosis from your practitioner. For example:

- Fever
- Cough
- Flu

Plan

Here you write the treatment plan for your child. It can be a remedy, home treatment, doctor visit, or even a wait-and-see. For example:

- *Arsenicum album* 30C
- Hot water bottle
- Call the doctor

Examples of Record Keeping

Let's take two examples: Olivia, a fussy two-month-old baby girl, and Jack, an eight-year-old boy, both suffer from tummy upset. When you are determining a remedy, you will want to take into account both the objective and subjective aspects of the illness, balancing what your child reports with what you see. One of the keys to finding the right remedy is to note every aspect that helps you to distinguish your child's condition, from the time of day her symptoms occur, to the possible causes, to temperature readings and mood swings. Once you have taken down the full spectrum of your child's signs and symptoms, Part IV provides you with a number of choices of remedy, varying according to the subtle differences among conditions. I have tried to simplify your search by providing several commonly used remedies for each condition, listing them with the symptoms they best treat.

Name: Olivia	**Date:** July 27, 2015 **Age:** 2 months
SUBJECTIVE	For the past several weeks, she has been crying and screaming with gas pains, that come in waves. Angry while nursing. Fidgety, can't find a comfortable position.
OBJECTIVE	Brings her knees up to her belly. Doubled over in pain. Feels better with firm pressure on tummy, better lying on tummy. Stools are jelly-like.
ASSESSMENT	Fussy Colicky Gas Pains
PLAN	Nursing mother's diet (omit common gas-producing foods) Infant massage which can be helpful for colic Swaddle, baby wear, and carry Hot water bottle *Colocynthis* 30C – chosen as it is a good colic medicine for gas pains associated with angry mood, doubled over in pain, and for symptoms that improve with firm pressure on the abdomen. Called practitioner who said it was common at this age. Will visit practitioner if the above measures to not help.

Name: Jack	**Date:** October 23, 2014 **Age:** 8 years
SUBJECTIVE	Comes home in an angry mood after going to a birthday party. Afterwards starts to complain of stomachache. Says, "My tummy hurts, I'm not hungry!"
OBJECTIVE	Feels better with warmth, worse being touched. Constipated.
ASSESSMENT	Stomachache, probably due to overeating sweets and birthday cake at the party.
PLAN	Hot water bottle Avoid eating Liquids, such as water and broth, as desired. *Nux vomica* 30C – good medicine for complaints from overeating. Visit practitioner if above measures do not help or condition worsens.

Buying Homeopathic and Natural Medicines

It used to be that natural medicines were only available in select health food stores, but today more drug stores are carrying homeopathic medicines, herbs and supplements. If you are unable to find a remedy locally, consider the Internet or homeopathic pharmacies which will ship orders (see Resource and Further Readings). Most of the products in this book can be ordered at www.drfeder.com.

Also available are homeopathic kits containing up to several dozen medicines. They come in different shapes and sizes for portability and are often more cost effective than buying one medicine at a time. Homeopathic medicines come in various potencies. The 'X' and 'C' come from the Roman numerals ten and one hundred. Hence, the 6X strength is weaker than the 6C. The lower potencies, ranging in strength from 6X, 6C, 30X, and 30C, are appropriate for use at home. The correct choice of medicine will work at any strength. In general, remedies in the strengths of 6 (6X or 6C) need to be repeated more often than the 30 (30X or 30C) potencies. Contrary to "rational thinking," a homeopathic medicine that is more diluted is actually stronger and deeper acting. Thus, although the 30C potency is diluted more than a 6C potency, it is stronger than a 6C potency. The

30C potency, which is commonly found, is my preference; however, the correct choice of medicine will work at any of these strengths.

Administering Homeopathic Medicines

Homeopathic medicines come as round, chewable pellets or as quick-dissolve tablets, depending on the brand you purchase. Both types are sweet and pleasant tasting, which makes it easy to administer to children. When possible, avoid touching the tablets with your fingers. Use a spoon.

Dosages. Take 3 pellets 3 times a day or as directed by your practitioner. In acute cases, take every hour until relieved. Doses are the same for all ages. If you see no improvement after 3 doses, discontinue the remedy. Adults and older children are encouraged to let the tablets dissolve under the tongue. Younger children can let them dissolve in their mouths. If your child is too small to take the medicine, place 3 pellets in ½ glass of water and let stand for 5 minutes. If you are using the hard pellets, they will not dissolve immediately, but the water will become medicated. Stir ten times, and give ¼ teaspoon (or dropperful).

Eating and Drinking. Avoid eating or drinking 10 minutes (if possible) before and after taking your homeopathic remedy. With a baby or small child this is not always possible. Not to worry!

Substances to Avoid. During the time period that you are taking a remedy, it is best to avoid coffee, chocolate, camphor, eucalyptus, mint, and other strong-smelling substances (mint toothpaste is okay).

Persistent or Worsening Symptoms. If symptoms persist more than three days or worsen, discontinue the remedy and consult your doctor.

Improving Symptoms. As your condition improves, take your homeopathic medicine less often (1 to 2 times a day). When you are substantially better, discontinue the medicine.

Storing and Traveling. Store your homeopathic medicines away from electrical appliances, strong-smelling substances and extremes of temperature. If possible, have your medicines be hand-checked at the airport, instead of going through the x-ray machine.

Administering Gemmotherapy

Gemmotherapy herbal remedies are diluted (1:10 strength) in a base of alcohol with glycerin and water. They are prepared in an amber glass bottle with a dropper. In addition to gemmotherapy, Bach Flower Essences are prepared in an alcohol base. If your child is sensitive to alcohol, place the open bottle in 1 inch of slow boiling water for 5 minutes. Cool the bottle before screwing on stopper. The shelf life without alcohol is approximately 3 weeks.

Gemmotherapy remedies are easy to administer. They can be given directly under the tongue, though most children prefer them in a beverage, such as water. Ideally, they should be taken one at a time in water. However, they can be taken together mixed in water or juice.

The dosage for infants is 5 to 8 drops. Give children ages 2 to 8 years old 12 to 15 drops, and older children and adults, 25 drops. The remedies can be used as often as 2 to 3 times per day during acute illness. Gemmotherapy is available through healthcare providers and selected pharmacies. Gemmos can be used in conjunction with each other (up to three at a time), with homeopathic remedies, and any other medicines. As with any remedy, use when needed, then discontinue.

Administering Essential Oils

Essential oils, such as lavender and chamomile, are highly concentrated and should not be used undiluted on your child's delicate skin. When prepared, they are mixed with a carrier oil, such as apricot, wheat germ, sweet almond, or other specific oils. If your child is allergic to nuts, avoid using preparations that contain carrier oils made from nuts. If you are not knowledgeable about using essential oils, I recommend that you consult with a qualified aromatherapy practitioner or use the commercially prepared brands for children. Babies and children have more sensitive skin than adults, so use only gentle oils in weaker dilutions. When using an oil for the first time, rub a few drops on the skin for a patch test. Wait one day. If your child shows no signs of reaction, like a rash, then you can use it as needed. To use, place a quarter size amount of oil in the palm of your hand. Rub your hands together to warm the oil and massage into skin as needed. Avoid applying on the delicate areas of the face, ears and bottom. Essential oils are not to be taken internally. Keep oils, herbs, and all remedies out of the reach of children.

External Healing Applications: Making a Compress, Poultice, Bath, or Inhalation

Learning about foot baths, compresses, head wraps, and soothing steam inhalations feels like traveling in time to the days of our great-grandparents, who relied on these healing applications as adjuncts to basic home healthcare. All of these modalities can be used in conjunction with other treatments. For this section, I am indebted to Wiep de Vries, R.N. and the Wellness Nurses of the Los Angeles Alliance for Childhood, whose practical workshops are an invaluable resource on basic home healing applications.

External healing applications are designed for application to the skin. As a living organism and the body's largest organ, the skin is immensely responsive to both external and internal stimuli: it breathes, protects, perceives, excretes toxins, and communicates with the brain. By touching your child, you can learn a lot about her physical, mental, and emotional state. If your child has a fever, different parts of the body may feel warmer or cooler than others; in a state of fear, you may see goose bumps and feel rigidity.

Through the skin, we are able to perform healing measures that will permeate deeply into the body. Therapeutic applications can bring down a high fever, comfort an earache, and alleviate sore muscles, cramps, and fatigue. Depending on the need, applications will be either cool or warm. Cool applications cause constriction of the blood vessels, decreasing circulation to the area. Typically, cold is useful for injuries with swelling and acute sprains, and for some headaches. Warm applications increase circulation to the local area by dilating vessels and are indicated for stiff muscles, menstrual cramps, earache, and backache.

For compresses, poultices, and wraps, you will want a cloth made of cotton (preferably organic) or another natural fiber. When in a pinch, I have cut a clean cotton rag to size, which also works fine.

Some substances used for external applications can also be prepared as a drink to augment the treatment. For instance, with lemon or chamomile applications, try serving a lemon or chamomile tea.

Compress

A simple way to apply herbs is with a compress applied directly to the skin. Pour one quart of water into a glass bowl. Use hot, warm, room temperature, or cold water, depending upon the desired compress. For compresses, use cotton or natural fiber material. Add the appropriate substance and soak the cloth in the bowl of water and wring it out, placing the compress over affected area. Wrap or cover.

For warm compresses (also referred to as fomentations), a hot water bottle can be placed on top to maintain its effectiveness; for cold compresses, an ice pack. Depending on the condition, keep in place for ten to fifteen minutes, or as tolerated. Common compresses include lemon, onion, chamomile, lavender, *Arnica,* or *Calendula.*

Poultice

In a poultice, the crushed fresh herb or substance is placed into a cloth and tied to make a pouch or folded into a flattened envelope and then placed topically. To prepare, place substance in the center of cheese cloth or natural fiber cloth. Fold up the ends, and secure with a string or rubber band. Poultices can be made from familiar items such as onion, lemon, potato, and ginger, and are especially effective in "drawing out" inflammation. For this reason, onion and potato poultices are also known as drawing poultices.

Wrap

Wraps can be used directly on the skin, such as a foot wrap, or used as an outer layer that secures an application, such as a compress, to the skin. They are similar in size to an ace bandage and are wrapped around the affected part. Foot wraps are especially useful for fevers and fatigue. Choose a cotton or natural fiber cloth to the dimensions given above (it can be shorter, if necessary) and saturate in the desired liquid preparation. Wring it out so it is damp and carefully begin to wrap the toes encircling the whole foot, ankle, and calf up to the knee as you would with an ace bandage.

Choose a cotton or natural fiber cloth that is up to 6 inches wide (15.2 cm) and 2 yards long (182 cm). To treat an area where you want to retain warmth, use long wool wraps. When I do not have the exact materials, I improvise with wool scarves.

Bath

Many of us already use baths therapeutically as a form of comfort and relaxation, but with the addition of healing herbs, oils, and other substances, baths can provide treatment and relief to a number of conditions. Depending on your child's needs, you can prepare either an oil dispersion or nutritional bath.

For general strengthening, improving circulation, and relaxing, oil dispersion baths can be done several times a week before bedtime. Use an aromatherapy preparation approved for children. Use according to directions and place in warm bath water. With your arm make a large figure eight motion to disperse the oil throughout the bath approximately 20 to 30 times. Your child is ready to get into the bath when the oil has risen to the top of the bath and makes a thin film.

Nutritional baths help with metabolism and digestion as well as fatigue, stress, and exhaustion following convalescence from a debilitating illness. Before your child gets in the warm bath, stir one cup of whole milk, one raw egg, and a lemon into the bath water. Cut the lemon in the bath, under the water. This allows the aromatic oils of the lemon to be dispersed in the water.

Avoid baths if your child has a fever or infection. In addition to preparing the therapeutic bath, have everything ready for your child after the bath so that she stays warm and comfy. This would include two towels and two hot water bottles already warming up the bed during the bath. After the bath, pat your child dry with one towel, cocoon wrap with the dry towel, then let her rest in the warm bed.

A soak involves submerging a body part, such as a foot or hand, in warm or cool water. Foot baths are among the most common soaks and can be made by adding an herb or remedy to water and immersing the foot up to the ankle. Warm foot baths increase circulation, and are good for colds, flu, and insomnia. Room temperature (or cool) soaks revitalize you from fatigue and stress. Soak feet for 10 to 15 minutes in a foot bath or large bowl.

Inhalation

An ear, nose, and throat doctor, my father routinely recommends steam inhalation for his patients with sore throats, hoarseness and sinus infections. After the water has boiled, pour into a bowl, and then place the bowl in a heavier bowl (i.e. ceramic) to prevent tipping and burns.

For safety reasons, both you and your child will do the steam inhalation together with large towel or sheet draped over your heads like a tent. To avoid dampened hair or chills afterward, keep head covered with a hat or towel during inhalation. Inhale for 5 to 10 minutes. Slices of lemon make an especially effective steam inhalation remedy.

You can also do a room inhalation remedy. In that case, oils (e.g., lemon, lavender) are placed in a vaporizer or non-flammable bowl on top of the radiator, which can be helpful in treating colds, sore throats, coughs and sinus infections.

Common Home Remedies

You already have in your home many of the ingredients for common home remedies. In fact, although you may not think of them for medicinal purposes, you may already use some of these remedies; perhaps they were taught to you by your parents, or perhaps you simply realized one day how soothing chamomile can be. Now, you can see how you can use these to help your baby.

The Hot Water Bottle

Warmth is key to effective healing for many conditions, though most of us do not make full use of its soothing, therapeutic qualities (on dressing for warmth, see "Dressing Your Child" in Chapter 10). Many of the compresses and poultices described in this chapter make use of heat, and you will find a hot water bottle indispensable in lengthening and improving the effectiveness of applications. We all have hot water bottles buried somewhere in a cabinet; now is the time to pull it out, dust it off, and if you cannot find yours, buy one! This part of our medicine chest gets used for most of our illnesses.

To prepare, fill the water bottle midway with hot water. Standing by a sink, I fold the hot water bottle in half to expel the air, with any excess water spilling into the sink, then I securely fasten. Expelling the air helps the bottle retain its heat. Never place a hot water bottle directly on the skin, but wrap it instead in a towel. The hot water bottle can be used anywhere for comfort, though its most common applications are next to a painful ear or on the chest, tummy, and feet. To warm feet, secure the water bottle around the feet with towels for at least five to ten minutes until they are warm. Hot water bottles can also be used to warm a cold bed before going to sleep. An electric heating pad is not a replacement for a hot water bottle. Avoid using an electric heating pad, as studies have linked exposure to low level electromagnetic radiation from these devices to cancer and other health conditions.

Chamomile

Chamomile, as a tea or remedy, is the great soother, and can be employed as a compress or poultice, especially to the belly. To make a tea, poultice, or compress, place 2 to 3 tablespoons of organic chamomile flowers (or 2 to 3 teabags) in a bowl and add hot water. Steep for 3 minutes. To make a poultice, use the soaked chamomile flowers; if making a tea or compress, strain before use. As an essential oil, use chamomile that has been diluted in a carrier oil and massage into the skin or apply an oil compress. In addition, a hot water bottle can be placed over the compress, poultice, or massaged areas to preserve warmth. Unfortunately, some children react to chamomile because of its similarity to ragweed. If this is the case, discontinue its use. Also, do not use chamomile applications if your child has a high fever.

Chamomile is useful for:

- Stomach upset, tummy aches, or colic
- Cramps (including menstrual cramps)
- Eye inflammation (including pinkeye)
- Chest congestion (bronchitis), stopped ears
- Soothing for ear, nose, and throat

Ear, Nose, and Throat. Chamomile steam inhalation is useful in treating chest congestion (bronchitis), irritable coughs, and stopped ears, and in general helps soothe the ears, nose, and throat.

Stomach Upset. For digestive trouble, liver problems, constipation, or diarrhea, try a chamomile abdominal compress after a meal. With severe stomachaches, however, you should see your practitioner to rule out appendicitis or other serious conditions.

Lemon

Hippocrates once said, "Nature is the healer of all disease," and perhaps no natural substance proves his point as beautifully as the lemon. In the healing application workshop, Wellness Nurse Wiep de Vries speaks of the unique vitality of the lemon tree, which blooms and bears fruit at the same time. The fruit itself has multiple uses, its sliced interior bearing witness to nature's lovely symmetry, while the skin holds an abundance of medicinally therapeutic aromatic oils and flavenoids.

Like its neat, segmental structure, the lemon's role is to organize and rearrange the conditions necessary to speed healing. For example, if a child has a fever and the majority of the heat is in the head, the lemon will help displace the heat, lowering the fever. Lemon's cooling and calming properties make it an excellent remedy for fevers and stress.

To prepare for compresses and wraps, cut a lemon (preferably organic) in a bowl of warm water. Cutting it in the water is important in capturing the aromatic oils from the skin of the lemon. Lemons can be sliced or, for the artistically inclined, starred. To make a lemon star, cut a lemon in half and place the halves in a bowl of warm water. Slice each half underwater five times from the center outwards. Press the lemon on the bottom of the bowl. This releases the juice and the lemon halves come to look like stars.

Lemon is good for:

- Fevers
- Bronchitis
- Tickle in the throat or chest (tickly cough)
- Watery runny nose or eyes (opposite of onion, which is good for thick discharges)
- Sore throat
- Allergy/hay fever
- Stress and fatigue

Try using lemon in a foot and calf wrap, throat and chest compresses (line up the lemons in a cloth), foot baths, or room inhalation.

Fevers. Lemon foot wraps are especially soothing for high fevers accompanied by hallucinations, lethargy, and glassy eyes. Often with this type of fever, most of the heat centers in the head (often with bright red cheeks), while the limbs are cooler. The lemon exerts a cooling influence and disperses the heat away from the head, making the child more comfortable. If the legs are cool, warm them up with a hot water bottle for 5 to 10 minutes before using the lemon wrap. If you do not have lemon, use vinegar. With a high fever, the wrap may dry in a few minutes. Repeat every 10 to 15 minutes as needed.

To prepare the foot wrap, dip a long cotton or natural fiber scroll in lemon juice and use as a compress, or line up the lemons in a poultice and secure, still dipping the scroll in lemon juice. Place on the feet and wrap up to the knee. Lemon slice poultices can also be placed in a sock and put on your child's feet.

Bronchitis. For bronchitis, lemon inhalation can be helpful. Slice lemon in a bowl of hot water, place towel over the head, and breathe for 5 to 10 minutes. For the wheezing, prolonged cough associated with bronchitis, a hot lemon chest compress can also offer relief. In addition, try placing lemon slices in a non-flammable bowl on the radiator so that the oils and aroma permeate the air.

Stress and Fatigue. For a child (or adult) who has nervous worry such as an upcoming exam or meeting, lemon can be used for relaxation and stress relief. Place a room temperature lemon compress or poultice around your wrists, or submerge feet in a room temperature foot bath with lemon slices or stars. The coolness of the lemon is calming and, if fatigued, will wake you before an important event. The lemon foot bath with floating lemon slices can be a wonderful treat for fatigued and tired feet in general.

Onion

Cutting up an onion causes a reaction in most cooks—eyes water and noses run, sending us hunting for a tissue. While the irritation in never pleasurable, it is precisely this reaction that makes the onion so versatile and useful as a healing herb. Onion improves circulations and breaks up thick mucus and congestion, making it a great remedy for colds. The high sulphur content in onion causes thick mucus to move outward toward the surface of the body.

Both the onion and its juice have important properties, so be sure to extract liquid from the onion in your preparation. To prepare an onion:

- Chop onions finely (white or yellow).
- To bring out the onion juice do one of the following:
  - Finely chop
  - Place cloth over chopped onion and smash under a cup
  - Put in blender for 5 to 10 seconds.
- Although onion can be used at room temperature, I am partial to the warm version. After you have the desired consistency, lightly sauté for a few minutes with a little water or olive oil until warm.

- Place onion into a rounded pouch or a flat envelope, if used for the ear, swollen glands, or feet.

Onion is good for:

- Colds
- Earaches
- Teething
- Bladder infections
- Swollen glands
- Boils and abscesses

Colds. For colds, an onion pouch in a child's room can help with congestion. Using a cloth or sock, make an onion pouch, securely tied. Place near the child on the nightstand, by the bed, or above the crib, and leave it overnight. You can also use sliced onion: simply place one to two slices on a plate by the bed. For chest colds, place an onion poultice on the chest and wrap with a scarf.

Onion poultices can also be applied to the feet by way of onion socks. To make one, put the prepared onion in small pouch and place the securely tied poultice in a sock. Fit the sock on your child's foot, so that the pouch securely stays in place on the sole of her foot. Let your child sleep overnight with the onion sock. In addition to treating colds, onion poultice socks can be used for earaches, teething, and bladder infections.

Earaches. When my son has an earache, he often requests an onion application, which can soothe and alleviate discomfort. I place one small onion envelope in front of the entrance of the ear, and another envelope behind the ear and wrap with a scarf, leaving the wrap on for ten minutes or overnight. Before putting on the applications, I take a little warm onion juice mixed with olive oil, and gently place it in the ear (do not do this if there is any pus, blood, or liquid coming from the ear).

Swollen Glands. Onion helps soften the lymph node, making it an ideal remedy for painful swollen glands. Place a cloth envelope of chopped onion over the swollen glands and wrap with a scarf. Onion pouches can also be placed over boils and abscesses.

Potatoes

Potatoes draw out toxins and break up congestion, which makes them useful in alleviating aches and pains. Potatoes are an excellent source for moist heat and retain temperature longer than a hot water bottle. Hot potato applications should feel comfortable, though, and not burn the skin. If the heat is dissipating, a hot water bottle can be placed over the preparation to lengthen its duration.

Potatoes are good for:

- Sore throat
- Cough
- Headache
- Neck ache
- Muscle pain
- Chilliness
- Boils and abscesses

Just when you thought you had experienced mashed potatoes every which way, the Wellness Nurses offer a wonderful recipe for preparing these hot potato poultices for any of the above conditions. Cook several whole potatoes (as many as 4 to 6) with the skin on. Allow them to cool for a few minutes, and place them in a sock or sleeve. Smash the potatoes, allowing them to further cool (6 to 8 minutes). Make sure the poultice is not too hot (monitor heat on your wrist or cheek first!) and close the open end with tape. When potatoes are still warm, place the enclosed potato poultice around the neck, chest or other body part.

Boils and Abscesses. Raw potato slices are also helpful in reducing inflammation associated with boils and abscesses. Place raw potato slices directly on the boil and wrap with cheese cloth.

Infant and Child Massage

Several nights a week, my seven-year-old son requests a massage: feet, tummy, hands, and face, and in that order. The term infant massage is a relatively new addition to Western culture and encompasses everything from a do-it-yourself approach to a visit with a certified infant massage practitioner and instructor to specific trainings that teach parents how to treat various conditions.

While infant massage is only now gaining mainstream popularity, it is hardly a new practice. My mother may not have been familiar with specific massage techniques, but she intuitively rubbed our bodies when we were sick with tummy aches, headaches, and fevers. In fact, parents have been massaging babies for centuries throughout the world. With massage schools beginning to offer training courses in infant massage for therapists as well as eager parents, this ancient practice is returning to the home. The advantages of learning infant massage are many: it promotes your baby's mental, physical, and emotional health and fosters a bond between you and your baby through the comfort and warmth of touch. Most people equate massage with pleasure, and same goes for your baby.

Infant massage:

1. Helps baby relax. During massage, the body releases chemicals and hormones in the body (endorphins and oxytocin), which offer pain relief and promote feelings of well-being.
2. Prevents certain illnesses. Daily massage may be helpful in preventing or minimizing conditions such as colic.
3. Strengthen the immune system. Infant massage combines the use of body movement, stretching and comforting touch, which promote sound sleep and help reduce stress. All of these help stimulate and strengthen the immune system.
4. Stimulates blood circulation, which is especially good for alleviating cold hands and feet.
5. Improves sleep. After massage, some infants are known to sleep more soundly and for longer intervals.
6. Aids the digestive system and particularly helps with gas pains, colic, and constipation. Specific motions that can offer digestive relief and aid in elimination may be performed by a trained practitioner or taught to parents and caregivers.
7. Alleviates discomfort from teething. Massage releases oxytocin and endorphins which help make baby feel better.
8. Helps treat infections by breaking up mucous in colds, sinus, and chest congestion.
9. Promotes bonding through touch, allowing parent and baby to spend one-on-one time together. This is not only helpful for the baby but calming for parents. In addition to supporting bonding, massage can build a parent's

confidence in his or her caretaking skills. Older siblings, family members, and caretakers can make great massage therapists, too.

10. In preterm infants, helps baby gain weight. In a study published in Pediatrics in 1986, massage was associated with as much as a 47% increase in weight gain in preterm infants.
11. In depressed mothers, helps alleviate depression and anxiety.

Basic Infant Massage Techniques

The following are basic techniques, though as you and baby become comfortable with this lovely experience, you will invariably make your own variations. Many massage tips for adults are also applicable with your baby. This time, though, you will be the massage therapist.

Before you begin:

- Wash your hands and remove bulky jewelry. Keep nails clipped.
- Put on gentle, calming music in the background if desired. Turn off any loud disruptive sounds (like your mobile phone).
- Keep lighting dim. Avoid direct sunlight in baby's eyes.
- Keep baby warm. Avoid cool rooms and open drafts. Drape areas of the body that are not being massaged.
- Collect any oils you may want to use for massage. Use cold pressed oils, pesticide- and petrochemical-free. Vegetable, nut or seed oils can be used, but my special favorites are sweet almond, jojoba, coconut, apricot, and avocado oil. Blended oils designed especially for baby massage are also available; choose one without any fragrance. There is no need to clean it off. Avoid olive oil.
- Ensure that you are in a comfortable position. Avoid leaning over and hurting your back.

Now you are ready to begin:

1. Begin with the feet and ankles, massaging one at a time. With your hands at the ankle, work your way up to baby's knee and thigh and down back to the ankle. Use two strokes: a gentle long motion and also a wringing action. Avoid light, feathery strokes, which can tickle baby.

2. Don't forget the feet. Foot reflexology recognizes that all the organs of the body are reflected on the foot, ball and sole. With gentle circular motion, begin with the heel, arch, and ball of foot. Gently massage each toe (from the base to its tip), including a little massage between the toes.
3. At the belly make gentle circles in a clockwise fashion (your left to right). Avoid massaging the bellybutton.
4. Slide hands up to baby's chest. Start at the central breast plate and simultaneously move hands upwards and outward toward the shoulders and under the armpits.
5. The arms are similar to the legs. I prefer to do one at a time. From the wrist begin in an upward motion, first with long gentle strokes and finishing with a wringing motion. Massage the palms and concentrate on one digit at a time to the tip of the fingers.
6. Now place baby on her tummy. Begin with the neck, shoulders, shoulder blades, and back all the way to the base of the spine (avoid massaging the actual spine). Finish with little circular motions on baby's bum. Finish with long strokes down the back of the legs to the Achilles tendon.
7. Turn baby on her back. On the face, begin at the middle of the forehead. Similar to the breast bone, gently move from the midline of the forehead out to the temples. Make a few light circles around the temple. Gently follow the curvatures around the eyes, nose and mouth. Be sure to include cheeks and chin. Avoid getting too close to eyes and mouth.
8. Massage the earlobes, including a circle around the outer ear. My son loves this!

Go with your baby's flow. If she is squirmy and fidgety, avoid making her stay in rigid positions. If she is letting you know that she is not in the right mood, or has had enough after a few minutes, respect that and discontinue the session. Be careful when moving your baby, as the oil will make her skin slippery. Watch your baby, not the clock. Enjoy the time together. Kisses are allowed before, during, and after.

For all its benefits, sometimes it's best not to give massages:

- After eating or hiccoughs, avoid massage to the belly.
- For infants under 4 or 5 months, avoid giving a bath and massage one after another, as they can be over stimulating. For older infants, you can do massage following the bath.

- Avoid massaging when baby has a fever, suspicious lumps (unless your practitioner has given an okay), open cuts, skin infections (i.e. impetigo), bruised or swollen areas, or other serious illness or injury. If your baby has recently had surgery, wait until the area has healed, inside and out.

SUMMARY

THE ABCS OF CASE-TAKING

In order to prescribe the correct treatment (be it a home remedy, medication, or visit to the doctor) for your child, go through the "case-taking" process using the acronym S.O.A.P. (Subjective, Objective, Assessment, Plan).

BUYING HOMEOPATHIC AND NATURAL MEDICINES

Homeopathic remedies come in various potencies; the lower potencies (6X, 6C, 30X, and 30C) are appropriate for home use. Also available are homeopathic kits containing up to fifty remedies.

ADMINISTERING HOMEOPATHIC MEDICINES

- Take 3 pellets 3 times a day. As the condition improves, take it less often.
- If you see no improvement after 3 doses, discontinue the remedy
- Avoid eating and drinking 10 minutes before and after taking the remedy. Avoid coffee, chocolate, camphor, eucalyptus, mint, and other strong-smelling substances (mint toothpaste is okay).
- If symptoms persist more than 3 days or worsen, contact your practitioner.
- Store your remedies away from electrical appliances, strong-smelling substances, and extremes of temperature.

ADMINISTERING GEMMOTHERAPY

Gemmotherapy herbal remedies are diluted (1:10 strength) in a base of alcohol with glycerin and water. The dosage for infants is 5 to 8 drops. Give children 2 to 8 years old 12 to 15 drops, and older children and adults, 25 drops. The remedies can be used as often as 2 to 3 times per day during acute illness.

ADMINISTERING ESSENTIAL OILS

Place a quarter size amount of diluted oil in the palm of your hand. Rub your hands together to warm the oil and massage into skin as needed. Avoid applying on the delicate areas of the face, ears and bottom.

EXTERNAL HEALING APPLICATIONS: MAKING A COMPRESS, POULTICE, BATH, OR INHALATION

With poultices, a crushed herb or remedy is placed in a cloth made of cotton (preferably organic) or another natural fiber and applied to the skin. With compresses, baths, soaks, or inhalations, the herb or remedy is added to water.

COMMON HOME REMEDIES

Many common household items and foods, such as hot water bottles, onions, lemons, chamomile, and potatoes, can be used for colds, aches, stomach upset, and many other conditions.

INFANT AND CHILD MASSAGE

Infant massage helps baby relax, prevents certain illnesses, strengthens the immune system, stimulates blood circulation, improves sleep, aids the digestive system, alleviates discomfort from teething, helps treat infection, promotes bonding, and alleviates mothers' postpartum depression. To massage your baby:

1. Work your way up from baby's feet and ankles to her knee and thigh with a gentle long motion and a wringing action.
2. With gentle circular motion, gently massage each heel, arch, and toe.
3. At the belly make gentle circles in a clockwise fashion (your left to right).
4. Slide hands up to baby's chest and move hands upwards and outward toward the shoulders.
5. For the arms, begin from the wrist with a long gentle stroke and a wringing motion. Massage the palms and concentrate on one digit at a time to the tip of the fingers.
6. Now place baby on her tummy. Begin with the neck, shoulders, shoulder blades, and back. Finish with little circular motions on baby's bum.
7. Turn baby on her back. On the face, begin at the middle of the forehead. Make a few light circles around the temple. Gently follow the curvatures around the eyes, nose, and mouth.
8. Massage the earlobes, including a circle around the outer ear.

chapter 10

Decorating, Clothing, and Bathing

Our life is frittered away by detail . . . Simplify, Simplify.

–Henry David Thoreau

Creating a Nontoxic Environment for Your Baby

Even before baby is born, many eager parents have dressed up a nursery, not realizing that everyday products can contain harmful toxins with deleterious effects. At birth, your baby is more vulnerable to her environment physically, through her skin, lungs, and digestive system, as well as cognitively, in her mental and emotional development. Particularly in these early weeks and months, it is vital to protect your child as much as possible from toxic exposure.

Take a look at your home: from the kitchen to the bathroom and even to the bedroom, most families are surrounded by products that are potentially toxic. Such everyday items as the paint, carpet, and crib that decorate your baby's nursery could negatively impact her health. At baby showers, many moms-to-be receive a baby bath tub filled to the brim with goodies. Chances are the products inside are filled with synthetics: diaper creams, baby lotions, shampoos, soaps, plastic bottles and nipples, pacifiers, and flame retardant pajamas. I am well aware that we cannot completely cocoon a baby from harmful chemicals but we can minimize our children's exposure.

You could easily find lists and lists of chemicals to avoid. In general, however, the ones to stay away from can be grouped into four families.

1. Brominated flame retardant chemicals are used to make items such as pajamas, furniture, and mattresses less flammable. One of these chemicals, known as Polybrominated Diphenyl Ethers (PBDEs), has been linked with the onset of learning disabilities and can cause thyroid damage and cancer. While PBDEs have also surfaced in farm-raised salmon, they are primarily found in polyester fabrics, plastics, and foam, including carpets, furniture, mattress and bedding, computers, and so on. PBDEs, although banned in Europe, are still being used in North America. PBDEs have also been recorded in breast milk.
2. Bisphenol A (BPA) is found in baby bottles and plastic food containers, and may be absorbed into the milk. It has estrogen-like effects in the body which can disturb the hormonal system, potentially raising the incidence of breast cancer. In addition to baby bottles, BPA is a component in the lining of canned foods.
3. Phthalates can be found in soft squeezy plastic toys, pacifiers, and teething rings. Children often put these items in their mouths, and this chemical is known to accumulate in the body. Phthalates are linked to abnormalities in the genitals of baby boys and are banned in Europe.
4. Organotin compounds are found in hard plastic toys. They are known to cause hormone changes according to tests on animals.

Here are some additional tips to minimize your baby's contact with these potentially harmful chemicals (and yours!):

- Avoid synthetic fabrics and plastic toys.
- Choose natural brands of cleaning products or make them yourself. Hydrogen peroxide has antiseptic properties and is considered a safe and natural cleanser. Vinegar has been used for thousands of years medicinally and for household purposes, including as an antiseptic that kills most bacteria, viruses, and mold. To make a simple cleaning solution, pour 3% hydrogen peroxide and 5% white distilled vinegar (or apple cider vinegar) into two separate clean spray bottles. Whether it be cleaning countertops, vegetables, or wood cutting boards, the paired sprays work well. Although any order can be used, I prefer the

vinegar followed by the hydrogen peroxide (the stronger odor of vinegar is then toned down by the hydrogen peroxide). Rinse food with clean water afterward.

- Steer clear of all fumes: glue, new carpeting and furniture, gasoline, finishes, and dry cleaners can all pose inhalation risks.
- Drink filtered water to reduce intake of chlorine and fluoride.
- Avoid antiperspirants (which prevent release of the toxins through the skin) and only use natural deodorants, if any.
- Use stainless steel, ceramic-coated, or iron cookware, and avoid aluminum, as it has been linked to Alzheimer's disease. Also, avoid Teflon-coated pans. Teflon contain chlorofluorocarbons (CFCs), which have been linked to ozone damage; trifluoroacetate (TFA), which is toxic to plants; and polyfluorocarboxylic acids (PFOs), which can accumulate in humans and animals where they are known to affect the thyroid gland.

See the Resources and Further Readings section at the back of the book for more information on safer products for the family.

Decorating Your Baby's Room

Most people rarely consider that the new paint, furniture, or carpeting in baby's room may be toxic. Fortunately, healthier options in décor are increasingly available, allowing you to decorate the nursery both safely and in style.

Flooring: People with allergies often rip up carpeting to minimize the exposure to mold, dust, and dirt. Hardwood floors or hard surfaces are easier to clean. If you do want carpeting, look for the "green label," which designates a product containing fewer chemicals.

Paint: For less toxic paints (low Volatile Organic Compounds, or VOC's), look for the environmentally friendly logos like Envirodesic. This certification endorses ecologically sustainable products and services in the areas of home and building. Also keep an eye out for "Maximum Indoor Air Quality," which specifies a low-toxicity brand. When choosing paints, I prefer the type that can easily wash away finger prints and crayon marks. There are now low and zero VOC paints as well as natural paints and stains and an asthma and allergy friendly brand of zero VOC paint.

Window Treatments: When curtains and blinds are exposed to the heat of the sun, they can release unhealthy chemicals. Curtains made of natural fibers are better than synthetics, and metal blinds are superior to plastic varieties, which release PVCs (Polyvinyl Chloride (PVCs) when exposed to sun or heat.

Bedding, Mattresses and Furniture: Avoid stain repellants (i.e. Scotchgard) on furniture and clothes as well as polyurethane foam in couches in beds. Scotchgard breaks down into fluorocarbon chemicals that are similar to banned, ozone-depleting CFCs. Watch out, too, for the popular memory foam mattresses, which can contain up to a pound of flame retardants known to cause cancer and brain damage. The healthier choice is to use mattresses, futons, mattress pads, and crib bedding made of organic materials. Consider wool as well it is naturally flame retardant and increasingly more popular for use in bedding and mattresses.

Feng Shui for Your Child

When you are decorating your child's room, consider Feng Shui (pronounced "fung-schway"), the ancientt Chinese system designed to create harmony and balance in our living spaces. Often life for our children can be hectic and overly stimulating, so it is all the more important that their homes be, indeed, "home sweet home." According to interior designer and Feng Shui specialist Suzanne Bank, the family's living space should have a calming, harmonious, healing influence. Especially in the bedroom, it is important to establish a peaceful quiet environment for your children. Your child's bedroom should be a place for rest, regrouping, and rejuvenation, away from the electronic, fast-paced stimuli around us. The interior of your house—including the paint color and placement of furniture—can influence moods, relationships, even school work.

As your child is the center of the family, the layout of the bedrooms should reflect this. When possible, it is best to have your child's bedroom at the hub of the house, the center of security, away from the front street or back of the house. The back of the house signifies the power position—the preferred location for the parents' bedroom.

Begin with a clean slate. When people live and work in a space, they bring their energy with it. When you move into a new home, the previous tenants' energy remains, although they are physically gone. Sometimes their energy is positive and sometimes not. Try "clearing the air" in a new space: some people clear the space with smudging (waving a sage plant through the space), salt, camphor crystals, or pendulums. If you are not sure what you are doing, consider hiring a professional which is what I did for both my home and office.

The position of the furniture in the bedroom is also important. When sleeping, the head of the bed ought to be facing the door, so the child can see the door while in bed. The bed should not be in line with the door. Having your child's back to the door promotes a subconscious awareness of the unseen, which translates to uneasiness. Want to increase creativity and freedom of thought? Avoid placing your child's desk up against a wall, which can promote a feeling of being mentally up against the wall.

Whether you live in a big home or a small space, your child needs a space that she can consider her own where she is allowed to express herself. A cork bulletin board allows your child to express herself through a changing gallery, letting her transform the décor at the press of a push pin. The bulletin board also gives your child a contained area to change and add pictures on a whim without the clutter all over the walls.

Wall color can also have an impact on the family. Yellow can be anxiety provoking. It is no accident that taxis are yellow, as the color that evokes an immediate response and attention, often with a sense of urgency. Red is the color of love, but also that of anger and passion. Softer shades of blue and green work well in a bedroom and can be more restful.

Dressing Your Child

Many of us are familiar with the benefits of eating natural and organic foods, but organic clothing? Clothing is just clothing, isn't it? Not necessarily, as it turns out. Standard cotton is heavily laden with pesticides and chemicals, which remain in contact with your skin, the body's largest organ, for hours a day. The residue on the cloth can be inhaled or ingested, a real risk for children who are prone to sucking, chewing, or biting their clothes. Synthetic dyed clothing poses similar problems. Made from acrylic, polyester, nylon, and spandex, these items contain formaldehyde and flame retardants. Chemicals are also found in standard detergents and fabric softeners.

When possible stay away from the following harmful products:

- Cotton with pesticides. Nearly half the world's pesticides are used on cotton crops.
- Dyes.
- Formaldehyde, which is widely used in waterproof fabrics, permanent press, anti-wrinkle finishes, and commercial brand detergents.
- Synthetic fibers made from plastic (nylon, polyesters, acrylic, spandex).
- Flame retardants which are found in some brands of pajamas. Up until recently the U.S. government required all children's sleepwear to be flame retardant.under the Flammable Fabrics Act. Some parents refused to use flame retardant sleepwear because, as we have seen, flame retardants (PBDEs) contain toxins that may cause developmental problems, cancer, thyroid conditions and immune system dysfunction. As a result, the U.S. Consumer Product Safety Commission amended the children's sleepwear standard to allow the sale of tight fitting cotton sleepwear for infants nine months of age or under even though it is not flame retardant. The commission concluded that tight fitting sleepwear is less likely than flowing nightgowns, oversize T-shirts, and other loose-fitting sleepwear to make contact with a flame and ignite. When your child is old enough, teach her about fire safety precautions including the "stop, drop, and roll" technique in case clothing catches fire and dress your child in snug fitting sleepwear.

Healthy Fabrics for Baby Clothing

As people become more educated about the health dangers posed by these chemicals and processing procedures, they are increasingly demanding healthier clothing for themselves and their children, made from fibers that are eco-friendly. In response, organic clothing sources are emerging that offer natural, dye- and pesticide-free alternatives to synthetic fabrics and standard cotton.

Hemp. Hemp has been cultivated for thousands of years for use in textiles and paper, and is considered by many an ideal plant fiber for clothing. An eco-friendly crop that uses little water, hemp requires no pesticides, is excellent for the soil, and grows in a variety of climates. Clothing made from hemp fibers is weather resistant, more durable than cotton, and can be blended with other fibers such as cotton or silk for textural variety. It uses also extend beyond textiles: hemp appears in skin care products, paper, food products, ropes, paints, and fuel. The Declaration of Independence and the first American flag were made from hemp fibers, and as recently as the 1920s, 80% of clothing was hemp-based. Currently, the Drug Enforcement Agency (DEA) classifies industrial hemp similarly to marijuana, as both are part of the cannabis plant family, despite the fact that hemp has been used for thousands of years and does not cause marijuana-like effects.

Wool. Wool is warm, durable, and the most absorbent of available fibers, which means it is excellent for keeping dry on damp days. Compared to cotton, which feels damp at 15% saturation, wool still feels dry at 30%. As a "breathable" natural fiber, wool can be equally comfortable in cool or warm weather and is helpful in regulating body temperature. When exposed to rain, wool can shed water while keeping the person warm; in warmer temperatures, light wool can cool the body. People who have allergies to wool will likely find that they are sensitive to the chemicals used in some wool, not to the wool itself. Buying untreated, natural wool products may alleviate these sensitivities. Look for clothing that is pure fine wool. Wool can be itchy next to the skin, but is useful over shirts. Wool clothing is easy to maintain, keeps its shape, and does not need to be washed frequently.

Peat. Since ancient times, peat has been employed for a variety of uses including fuel and electricity. As an absorbent fabric, it can be made into cloth diapers, surgical dressings, and home insulation, and even seems to be helpful in alleviating the effects of radiation exposure. A vegetative material grown on raised bogs, its fibers can be thousands of years old. Peat is frequently incorporated with other fibers like wool or silk and made into a light-weight fabric that works almost like a second skin. Peat is made into clothing for children and adults.

Other Considerations When Dressing Your Child

One of the most important considerations when dressing your child is to dress for warmth. According to the Wellness Nurses of the Los Angeles Alliance for Childhood, warmth is vital in promoting healing and keeping illness at bay. Before nine years old, your child will not be able to appropriately gauge temperature and will rely on you to ensure that she is comfortable throughout the day. Your infant in particular will need to be dressed more warmly than you. This is because your baby's body surface-to-body weight ratio is higher than yours, meaning she loses more heat than she can generate.

Parents can use their own body temperature and comfort level to decide how to dress their toddlers and older children. As my mother used to say, "I'm cold, so put on a sweater." If you want to test your child's temperature, place your hand over your child's forehead, belly, and feet. If she is adequately dressed and warm, the areas should be warm to touch. Be sure to cover or layer any area that is cool to the touch. This is especially important if she is feverish, when it is common that much of the heat is concentrated in the head area and less in the limbs, leading to a hot head and cold feet. Over 50% of body heat is lost through the head, which is why it is important for children and adults to cover their heads during cooler weather. Babies and toddlers are especially vulnerable and should always be given a hat in the winter. Throughout the rest of the year, place a cap or bonnet on your baby to protect her head from air conditioning and the sun. Year-round, feet should be adequately covered with socks or natural foot coverings.

During the autumn and winter seasons (at least seven months out of the year, even for those of us who live in places like "sunny" Southern California), our boys wear undershirts underneath their clothing. Layers are great for kids since they can be removed if a child grows too hot. Ideally, a child should wear two layers on the legs, and three above, with the belly always covered as drafts can affect the liver. Additional warming paraphernalia include scarves, mittens, blankets, masks, and adequate waterproof rain clothing. Outdoor clothing such as jackets should be removed once indoors.

Of course, you also don't want to dress your child too warmly. You know your baby is overdressed when she has beads of sweat above the lip or on the forehead.

Other things to keep in mind when you dress your child:

Dress for safety. Especially with infants and small children, be cautious with clothes that have buttons or decorative appliqués that can easily fall off and be swallowed. It is better to use snaps. Cut ribbons, strings, or strands that are longer than eight inches (20 cm) as they can strangulate.

Dress for comfort. Although each child grows at a different rate, I found that my sons were always dressing in sizes larger than their corresponding age. When they were three months old, they were fitting into clothing closer to the six-to-nine-month size. We found it worked better for us to buy on the slightly larger side, since even items that were too big at the time would fit soon enough. In any case, too tight clothing is neither comfortable nor healthy for your child. In the beginning few weeks, I skipped the fancy formalwear and opted for practical 100% cotton onesies.

Dress for easy diaper-changing access. Full-length clothing that did not provide easy snap access for diaper changing rarely got used in our house. Especially when on outings, easy access for changing a diaper is essential.

Dress for sleep. Unless it is bitterly cold outside or scorching hot, I recommend that your family sleep without air conditioners or heaters. The body usually adapts to the local climate during the night.

Dress up. As the mother of boys, I swore that I would not be left out of the adorable clothing-for-girls pageantry. Boys can look great in mix-and-match outfits, if you are a little creative. My son Étienne was four months old for his first Christmas, and I put him in a cotton red beret with cotton plaid jacket and full-length onesie, complete with red knit booties.

The Family Bath

I recently received a call from a concerned mother of a six-day-old who anxiously asked, "Do I have to bathe her every day?" What's the rush? I wondered. Americans in general tend to bathe too often, babies included. The average baby does not get dirty, especially compared to a busy, active toddler, but most parents like to bathe their baby frequently, often as part of the pleasurable nighttime ritual, rather than because of hygienic concerns. Contrary to our own habits, babies generally need a bath a couple of times a week, with shampooing once a week. Washing too frequently takes off a baby's natural oils, leaving the skin dry or irritated. Instead of a full bath, focus on cleaning specific body parts like the diaper and groin area, hands, face, and in creases (for instance, under the neck and behind the ear) as needed.

At birth, your baby is born with a white creamy coat on her skin called vernix caseosa. Even now, I still remember the smell of this protective coat on my babies. In the few hours following their births, my midwife gently patted them dry and swaddled them. In the hospital, however, the vernix is typically washed off, as if the baby is "dirty." Quite to the contrary, the vernix provides protection in utero, and should be left on after birth, too. Let it absorb naturally.

After my babies were several days old, I knew it was time for a warm sponge cleaning. I prefer to avoid immersing babies until the bellybutton cord has fallen off and is healing. If your baby was recently circumcised, discuss bathing protocols with your practitioner. We were given a portable plastic baby bath at my baby shower. Although I prefer not to use plastic materials, I realized early on in motherhood that I would not go crazy in search of all things natural. Initially, we placed the portable plastic baby bath in the kitchen sink, making it easier to reach our baby and easier on our backs, too. René attached a long hose to the faucet for easy and continuous sprinkling. My son was given a lovely monogrammed pink-hooded towel (the name Étienne was mistaken for a girl's—oh well) that we used for both boys. They did not mind, and neither did we.

Initially, newborns may not appreciate the bath. However with time, most parents and babies find bath time pleasurable. I have wonderful memories of taking a bath with my grandmother and how soft her skin felt. Many parents get in the tub with their baby, if not occasionally then with each bath. The family bath can be lovely shared time with your child and is especially comforting for a baby who is cautious or fearful of the water.

How to Bathe Your Baby

Never leave baby alone in the water, so forget about the answering the phone. In fact, turn off all your phones. Remember to keep the room warm, and avoid drafts. Make the bath quick to prevent your baby becoming chilled, and organize your bathing and drying paraphernalia ahead of time, keeping it next to the tub.

Bathing supplies should include:

- Soft washcloth.
- Cotton balls to clean around the eyes and around the ear. As my father, an ear, nose, and throat specialist, taught me, "Never put anything smaller than your elbow inside the ear." As much as you would like to, avoid placing q-tips inside of baby's ear canal (or your ear, too, for that matter).
- Natural baby soap and shampoo. Often warm water is enough to clean

your baby, so don't feel obligated to use a variety of different products. Use the natural brands without chemicals and avoid commercial preparations that contain mineral oil and chemicals.

- Clean clothes.
- A fresh diaper.

You also might want to consider an infant baby bathing seat for newborns to six months old that offers support while bathing in either a baby tub, standard tub, or kitchen sink.

There are numerous variations on the infant tub. We used a plastic inclined tub that also could be secured on top of the kitchen sink. You can forgo buying the separate tub and simply use the kitchen sink by lining the bottom with a rubber mat to prevent slipping and the sides with a towel for comfort. Inserts, tubs, or inflatable tubs are all available for converting the sink into a baby bath. As your baby gets bigger and grows out of the plastic tub, you will have to become creative for the next step. Once they were sitting upright, our boys liked the upright bath chair.

Sponge cleaning is useful for newborns or a baby who is not able to be immersed. Place baby in a comfortable position for both of you. She can be on top of a towel on a firm surface (like the kitchen countertop). Keep baby covered except for the section that you are cleaning. After cleaning parts of the body, immediately dry and cover, then go onto next body part. Avoid rubbing the skin too hard, as baby's skin is sensitive.

Shampoos and Soaps

When shopping around for a good baby shampoo and soap, I prefer to avoid the standards. Shampoos in particular often contain harmful substances, including detergents, chemicals, and carcinogens. Babies are especially vulnerable to these substances, because they are often accidentally swallowed in small amounts. Some of the common ingredients in shampoos (and other health and beauty care products) to avoid include:

- Cancer-causing ingredients such as sodium lauryl sulfate/sodium laureth sulfate. Common in shampoos, toothpaste, and creams, these substances are produced from petroleum and can be irritating and drying to skin.

- Monoethanolamides (MEA), diethanolamides (DEA), Triethanolamine (TEA), all known cancer-causing agents.
- Quaternium-15 formaldehyde-releasing preservative, which can cause severe skin irritations, allergies, and cancer.
- Propylene glycol, a neurotoxin linked with skin irritation and kidney and liver damage.

Ingredients to avoid when choosing soaps include:

- Ammonia
- BHA/BHT
- Dye
- Formaldehyde
- Glycols
- Mineral oil
- Perfumes and fragrance
- Petroleum products
- Phenols

These common substances dry skin, cause local irritations, and block the pores. Standard bubble baths can also be irritating to the skin and should be avoided. Instead, use natural soaps made from plant or animal fat.

Many parents have also looked to antibacterial soaps to help prevent colds and other common conditions. The exponential rise in antibacterial soaps and cleaning products in recent years indicates our current "bacteriophobia"—our deep fear of encountering unseen, unhealthy bacteria. But our attempts to avoid and eliminate bacterial exposure lead only to stronger, more resistant strains, compounding the problem as future generations of bacteria become harder to fight. Antibacterial soaps are not the answer to preventing infection, nor are they particularly healthy. A common antibacterial agent triclosan, derived from an herbicide, is also carcinogenic and irritating to the skin.

Until the teen years, sweat glands and oil glands are not terribly active. Because of this, it is advised to bathe your child with water and little to no soap. Unless your child gets very dirty, soaking in a bath should be enough and for older children a quick rinse should be sufficient cleaning. Even children with healthy and wholesome diets will get skin infections if they are too frequently bathed. This is typically because the oils are washed off and the layers of unsloughed skin are washed off, leaving a thinner protective barrier.

Sun Safety

We are all aware of the links between sun exposure and skin cancer, and more people are making sunscreens, hats, and other protective clothing a regular habit. Media and health campaigns in recent years have convinced many of the necessity of applying sunscreen prior to any sun exposure, and in fact, many people wear sunscreen all year round in an effort to protect against skin cancer. But emerging research suggests that the chemicals in standard sunscreens may increase the risk of cancer, and that some exposure to the sun is beneficial.

The radiation from the sun contains both visible and invisible rays. The latter, called ultraviolet (UV) light, can increase the risk of skin cancer when an individual is exposed for prolonged periods and at high doses. People can be exposed to UV rays on cloudy days as well as on a sunny one. UV light is divided into ultraviolet A (UVA) and ultraviolet B (UVB). UVA provides most of the sun rays and are longer and penetrate deeper into the skin's layers. UVA rays are known to cause leathery skin and wrinkles. UVB rays are shorter, and only reach the superficial layers of the skin and are responsible for sunburns and skin cancers. The Food and Drug Administration (FDA) distinguishes sunscreens on two main factors, the sun protection factor (SPF) and UVA and UVB protective actions. An SPF 30 means that it takes 30 times longer to burn with the sunscreen than if you were in the sun without sunscreen.

In an article on sun exposure in the *British Medical Journal*, the writers concluded that sun exposure without sunscreen was sensible in moderation. Every body needs sun to maintain good health: vitamin D is made in the body through exposure to the sun, and the sun may be helpful in treating depression, alleviating Seasonal Affect Disorder, and protecting against certain cancers and diseases like multiple sclerosis.

Old-fashioned sunblocks create a physical barrier to the sun's rays by using titanium dioxide and zinc oxides to block UV rays.. These ingredients are not absorbed into the skin but rather leaves a whitish gleam to the skin. Sunblocks provide a broad spectrum to protect against both UVA and UVB rays. On the other hand, sunscreens are absorbed into the skin creating a chemical sun barrier which are usually invisible when rubbed into the skin. The sunscreens act to filter the UV radiation, and are considered the unhealthier choice. Sunscreen ingredients are linked to cancer due to their free radical generation and similarity to estrogen, known as toxic estrogenic chemical sunscreens. In addition, the latter may affect sexual development, birth defects, and lower sperm count and penis size in men. When using sun protection, the one that provides a physical barrier is preferable. I prefer the more natural varieties that are chemical free and PABA free. PABA (para-aminobenzoic acid) is known to cause allergy and is rarely used these days.

In addition, emerging research suggests sunscreens may not be enough to prevent skin cancer, since they do not offer protection against the formation of moles, which have been implicated in skin cancer, including the common and sometimes fatal form, melanoma. Only clothing can prevent moles from forming on the skin.

Most sun damage occurs during childhood, so it is particularly important to take precautions in these early years. Children and babies are more vulnerable to the effects of the sun and should be well covered, whatever the weather. Dress your child in a long white t-shirt (an adult sized t-shirt can be used to protect legs) and hat. The hat should also protect the eyes. If this is not sufficient, consider sunglasses with 100 % UV filtration. Clothes provide minimal protection with an SPF of 5.9. Sunscreen should not be used on babies less than six months old.

At the beginning of your outdoor season, take your child out for ten minutes a day, preferably in the morning hours before 10 A.M. and increase exposure time gradually. Avoid the noon hour outside. Gradual exposure allows her skin to become accustomed to the sun, and within several weeks, she will be at less risk for sunburn. If skin ever appears too red, go inside. When outside, drink plenty of water and eat vegetables (the antioxidants in vegetables help protect against sun radiation). Be sensible and avoid excess exposure.

SUMMARY

CREATING A NONTOXIC ENVIRONMENT FOR YOUR BABY

To minimize baby's exposure to harmful toxins in common household objects and products, stay away from synthetic fabrics and plastic toys, use natural brands of cleaning products, drink filtered water, steer clear of fumes, and use stainless steel, ceramic, or iron cookware. When decorating baby's room, consider nontoxic flooring, paint, and bedding. You may also be interested in learning about Feng Shui, the Chinese system designed to bring balance to our living spaces.

DRESSING YOUR CHILD

To minimize baby's exposure to harmful toxins in clothing, stay away from cotton with pesticides, dye, formaldehyde, synthetic fabrics, and flame-retardant pajamas. Instead, look for hemp, wool, or peat. In addition, it is important to dress baby for warmth, safety, comfort, and easy diaper-changing access.

THE FAMILY BATH

To keep bathtime pleasurable for you and baby, keep the room warm and have supplies (including a soft washcloth, cotton balls, natural shampoo and soap, clean clothes and diapers) handy. Avoid shampoos and soaps with mineral oil, petroleum products, dyes, fragrances and perfumes, and ammonia.

SUN SAFETY

Most sun damage occurs during childhood, so it is particularly important to take precautions in these early years. However, sunscreens (which are not suitable for babies under six months old) may include toxic ingredients and some sun exposure is beneficial. Dress your child in a long white t-shirt (an adult sized t-shirt can be used to protect legs) and hat, which should also protect the eyes. Take your child out for ten minutes a day, preferably in the morning hours before 10 A.M. and increase exposure time gradually.

chapter 11

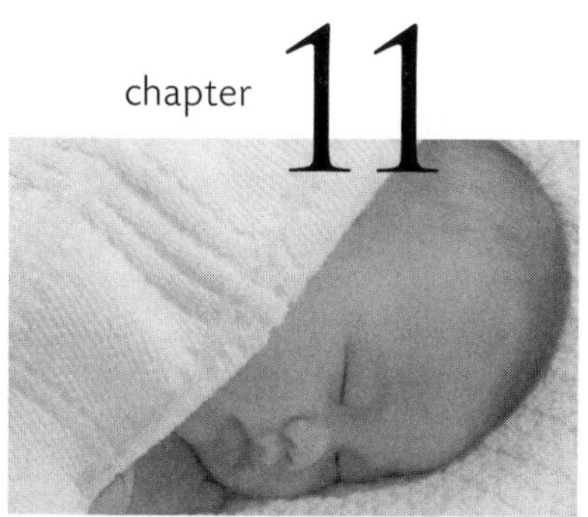

Sleep

A well-spent day brings happy sleep.

–Leonardo da Vinci

WE SPEND NEARLY ONE THIRD OF OUR LIVES in slumber, making sleep one of our body's most important and time-consuming activities. When I was pregnant with my first child, I worried, like many new parents, whether I would ever get my cherished eight hours of peaceful sleep again. I knew that my baby would come first, but I also hoped I might once again get an uninterrupted night's sleep. I wanted the best of both worlds, assuming that I would have to settle for long stretches of sleep deprivation as one of the prices of parenthood. Uninterrupted sleep was indeed difficult to come by in my early years as a parent, but I also learned that attending to my children's sleep needs helped me better attend to mine as well. By looking for effective and efficient ways to foster my sons' energy and restfulness, I simultaneously improved my own sense of wellbeing.

Many of our frustrations with children and sleep stem from our assumption that babies should "learn" to sleep through the night at as early an age as possible. We place high expectations on our children, even as newborns, when we anticipate that they should sleep for a full eight hours. I am not convinced, however, that this is the healthiest approach, as currently more than 30% of American adults suffer with insomnia. Did the roots of this common occurrence begin when we were infants and taught the sleep habits that follow us through to adulthood? If so, is there anything we can do as parents to build foundations for our children for healthier sleep now and later on when they are adults? By revisiting the sleep expectations and habits we develop in our children, we might begin to better understand how to prevent and even treat the chronic sleep problems of adolescence and adulthood.

Sleeping well is among the most vital components of your health and your baby's, and the objective of this chapter is for you to find an arrangement that is flexible and beneficial for both you and your infant. The goal is to help both of you get a restful sleep that leads to an energetic productive day, and, fortunately, you have no shortage of options and choices.

Your Baby's Sleep Patterns

We all know the feeling after a good night's sleep. In addition to providing rest, sleep boosts the immune system, helps concentration and memory, and generally makes you look and feel better. The same holds true for infants, but as a newborn, your baby will have different sleep needs that you do. Adjusting to the pattern of your baby's sleep cycle will be one of your first challenges as a parent: by learning about your child's sleep needs, you will be better able to gauge your expectations and will find yourself more accepting and respectful of baby's natural phases. Keep in mind that no baby sleeps in exactly that same way as another and a wide variety of sleep patterns fall within the bounds of normal, healthy infant behavior. Some babies sleep through the night, and some do not; both tendencies are perfectly normal. Sleeping patterns can also change during phases of teething, illness, and growth spurts.

In general, humans experience different stages and cycles of sleep during the night, oscillating between active and quiet sleep. REM (rapid eye movement) is the active sleep cycle and the phase where most of the dreaming occurs. During this cycle, the brain is active and working, making it also the easiest time to wake or rouse your baby or child. NonREM (NREM) sleep, on the other hand, is the quiet sleep cycle. The deeper sleep experienced in this phase helps replenish energy and strengthen the body.

An adult can get into bed and fall easily into a deep, sound sleep, or NREM sleep. After approximately ninety minutes of deep sleep, the cycle shifts to lighter REM sleep, in which the brain becomes more aroused. An adult may spend approximately six hours in quiet sleep and two hours in active sleep. As we age, deep sleep lessens in proportion to active sleep.

While you may be able to enter deep sleep immediately upon going to bed, your baby is different, initially falling into an active REM sleep cycle that lasts approximately 20 minutes. Signs that she is still in this active sleep phase include movements like muscles twitches, startling, and sucking. Some babies will easily arouse if they are put down too early while in this phase. For those babies who awaken while being put to bed, try a calming bedtime ritual: this may include nursing her to sleep, singing a lullaby, or rocking her for a long enough period to allow baby to enter the deeper sleep cycle. You will know she is in deeper sleep when the body is less active, the arms and legs are limp, and she is less easy to arouse.

Newborns sleep as well as feed in two- to three-hour cycles. In these first few months, their sleep cycles are shorter, which means they have more periods of active, light REM sleep than adults and are more likely to be aroused or awakened. Fully half of your baby's sleep cycles are spent in the lighter REM sleep, compared to twenty percent of an adult's cycle. Given this, it is little surprise that babies wake more frequently than you—from birth to six months, as often as two to three times a night. From six months to one year, they may wake once or twice a night, and then once a night until two years old. In general, breastfed babies wake more easily and frequently than formula-fed babies because breast milk is digested and absorbed quicker and more efficiently.

Particularly in the first six months of life, your baby's breathing will have an important impact on her sleep. In infancy, a baby's breathing organs are still young and not fully developed, and it is not uncommon for her to have irregular breathing patterns during sleep. This is known as periodic breathing, in which there can be several pauses in breathing lasting more than three seconds. They can occur at least three times in a row; this is considered normal. Your baby usually senses she is not getting enough air and wakes up. Typically, she then automatically starts breathing again without any problems. By six months old, your baby breathes at a regular rate and the periodic episodes lessen. Periodic breathing is more common in premature infants.

According to researcher Dr. James J. McKenna, "New research suggests that co-sleeping affects infant physiology and patterns of arousal." These early breathing habits with ability to arouse may be important survival mechanisms for your child and may help to prevent devastating occurrences like SIDS. If you are concerned about your child's breathing patterns, or your child is experiencing pauses longer than 20 seconds contact your practitioner immediately. For more information on SIDS, see Chapter 5.

How Much Sleep Does My Child Need?

The following is a suggested sleep guideline for your child. Every baby is an individual, and her sleep needs will vary as well. In general, the younger the child, the more sleep she needs.

- **Newborns:** 15 to 18 hours. Newborns sleep day and night, approximately two thirds of the time, or fifteen to eighteen hours a day. They sleep in short periods of two to three hours.
- **3 to 6 months:** 14 to 16 hours. As babies get older, their sleep habits start to change. From three to six months, babies begin to sleep longer stretches during the night (six to eight hours) and spend more awake time during the day. A three-month-old may sleep eleven hours a night with several interruptions for changing, feeding, and comfort. At this age, baby will sleep a total of fourteen to sixteen hours including two to three naps (one to two hours each).
- **6 to 12 months:** 12 to 15 hours. A child between six months and twelve months old will usually sleep a total of twelve to fifteen hours. She may sleep eleven to twelve hour stretches at night (including interruptions) plus two naps of one to two hours each.
- **1 to 2 years old:** 11 to 13 hours. From one to two years old, your child will sleep from eleven to thirteen hours including two naps (one to two hours each).
- **2 to 5 years old:** 10 to 12 hours. From the ages of two to three years old, your child will sleep from ten to twelve hours with one nap. Preschool age children will sleep from ten to twelve hours, often without a nap.
- **School aged children:** 10 to 12 hours. Children under age twelve need anywhere from ten to twelve hours of sleep at night.
- **Teens:** 9 hours. Teens need approximately nine hours of sleep, and adults eight hours.

If you are concerned whether your child is getting enough sleep, use the following questions as a guide:

1. Does your child fall asleep easily?
2. Does she sleep well through the night allowing for normal interruptions?
3. Does she wake up relatively easy in the morning?
4. Is her energy good during the day?

If you answered yes to these questions, then your child is probably getting enough sleep. Signs of sleep deprivation in school-aged children include extreme difficulty waking up in the morning, a tendency to fall asleep in class, and a strong urge to take naps. Younger babies can be irritable and fussy if they have not slept enough.

Napping

Throughout the day, your child's energy (and yours, too) will flag, leaving her feeling tired, restless and irritable. Your baby has eaten, has a clean diaper, and is not in pain; it must mean it is time for a nap. Especially in the early months when parents are recovering from the physical, mental, and emotional changes of a new baby, naps for both infant and parents are important opportunities to restore one's energy, mood, and productivity. Napping is especially important in children under five. During the day is when they get the additional hours to sleep, and children who fight naps or are hard to put to bed will benefit from osteopathy and/or homeopathy.

Naps are most effective when they follow a predictable pattern, becoming an integral part of the day rather than an as-needed interruption to the usual schedule. Routines in eating, sleeping, and napping help enforce habits that will stay with your infant throughout childhood, so especially in the beginning, try to adhere to an established naptime in the morning and afternoon. Similar to nighttime rituals, naptime might include darkening the room, using music, and nursing and rocking her to sleep. Naptime also evolves, and you will probably need to adjust the hours and amount of time your child sleeps according to their age and developmental phase. By around age two or three, your child will probably need only one nap and by four years old may stop napping altogether.

Research shows that naptime can be beneficial for nighttime sleeping. Far from decreasing the amount your child sleeps at night, regular naps can aid her in sleeping consistently and for longer periods of time. The timing of naps, however, is important. When our sons were toddlers, I had to be careful not to let them nap too late in the day as it was harder to put them to sleep at a reasonable time at night. An earlier nap helped remedy the situation. For babies who take one to two naps a day, the afternoon nap is best taken in the early afternoon. Ideally, your child should be allowed to nap or go to sleep when she shows signs of sleepiness. If you wait too long, she may get a second wind and be unable to fall asleep.

The Bedtime Ritual

Putting your baby or child down to sleep can often be the most intimate and special time you spend together in the course of the day, so nighttime rituals are more than just habits—they allow for vital bonding between parent and child and help to establish familial rhythms that will be in place for a lifetime. While bedtime rituals are unique to each family, many households make use of baths, books, singing, or massage as ways of readying a child for sleep. Keep in mind, too, that bedtime is not just for mothers: fathers offer a warm set of arms and hands for carrying and a large chest for lying on, making them wonderful natural soothers.

Certain end-of-the-day habits will help to ensure your child gets sufficient rest. Consistent bedtimes are important for young people, and since many bodily and hormonal functions work best while the body is at rest, earlier bedtimes tend to be better for children than later. This is especially important on school nights. Overeating before bed can also cause your child to be restless or unable to sleep. She should be neither too full nor too hungry, and sugar or caffeine late in the evening is always a bad idea.

For both infants and older children, atmosphere cannot be underestimated in helping to aid rest. I recommend surrounding your children with calming influences prior to going to sleep, including peaceful music, a warm bath, or aromatherapy and essential oil preparations for babies and children using lavender and clary sage. The room should be protected from bright, direct light and extreme temperatures. 60 to 65 degrees Fahrenheit is best for sleeping, so you will want to avoid keeping the room temperature much higher or lower; an over-warm bedroom (over 70 degrees) will often cause sleep difficulties. In this age of artificial heating and cooling devices, even temperatures and good ventilation are especially important, since artificial heat in particular can cause dryness in the mouth and nose. Avoid stimulating, upbeat music, television, and social activities right before bed, and try to choose bedtime stories that are soothing and calming.

Putting infants to sleep can include many of the same rituals you use for an older child, including warm baths, singing, or soothing reading. Babies also appreciate gentle motion, and many parents find success rocking their infant to sleep either in the arms of a walking parent or while in the lap in a rocking chair. Sometimes simply driving around the block in the car will work, too. Among the best and most underutilized methods of relaxing infants and children before bed is massage. For techniques on child and infant massages, see "Infant and Child Massage" in Chapter 9.

One of my favorite bedtime rituals when my boys were infants was breastfeeding. Nursing my child to bed allowed me to have special time alone with my baby and proved an excellent way to gently ease him into sleep. The age-old advice to drink warm milk before bed is even truer for breast milk. The calcium in milk is known to soothe the nerves and help one relax, another reason to keep breastfeeding. Along with eggs, cashews, chicken and turkey, warm milk also contains the amino acid L-tryptophan, known for its powers as a soporific.

Other tips for good sleeping:

- Proper dressing should be neither too cool nor too warm. If your baby or child kicks off the covers, make sure baby is adequately covered since feet can easily become cold. Dress baby in pajamas with foot coverings; older children and adults could also benefit from keeping the feet warm to help improve the body's distribution of heat.
- Daily fresh air and daytime exercise improve sleep. When weather permits, most babies enjoy being outside and exploring life around them. Older children, of course, benefit greatly from active playtime outdoors.
- Prescription drugs and other over-the-counter medicines can interrupt sleep. In my practice, I've seen some children suffer sleep problems including nightmares following antibiotics and vaccines. You may want to consider natural and holistic alternatives for everyday use, especially if your child is experiencing particular troubles with bad dreams or restless sleep.
- Avoid caffeine! I've seen many babies with cola in their bottles. Avoid this routine not only before bedtime, but all the time!

- Electromagnetic fields can interrupt sleep patterns. Avoid placing electric alarm clocks or baby monitors near the bed.. For more information, see the chapter on electromagnetic fields.
- Most children need the comfort of a nightlight to fall asleep. It is okay to use a nightlight initially, but make it a habit to turn off all lighting so that their sleep is more restful. If you need hallway lighting for the nighttime wake ups, keep a nightlight on in the hallway, in the bathroom, or keep an adjacent room dimly lit.

Poor Sleep

It's natural for newborns and infants to wake several times a night, but in addition to these regular interruptions, they may awaken for other reasons, depending on health, developmental stage, and sleeping arrangements. Colicky babies are particularly difficult to get to sleep and are prone to frequent waking, often accompanied by sudden screaming and anger at the gas-like pains that keep them up. Unfortunately, colicky symptoms, while a passing phase, cause great stress to already stressed-out new parents. For more information on soothing a colicky baby, see "Colic" in Chapter 5.

Just when you thought you had made it through the colicky phase, teething begins, which can again have your infant waking throughout the night. Teething can start as early as three months, and will be accompanied by its common signs—the fist in the mouth, drool rash, and swollen gums. Some babies suffer more discomfort than others, and if teething is posing a real problem for sleep, you may want to refer to "Your Baby's Teeth" in Chapter 5.

Among older children, poor sleep can just as easily result from developmental changes, such as growing pains, and environmental stresses, such as adjusting to school. Nightmares, night terrors, bedwetting, sleepwalking, and talking in your sleep are also not uncommon from the ages of five to ten. You can learn more about these conditions in "Bedwetting, Sleepwalking, and Nightmares" in Chapter 7.

Conventional Sleep Training Methods

Most conventional advice on sleep training emphasizes precisely that, training. Parents are taught that they should detach from their infant in order to make him or her independent and self-sufficient. Fussy or irritable babies need simply to learn not to fuss; crying babies need to learn that crying will not answer their needs. Sleep training experts advise putting baby to bed while she is still awake, waiting progressive periods of time before going in to check on your crying baby, and soothing without touch. Parents are also encouraged to follow the hands of the clocks rather than the cues of their babies. In this way, babies are "trained" to soothe themselves through behavioral conditioning and parents are trained to distance themselves from the distress of their child.

Conventional sleep training teaches that most babies do not need a nighttime feeding by three months of age, and that, by six months, no baby needs a night feeding at all. These recommendations are based upon research done with formula-fed babies, and may not apply to breastfed babies. Breast milk is relatively low in fat and protein, so breastfed babies usually need to be fed more often than formula-fed babies and awaken frequently. But with time, they begin to sleep for longer periods of time.

For some families, conventional sleep training works well. The approach, however, is the antithesis of the natural parenting philosophy, which recognizes that babies' sleep patterns differ from adults', and that they wake during the night for feedings, diaper changes, comfort, and a variety of other reasons. The natural parenting approach emphasizes listening to your child, rather than sticking to a schedule; she is trying to tell you what she needs, and as her parent, you are best equipped to respond.

As a mother, I intuitively felt the need to soothe my baby once he began to cry, and, as a doctor, I believe a baby has a right to be able to rely on her parents for comfort and attention, even (and especially) in the middle of the night. When an infant's cries are ignored, the parents inadvertently introduce an element of insecurity into their child's life, signaling that the primary caregivers cannot be relied upon for comfort, security, or a loving touch. To deprive your baby of cuddling, reassurance, and support may contribute to larger emotional problems for her as a child and later on as an adult. I have never heard my adult patients complain that they were cuddled or held too much as a baby. On the contrary, many are in therapy for not having had their needs met early in life.

Expectations that babies are supposed to sleep through the night—and that letting them cry is a way of instilling that behavior—are contrary to both an infant's and a mother's physiology. A baby's cries affect a mother's hormonal and body chemistry levels, translating into an instinctual urge to go and pick up the crying baby. The popular "let the baby cry it out" approach thus runs counter a mother's natural intuition and set up an all-too-common parenting phenomenon in which parents no longer trust their judgment and insight.

Although we humans possess a highly developed intellect, our babies' needs operate on a more instinctive plane. Babies communicate to us when they are hungry, uncomfortable, scared, or in pain, and we communicate back to them by providing love, attention, and emotional and physical care. Building a foundation that begins with the compassionate care of your infant will lead to a happier, more well-adjusted future for your child, as well as happier and more well-adjusted attitude for you.

The Family Bed

When I was eight-months pregnant with my first child, I remember shopping for cribs at different boutiques. I looked at convertibles, bumpers, mattresses—there seemed no end to choices, which left me feeling only more confused. Around the same time, I was introduced to the old-fashioned notion of the *family bed*, also known as co-sleeping. My initial response to the idea of families sleeping together was negative—the concept seemed entirely foreign to me. However, I soon learned that co-sleeping has a long history, even in the West. It was only in the 19th century that the notion of separate bedrooms began, when childcare experts decided that children who slept with their parents would become dependent and suffer psychological problems. The Victorians also attached moral value to the notion of the family bed, suggesting that it was simply wrong to sleep with one's baby.

In my quest to make the best choices for our new family, I decided that I needed to research co-sleeping further. It hardly made sense to me that I needed to sleep separately from my child. Other animals slept with their young, so why shouldn't I? I also knew that I would be going back to work after six weeks and wanted to be able to provide comfort and closeness, and to nurse with ease—all while getting a good night's sleep. It seemed logical to my husband and me. Needless to say, we never bought the crib!

I soon found out we were not alone. According to surveys, 30% of families sleep together either all or part of the night. Most parents in my office practice some form of co-sleeping. In fact, I have never met a family that hasn't at one time or another played the game of musical beds, all in the name of getting a better, more restful night's sleep.

The Benefits of Co-Sleeping

We have many names to refer to children sleeping with their parents—family bed, co-sleeping, attachment parenting, and natural parenting. All of these terms suggest that parenting does not stop at bedtime; it is a 24-by-7, around-the-clock job. Paradoxically, though, being close to your child makes your job as a parent easier. Whether you are a stay-at-home parent or a busy executive, co-sleeping is excellent for bonding, breastfeeding, and minimizing sleep disturbances, since your baby is right next to you.

Co-sleeping promotes bonding. During sleep, baby and mother's sleep cycles become harmonious: research has shown that nursing mothers and their babies dream in the same cycles from twelve weeks of age to weaning. This phenomenon does not occur in bottle-fed babies.

Co-sleeping makes breastfeeding at night easier. The ease of breastfeeding during the night cannot be overemphasized when your baby is right next to you. It is natural that your baby will want to feed several times a night the first several months of life, and having baby right next to you allows minimal interruption from sleep so that both baby and mother can easily go back to sleep. According to researchers, mothers who sleep with their babies and breastfeed seem to be better able to "welcome the day." This may be due to the fact that prolactin, the hormone that makes milk, is also known for its calming effects. Prolactin increases with touching and during sleep.

Co-sleeping minimizes sleep disruptions. Because you do not need to get up to soothe your baby if she is fussy for any reason, it is easier to get back to sleep afterwards.

Co-sleeping may help prevent Sudden Infant Death Syndrome (SIDS). It is not known exactly what causes SIDS but studies have shown that baby's ability to monitor parental sounds while asleep (which is of course easiest to do when she sleeps with you) may be correlated with a lower risk of SIDS. (See Chapter 5 for more details.)

Co-sleeping may boost baby's self-esteem later in life. Many parents also emphasize the comfort of feeling and hearing their baby right next to them. According to anthropologist and sleep expert Dr. James McKenna, adults who co-slept with parents when they were infants show greater self esteem and are more secure, independent, and self-reliant as adults.

Myths about Co-Sleeping

Co-sleeping promotes bonding, lets families get more sleep, makes breastfeeding easier, and protects against crib death. All of these positive points verify a practice that we intuitively felt to be the best decision for our family. Although my husband and I felt confident with our decision, people offered their concerns about our baby sleeping with us. In fact, there are many misconceptions and myths about children sleeping with their families.

Co-sleeping makes the baby dependent. He will never want to leave your bed, concerned people told me. The truth is that babies are dependent. According to researchers, human babies are the least neurologically mature primate at birth. Nevertheless, we expect them to be independent, perhaps at too early an age. Both of my children slept in our bedroom for the first four to five years, and we loved every minute of it. Even now that they are school aged, my boys sleep with us whenever they are sick or have a bad dream. Our bedroom is a refuge for comfort—with an open door policy.

Co-sleeping encourages nursing at night. In the first few months, breastfed babies often nurse in cycles of every two to three hours. In order to gain their necessary weight, they need to eat night and day. This occurs whether they co-sleep or not.

Night nursing causes cavities. Baby-bottle tooth decay occurs when a baby falls asleep with a bottle filled with formula, juice or any sweetened drink. Many practitioners are not familiar with breastfeeding especially in toddlers, and often lump breast milk in with these same groups of liquids. There is no doubt the issue is disputed among dentists and researchers. According to Dr. Constantine Oulis and colleagues, breastfeeding may "act preventively and inhibit the development of nursing cavities in children." Anthropologists studying the skulls of prehistoric babies and toddlers—all most likely breastfed—found most to be relatively free of tooth decay. Only more recently did children begin getting cavities. If your child is susceptible to decay, consider brushing the teeth several times a day, including first thing in the morning.

Co-sleeping ruins your sex life. Parents learn to be creative in finding the place and time to be intimate. Use your imagination, as there are other rooms in the house that offer possibilities. Some parents sneak time together while baby is being taken on a walk with grandparents or another caretaker. In general with the arrival of a new baby, this is an issue for most parents, not just those who are co-sleeping.

You could crush your baby and co-sleeping is unsafe. Safe sleeping guidelines address these concerns by helping parents take basic precautions to ensure their child sleeps comfortable and securely.

Safe Sleeping Suggestions for Co-Sleeping

To ensure that your baby sleeps comfortably and safely:

1. Your baby should be comfortable in bed on a firm surface, and free of anything that could interfere with breathing or entangle the body.
2. Newborns should sleep between the bed rail and the mother. A baby should not sleep in between parents or next to an older child.
3. If parents are substantially overweight, allow baby to sleep in a sidecar next to mother.
4. Do not sleep with baby if you are under the influence of alcohol, prescription or recreational drugs that would inhibit your responsiveness and alertness.
5. Avoid any situation that would allow for baby rolling off of the bed, or to fall in between the bed and wall.
6. Avoid soft surfaces, overloaded beds full of pillows, or fluffy bedding. This means no waterbeds, featherbeds, sofas, or beds with too many people in them or too many stuffed animals on them.

When Co-Sleeping Doesn't Work

Although I find most babies sleep better close to mom, there still are some that prefer to sleep solitarily. I am in favor of co-sleeping, but it does not work for all families. Parents have numerous choices in how they want to design their sleeping arrangements and the most common is the crib with baby sleeping in her own room, often with a baby monitor. Some parents find they sleep better, and, after all, a better night's sleep is of utmost importance in functioning well the next day. If you are looking for a compromise between a single room for your infant and co-sleeping, you might consider the side car or side crib, a standard crib pushed against mother's side.

Cribs have varying levels of safety. Avoid cribs made before 1982 as some have been known to be dangerous. In older cribs, avoid those with lead-based paints or missing screws. In arranging the crib, use lightweight blankets and avoid too many stuffed animals or objects. (See "Cribs, Playpens, and Walkers" in Chapter 5 for more details on safe cribs.)

Sleeping Tips for Parents

It is not uncommon to be exhausted after giving birth. Mothers have a better chance of regaining their strength and energy if they follow the age-old tradition of staying around the home for the first 40 days. During that time, I recommend that mothers get eight hours of sleep, albeit over a 24-hour period. Parents often have the urge to try to get things done while the baby is asleep. During the first few months, I encourage parents, especially nursing mothers, to take frequent naps, when baby naps, mother naps.

For fathers, too, poor sleep can lead to irritability, grumpiness, poor concentration, and a lack of energy and motivation during the day. To make matters worse, sleepiness during the day can provoke wakefulness at night, repeating the cycle for both parents and child. We all know the effects of a bad night's sleep. It is normal for baby to wake frequently and want to feed during the night: she may be perfectly content, and it is the poor parents that suffer the most. Sleeping close to your infant and napping when she does allows you to catch up on your own rest as your baby catches up on hers. Following the birth of both of our children, my husband and I quickly realized that there was no point in both of us getting a poor night's sleep. So he slept in the other room for approximately the first six weeks. Throughout different phases of our baby's lives, such as a difficult teething phase, sometimes we would switch roles and he would offer the comfort in the middle of the night.

SUMMARY

YOUR BABY'S SLEEP PATTERNS

Newborns sleep in two- to three-hour cycles for about 15 to 18 hours a day. From birth to six months, babies wake as often as two to three times a night. From six months to one year, they may wake once or twice a night and sleep about 12 to 15 hours (including naps). Then they will gradually sleep and wake less.

NAPPING

Naps are most effective when they follow a predictable pattern and can be beneficial for nighttime sleeping. The timing of naps, however, is important; don't let baby nap too late in the afternoon.

THE BEDTIME RITUAL

Bedtime rituals allow for vital bonding between parents and children, and help ensure that children get sufficient sleep and establish healthy habits for a lifetime. While bedtime rituals are unique to each family, many choose to make baths, massages, reading, or singing part of the ritual.

POOR SLEEP

Poor sleep may result from health or developmental issues such as colic, teething, growing pains, or nightmares.

CONVENTIONAL SLEEP TRAINING METHODS

Conventional sleep training teaches that most babies do not need a nighttime feeding by three months of age, and that, by six months, no baby needs a night feeding at all. Parents are taught that they should detach from their infant in order to make him or her independent and self-sufficient. For some families, this works well. But it is the antithesis of the natural parenting philosophy, which emphasizes listening to your child, rather than sticking to a schedule.

THE FAMILY BED

Co-sleeping has many benefits, such as promoting bonding, making breastfeeding easier, preventing Sudden Infant Death Syndrome, and boosting self-esteem. To ensure that baby sleeps safely, place her between the bed rail and the mother and avoid soft surfaces or situations where she may roll off the bed.

SLEEPING TIPS FOR PARENTS

During the first few months, I encourage parents, especially nursing mothers, to take frequent naps. In addition, parents may want to switch off being "on duty" during the night.

chapter 12

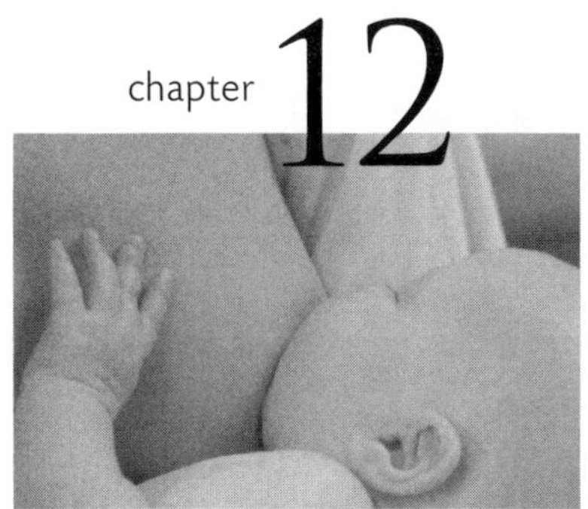

Breastfeeding: Nursing Your Newborn . . . and Beyond

A man's work is from sun to sun, but a mother's work is never done.

–Author unknown

When I was born, my mother assumed she would be breastfeeding. To her surprise, her doctor told it was not necessary. She was given a shot to "dry up the milk," and we were sent home with bottles and formula. As a strong advocate of breastfeeding, I view this attitude with a sense of loss. Breastfeeding is not only vital to your child's well-being and development, it offers mothers one of the richest and most satisfying experiences in childrearing. Fortunately, the conventional wisdom that governed my parents' generation has undergone a major transformation, and breastfeeding is seeing a resurgence in popularity: we are "rediscovering" the innate wisdom of a practice that spans thousands of years of evolution. Even so, the United States currently has one of the lowest breastfeeding rates worldwide. According to the Surgeon General, only 29% of mothers are still breastfeeding when baby is six months old.

In an effort to correct the formula "norm" established in the 20th century, breastfeeding support groups such as La Leche League, a nonprofit organization begun in the 1950s, have taught millions of mothers worldwide about the benefits of breastfeeding. To compensate for my mother's lack of breastfeeding experience, I had the pleasure of breastfeeding my two sons a total of nearly nine years (you do the math). I felt akin to mothers around the globe, as the average age to wean is approximately four years old.

What Is In Breastmilk?

Many mothers report that it "just feels right" to breastfeed their baby. This intuitive attraction to breastfeeding is backed by a great deal of scientific evidence indicating that breast milk is indeed the ideal food: packed with nutrients and antibodies, breastmilk protects your child as much as it nourishes her.

Breastmilk is the perfect food, formulated specifically to meet your baby's needs at various stages of development from newborn to toddler. The nutritional content of breastmilk is species specific—meaning it is designed for the developmental and nutritive demands of humans—and changes over time, adjusting in composition as your baby grows. Breastmilk is particularly suited to brain development, as a baby's brain grows faster than a baby's body.

Following birth, a mother generates her first milk, known as colostrum. Common to all mammals, colostrum is an antibody-rich first milk formulated to build a strong immune system. Known as nature's immunization, colostrum is rich in IgA. Secretory IgA is an antibody that has anti-infective properties that lines and protects baby's throat, lungs and gut. It is especially important at the time when the newborn is first exposed to the outside world and needs protection from germs and foreign substances entering her body. Colostrum also contains higher amounts of white blood cells and infection-fighting substances than does mature milk. It is easy for your baby to digest, high in proteins and carbohydrates, and low in fat. The natural sugars in colostrum help regulate baby's blood sugar level. Colostrum also acts as a natural laxative, helping baby pass early stools and eliminate bilirubin, which causes jaundice. It coats and seals a newborn's permeable intestines, protecting them from penetration by harmful substances.

Colostrum is thicker and more yellow in color than mature breastmilk, like melted butter or syrup. In the first few days of your infant's life, you will want to nurse often—at least 12 times in a 24-hour period. In addition to providing your baby colostrum, the nursing will stimulate the breasts to produce breast milk.

Following the colostrum, the first milk that a mother makes is referred to as transitional milk. It is yellowish in color and contains less fat and lactose and more protein than mature milk. A mixture of colostrum and mature milk, transitional milk appears within a few days to a week postpartum, and is followed in several weeks by mature breastmilk (mature milk can occur earlier in mothers who have breastfed before). Mature breastmilk is thinner in consistency than cow's milk, and may have a bluish hue.

Your breastmilk will change to meet your baby's needs and is based on supply and demand. During a nursing session, a mother generates two types of breastmilk: foremilk and hindmilk. The foremilk, which happens at the beginning of a session, is more watery and free flowing, higher in carbohydrates, and lower in fat. Foremilk comes during letdown. Hindmilk is the milk that comes when you are ending a period of nursing, and is two to three times higher in fat and slightly higher in protein than the foremilk. The latter is more filling and satisfying. In other words, the longer you feed on one breast in a session, the greater increase fat and protein. Feedings during the morning are higher in fat than later in the day. During feedings, remember to empty your breasts, so baby gets the right amount of hindmilk for energy and growth.

The primary energy source for a nursing baby is milk fat. When my son was five weeks old, my parents took a trip with us and were astonished to discover that he was breastfeeding at least every two hours. "He's eating again!" exclaimed my dad. Growing up in a generation that did not promote breastfeeding, they were not familiar with the feeding patterns of breastfed babies. One of the reasons my son ate so often was because of an enzyme called *lipase,* which breaks down milk fat quickly to allow it to be better digested and absorbed. Milk fat also contributes to healthy baby fat. As baby gets chubbier, she becomes more insulated. The fat stores can also be used for energy. In order for your baby to double and triple her weight the first year, she needs lots of calories, many of which are supplied by milk fat.

Another essential component of breastmilk are fatty acids, and particularly DHA (docasahexaenoic acid), an omega 3 fatty acid vital for infants and children in the development and growth of their brains. The brain is approximately 60% fat by weight, of which DHA is a primary element. It aids in concentration, vision, and intelligence. Imbalances or deficiencies in essential fatty acids are connected with attention deficit disorder, Parkinsons, depression, Alzheimer's, and schizophrenia.

The main group of milk proteins, casein, is rich in calcium, vital for growth and development. Also a protein in breastmilk, whey is watery and clear, and contains immunoglobulins (to fight infection), as well as high amounts of taurine, an amino acid important for the development of brain and eyes. Taurine is now added to baby formula.

Breastmilk also contains a number of vitamins and minerals, including calcium and phosphorus, both of which contribute to healthy bone and tissue development. Iron is also an important mineral in breastmilk. Interestingly, breastmilk contains less iron than formula. Because your baby's body more efficiently absorbs and utilizes the iron in breastmilk than in formula, less is needed in mother's milk. The principle, called bioavailability, reminds us that sometimes it is not quantity, but quality, that counts.

Finally, breastmilk is full of antibodies, which help strengthen a baby's immune system. When a mother is sick, her body will produce antibodies that will also transfer to baby. If a baby becomes sick, a mother will receive the organism through the breast from her saliva, and if she has not yet been exposed to it, will make antibodies and transfer them back to baby via the milk. Through mother's milk, baby may have additional protection from diseases such as measles, German measles, flu, ear infections, pneumonia, and botulism. Milk even changes seasonally. During the flu season, mother produces antibodies specific for the organism.

Breastmilk in mothers who give birth to premature babies is suited for the needs of an immature infant. This milk is higher in protein, anti-infective elements, specific fats and fatty acids helpful for premies, as well as in lactose, making it easier to digest.

The natural parenting approach favors on-demand nursing when possible. If a baby needs to feed more, it is generally because he or she is growing or in need of comfort. Maintaining a rigid schedule, which often includes longer intervals between scheduled feedings, fails to recognize that a baby is quite intuitive to its needs. By not listening to your baby's cues, you may be depriving him or her of vital nutrition.

Benefits of Breastfeeding

As we've seen, breastmilk gives your baby many advantages.

Breastmilk strengthens the immune system, assuring greater resistance to infections. In infancy, your baby's immune system is still young and immature, and one of the primary ways it develops resistance to various illnesses is through the antibodies provided in mother's milk. Studies indicate that the immune systems of breastfed babies develop earlier. As a result, they have lower incidence of infection—and less severe infections—than formula fed babies, including fewer occurrences of diarrhea, colds, ear infections, and bladder infections. In addition, breastmilk is known to protect baby against allergies, pneumonia, gastrointestinal disorders, allergies, meningitis, and SIDS (sudden infant death syndrome). Babies who gain the best immunological protection are those who are given only breastmilk (no formula) and those who are breastfed for a longer period of time.

Breastfed children suffer fewer chronic illnesses. Research shows that breastfeeding affords lifelong protection to your child's heart and blood vessels, as well as benefiting weight, glucose tolerance, blood pressure, and cholesterol levels later in life. In addition, studies suggest that it lowers the risk for chronic diseases such as diabetes, celiac disease, juvenile rheumatoid arthritis, eczema, inflammatory bowel disease, childhood cancer, and allergies. Breastfed babies also have fewer ear infections, and studies show that as breastfeeding decreases, the rate of ear infections increases.

Breastfed infants are less likely to be obese. Studies show that a specific protein in breast milk affects the body's ability to process fat. Breastfed infants tend to be leaner than formula-fed babies, and the longer a child is breast fed, the lower the rate of obesity.

Sucking at the breast helps babies develop oral muscles and facial bones. In addition, babies who breastfeed for more than one year are reported to have better alignment of their teeth and jaws, which means less need for orthodontic care later on. From the osteopathic perspective, breastfed babies have a flatter, wider palate because the coordinated muscular actions open up the bones and tissues of the face, mouth, jaw, and neck that were compressed during the birth process. These are also consistent with the findings of dentist Weston A. Price who found that cultures that breastfed and ate the whole foods of their culture (instead of eating processed foods) had fewer cavities and less crowding of teeth.

Breastfeeding affords better vision. Babies who are breastfed see better, and their strong visual acuity may be in part a result of DHA (omega-3 fatty acids) in breastmilk, which is important for the retina of the eye.

Breastfeeding fosters improved brain growth and development. The DHA present in breastmilk may also be responsible for benefits to your child's brain and IQ. A study of children ages 7 to 8 who breastfed eight months or longer showed that they had significantly higher verbal and performance IQ scores. Similar research also points to higher intelligence and improved academic achievement among children who were breastfed.

Breastfeeding offers vital health benefits to mothers as well as children.

Breastfeeding is ecological, economical, and efficient. Even including the supplies for pumping and extra food for mom, breastfeeding is easier on your pocketbook than formula feeding. Also, breastfed babies are generally sick less often, meaning fewer doctor visits, lower medical bills, and fewer parental absences at work. Employers take note: Encouraging and facilitating breastfeeding and pumping at work offers companies economic advantages, since employees are home less often with sick children.

Breastfeeding offers comfort and security and promotes closeness. No discussion of breastfeeding would be complete without emphasizing the psychological and emotional benefits provided to both mother and child. The interaction that occurs during breastfeeding promotes mother-infant bonding at a hormonal level. The hormone oxytocin, released in a mother as she feeds her child, offers a strong sense of well-being and attachment. Studies have shown that mothers who breastfeed suffer less of the baby blues than women who formula feed.

Breastfeeding after birth helps contract the uterus back to its normal size, which aids in minimizing blood loss and anemia at the time of childbirth. The hormone oxytocin, released while breastfeeding, speeds the release of the placenta and causes the uterus to shrink following birth, which results in less bleeding.

Breastfeeding enhances the mothering instinct naturally. Prolactin, the hormone that produces milk, relaxes the mother and promotes bonding with her infant. Skin-to-skin contact with your infant is important. Whether you are a stay-at-home mom or working mother, taking time to breastfeed your infant and hold him against you offers a strong sense of intimacy and fulfillment.

Research shows breastfeeding can lower the risk of certain cancers. Breast, endometrial, and ovarian cancers are less likely to appear in mothers who breastfed.

Breastfeeding prevents osteoporosis. Studies indicate that breastfeeding strengthens women's bones, helping to prevent osteoporosis after menopause.

Exclusive breastfeeding delays ovulation and fertility. Breastfeeding is nature's birth control, allowing you more time your little one before another child is possible. Caution: This is not 100% fool proof. Ask parents of Irish twins!

Nursing mothers usually have an easier time losing weight after pregnancy. Making milk requires calories, which helps mom reduce any fat she accumulated during pregnancy.

The Best Diet for Nursing Mothers

The day after my son was born, my husband made me an elaborate platter of food, telling me, "Now you are feeding for two." It is both an honor and a responsibility to be able to provide complete nourishment for your baby. Healthy nutrition based on a variety of foods provides an excellent foundation for both you and your baby. If mother and baby are healthy following birth, a mother can eat a varied, non-restricted diet, avoiding junk foods and other high-calorie, low-nutrient products. Milk production derives from the foods a mother eats as well as her stored body fat, so breastfeeding requires more calories a day. The good news is that the energy required to produce milk makes it easier to lose those extra pounds you gained during the pregnancy.

If you are nursing, you will want to be sure to get enough calcium in your diet. Many of my patients are more inclined to prefer the nondairy sources of calcium rather than the standard milk, yogurt and cheese. Nondairy sources include broccoli, dark leafy green vegetables (kale, collard green, turnip greens, Chinese greens, okra), hummus, figs, kelp, sesame, fortified soy milk, flaxseed, almonds, soy, and beans (navy, white, Great Northern). Nursing mothers are also encouraged to eat foods high in DHA or other omega-3 fatty acids which are important for the cells, especially in the brain and eye. Breastmilk is rich in DHA. Omega 3 fatty acids are found in coldwater fish and cold-weather plants: walnuts, pumpkin seeds, canola oil, wheat germ, eggs, flaxseed, green leafy vegetables, and soybeans. DHA is found in bluefin tuna, wild salmon, sardines, shellfish, herring, and mackerel. Eggs, chicken and turkey contains less amounts of DHA.

As you get to know your baby, you will become attuned to her every stirring, physically, mentally, and emotionally. You may notice that your baby may become more fussy, irritable, or gassy after you eat certain foods. If this happens, attempt to isolate the culprits and simply eliminate them from your diet for the time being. Common foods that may cause reactions include soy, fish, dairy products, eggs, corn, nuts, chocolate, caffeine, and citrus fruits. In addition, some babies may respond to a strongly flavored food or to spices. Signs of sensitivity to caffeine in your baby include irritability and difficulty with sleep. If there are family members that are sensitive to these foods, slowly introduce them into your diet and observe for any changes.

If your baby was sensitive to a particular food when she was a newborn, she may have no reactions when she is a little older. Wait and re-introduce. If she still is reactive, avoid consuming this food, and do not use it when introducing solids. Moderate and infrequent intake of alcohol is usually tolerated. For more information on dietary health for you and your baby, see "Nutritional Building Blocks 101" in Chapter 13.

How to Breastfeed

Breastfeeding is an innate and natural experience for mother and baby, yet I cannot overemphasize that it is also a learned skill. Some women are surprised to find out that breastfeeding in the beginning days and weeks can be a trying experience. They soon realize that it takes time, patience, and sometimes as long as six weeks (occasionally longer) to breastfeed smoothly. Other mothers and babies immediately begin breastfeeding without any problem.

Proper guidance and advice make the difference between easy breastfeeding and frustration and sore nipples. I dutifully read books and pamphlets, watched videos on proper positioning, and attended the many hours of instruction on breastfeeding provided by my birthing class. When my son Étienne was two weeks old, we met with a lactation consultant. She was extremely helpful with her suggestions and I encourage all mothers, both new and experienced, to seek out the counsel of lactation experts if needed.

In earlier times, before the formula fad, we would have looked to our mothers, aunts, and grandmothers for guidance on breastfeeding. But while our family systems may now lack this kind of knowledge, women in our communities have stepped in to provide advice and support. These days, many hospitals offer breastfeeding information and classes, while La Leche League, an international breastfeeding organization, has groups and chapters around the world. From lactation consultants to doulas to La Leche League leaders, numerous women have made it their mission to continue the mothering traditions that predate the 20th century.

The breasts begin preparing for milk production early in pregnancy. Often, one of the first signs that a woman is pregnant is breast tenderness and swelling. Throughout pregnancy, your breasts will change in shape and size, expanding along with your bra size. As your breasts change, your nipple and surrounding areola also enlarge and darken in color. Some lactaction consultants refer to this as a way to facilitate a baby's latching on, or getting *on target.*

There are about 15 to 20 openings in the nipple that allow milk to flow. Upon nursing, a baby creates suction, causing the milk to be released out of the nipple. Like so many bodily processes, this milk flow is made possible through a series of amazing hormonal communications. Baby's sucking action on the nipple and areola sends a message along the nerves to the pituitary gland in the brain, which then releases the hormones prolactin and oxytocin. Prolactin stimulates the breasts to grow and to make milk following childbirth. Oxytocin stimulates the milk glands to contract and squeeze the milk out, in what is known as let-down or milk ejection reflex. Oxytocin is also released during labor contractions, sexual intercourse, and in response to a warm, loving touch.

Breastfeeding includes the areola as well as the nipple. Since the areola contains the stored milk in the sinuses, it is important that baby latches on at least an inch beyond the nipple to ensure she gets the proper amount of milk. The nipple, including most of the areola, goes far into the back of baby's mouth, with her tongue under the breast and forward. Baby's sucking action will compress the breast and milk is expelled. Her upper and lower gums press on the milk stores (sinuses) that are an inch past the nipple. When I was first shown this placement, my initial thought was that I would be stuffing too much breast into my poor baby's mouth. This is not the case, however, and one of the first mistakes we make is not positioning baby high enough on the breast. Sore nipples occur when the infant slips back and only sucks on the nipple.

Here is a step-by-step guide to help you and your baby into the right placement for breastfeeding:

1. Comfortable breastfeeding begins with you, so take time to find a position and place in which you can be relaxed and focused. This may be a bed, couch, or chair. Use pillows and other props to help support your arms, back, and knees. If you are sitting in bed, use pillows under the knees for extra support and to avoid back strain. If you don't take the time to get comfortable at this beginning stage, it can lead to sore neck, shoulders, back, arms, and nipples.
2. Make sure the baby is comfortable too. If too groggy or drowsy, gently stimulate her. Call her name or stroke her cheek. If she is irritable or fussy, calm her down before introducing your breast.
3. To begin, place the breast into baby's mouth. This sounds simple, but it may take a bit of practice. The right amount of breast tissue is key to a proper latch on, but this will only happen if baby's mouth is open wide enough. As your nipple touches baby's mouth, she will instinctively open her mouth. If your baby has not opened her mouth wide enough, she needs a little bit of gentle coaxing. Gently place your nipple along baby's lower lip; this stimulates her to open her mouth wider. Since babies can imitate adult expression, try opening your mouth wide to model for your baby the ideal position. When baby's mouth is open at its widest, place the breast into her mouth. Remember: baby to breast, not breast to baby. Pull your baby to you. Whichever position or side you choose at the feeding, you will use your free hand to hold, support, and offer the breast for proper latch on.
4. If you are not satisfied with the latch on, or there is pain, start again. Gently place your finger at the corner of baby's mouth. This will break the suction and minimize tension on the nipple as you release your breast from the mouth to start again.
5. As you breastfeed, baby's nose should be nestled and pressed against the breast. It looks as though baby is not able to breathe, but be assured that she is able to breathe along the sides. If she was not able to breathe she would let you know. Be patient. It is not uncommon to feel that you are not getting it exactly right the first few times. Practice makes perfect, and be sure to ask for help!

It is one thing to read it all in a book, and it is another to experience breastfeeding firsthand. Initially, the feeling of the let-down can be unpleasant: your breasts are swollen, heavy, and can hold no more. Warmth, tingling sensations, and fullness are other ways to describe this feeling. The breasts can begin to leak at the mention or thought of your baby, or at hearing her cry. Some women never experience the let-down sensation. Initially, the let-down can be uncomfortable, but as you and your breasts become conditioned to this new experience, it becomes easier and easier. Some women may also have an abundance of milk that initially sprays in every direction upon release—this too is normal. At the beginning of a feeding, your breasts contain more milk and are heavier and fuller. By the end of the feeding, your breasts will empty, feeling softer and lighter.

Breastfeeding Positions

Before the big day, I knew that proper positioning was one of the keys to successful breastfeeding. "Position, position, and position," I heard the midwives and lactation consultants say. The key, they told me, is properly latching on. When your baby latches on correctly, she will get the right amount of milk. The first time my baby latched on, just after birth, it felt awkward and a little uncomfortable. I had seen so many moms breastfeeding their babies and toddlers and they seemed to accomplish it with such ease. I, on the other hand, needed to devote pure concentration and attention to the matter. How did they do it so easily? What was wrong with me? Would I ever be good at breastfeeding? For several weeks, I struggled. Finally, I visited a lactation consultant who offered advice on proper breastfeeding positions. Within four to six weeks, it was smooth sailing.

The best way to learn to breastfeed is to be shown by a professional lactation consultant. The breastfeeding positions given below will not replace the hands-on expertise of a lactation consultant, but are meant to enhance the breastfeeding experience and help you get started.

Cradle Hold

The cradle hold is considered one of the easiest and most comfortable breastfeeding positions. Sitting in a chair or rocking chair is preferable for this position, and you will want to get comfortable as you may be there 20 to 30 minutes or longer. Place the

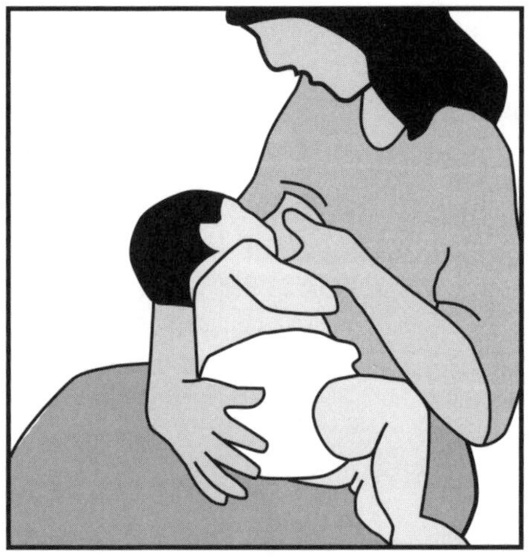

baby in your arm on top of a pillow resting on your lap so that baby is at breast level. Rely on pillows and other supports to keep baby at the proper level. Your baby's neck should be supported at the bend of your elbow, while her back rests along your forearm with her bottom in your hand.

In this alignment, she is placed on her side facing you—her chest to your chest. Her mouth should easily be within reach of your breast. Keep her body in line, assuring that the head and bottom remain on a level plane.

Clutch Hold

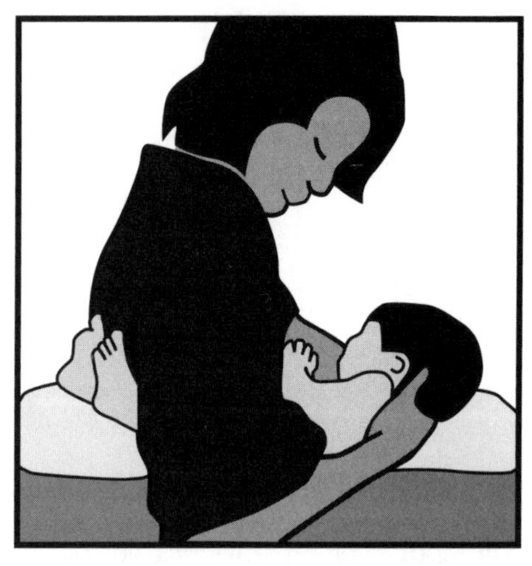

The clutch hold is a useful position following a cesarean section or if a baby is having difficulty latching on as it avoids putting pressure on the mother's belly. Also called the football hold, this position keeps the baby to the side of the mother's body, supported by the forearm—much like a football player tucks a football to his side. As with the cradle hold, you will want to find a comfortable place to sit, using pillows to bring the baby to the height of your nipple. Lie your baby next to you, supported with pillows. Your hand will support her head, while her body and back will lie along your forearm, and her feet behind you.

Cross-Cradle Hold

The cross-cradle is useful for mothers learning to breastfeed in the early weeks. The rule to remember with the cross-cradle position is that opposites attract: you will use your left arm and hand to support your baby at the right breast, and vice

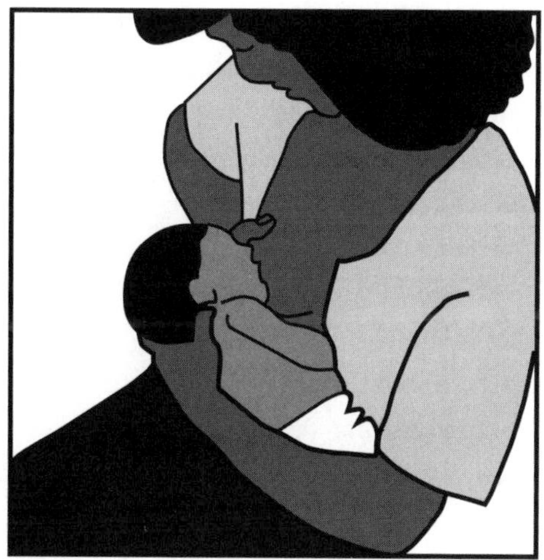

versa. Make sure you have adequate pillows to support the weight of your infant and to keep her at breast height. To nurse at the right breast, use your left hand to support the baby's neck, allowing the back of the head to rest in the webbing between your thumb and index finger. Her back should rest along your arm, remaining level with the head. Your right hand will support the right breast and guide it to your baby's mouth. In this position, your baby's stomach will be facing your stomach, offering both you and your infant greater stability during nursing. Other names for the cross-cradle position include the crossover hold, transverse hold, and transitional hold.

Side-Lying Position

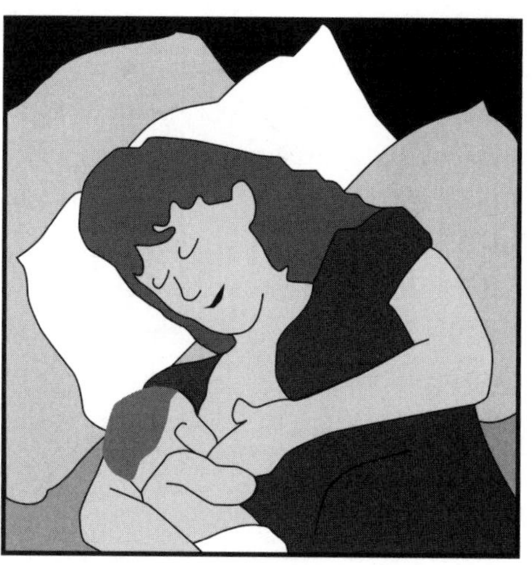

The side-lying position is one of my favorites as it allows you to lie down with your baby, facilitating nursing during the night. For this position, both you and the baby will face each other on your sides, with your arm cradling to support her back. Make sure that baby's body remains aligned with hips slightly flexed. This position is most comfortable when both you and the baby are well supported with pillows. You may want one under your back and between your knees for support, while baby should have a pillow or blanket at her back for stability.

Supporting the Breast

For all of the above positions, you will want to support your breast with your free hand. This relieves pressure from your baby, allowing her to nurse more easily.

Depending on the hold and what is most comfortable, you can support your breast with either a "C" or a "U" hold. With the "C" hold, your will place your thumb on top of the breast, back from the nipple, with your other fingers resting beneath the breast. For the "U" hold, your fingers lie flat against your ribcage under your breast, with the thumb along the outer or inner side.

Breastfeeding for Special Needs: Cesarean Birth, Premature Baby, Twins, and Augmentation

If you have had a cesarean birth, a premature birth, twins, or breast augmentation, you can still nurse. However, it is important that you find an obstetrician and pediatrician who are knowledgeable about breastfeeding and can support you, given your special considerations.

Breastfeeding after Cesarean Birth

Usually cesarean births are not a planned event. For this reason, it is best to include in your birth plan how you will handle activities such as breastfeeding in the event of a cesarean. With any birth, you are encouraged to breastfeed as soon as you are able.

Due to the fact that you have just had abdominal surgery, however, you will not be able to move as freely; your belly will be bandaged and you will have to contend with monitors and IV wires. Family, nursing staff, or lactation consultants will be able to make you comfortable with pillows for support and proper positioning so that you can begin breastfeeding as soon as possible. You will also need help with lifting the baby and changing diapers. Breastfeeding positions such as the side-lying position, and the clutch or football hold position are helpful following a cesarean.

Obstetricians prescribe pain medication following surgery. Homeopathic medicines can be started as early as possible to speed the healing process and reduce the amount of pain medication you will need (see Part IV, *Surgery*).

Breastfeeding the Premature Baby

A baby is designated premature if he or she is born before 37 weeks. Depending on birth weight and age of birth, each baby may have a variety of health considerations, but it is because—not despite—of these special needs that breastfeeding is of the utmost importance for your premature baby.

If your baby has to spend time in the nursery in the hospital, you will be deluged with a team of specialized doctors and nurses who may not consider breastfeeding a priority. It will take patience and perseverance to argue for your right to breastfeed, but I encourage you to do so. In addition to the warmth of bonding, your baby needs your nutritious milk! In fact, your milk production provides your baby with the right amount of nutrients according to her age—this is true for premature as well as full-term infants. Human milk for a premature baby is higher in nutrients and protein than milk for a term baby. Your milk will aid her development and pass on immunity to protect her against infections. If you are unable to provide milk for your baby, donor milk is a better alternative than formula.

One of the biggest challenges facing parents of premature infants is getting enough contact with their babies. In most premature infants born more than 32 weeks gestational age, the technology in the neonatal intensive care unit can be complemented by "intra-hospital maternal-infant skin-to-skin contact," also known as "kangaroo care." The notion of kangaroo care derives from Dr. Nils Bergman, Senior Medical Superintendent of Mowbray Maternity Hospital in Cape Town, South Africa who has worked on the biological concept of "habitat and niche." He argues that all animals—humans included—have four basic needs: oxygen, warmth, nutrition, and protection. A newborn's needs are met through skin-to-skin contact with the mother and breastfeeding.

While any amount of time in contact with the mother is helpful, ideally it should be day and night. Physical, bodily contact with the mother, through breastfeeding, being held or carried, or co-sleeping, is thus vital to healthy infant development and growth. A premature infant is no exception—in fact, their vulnerability means they need your bodily warmth and protection even more—so be sure to talk to hospital staff about ways to hold, breastfeed, and bond with your child during his or her stay in the neonatal ward.

Breastfeeding Twins

With the rise in fertility treatments, more and more families are having twins, an event that presents a number of rewards and challenges, not least among them breastfeeding. Fortunately, support and information abounds to help you enjoy a satisfying breastfeeding experience without needing to rely on supplementation.

The most common concern is about a lack of milk production for two or more babies. It is important to remember that your body makes as much milk as is needed, and if you have two or more hungry babies to feed, your body will respond to meet the demand.

As with any birth—singleton, twins, or more—it is best to begin breastfeeding as soon as possible. Because it is not uncommon for twins to arrive early or by cesarean section, familiarize yourself with pumping breastmilk before the day arrives. In the event of any separation from your babies, you will be able to provide them your own milk. If there are no complications, it is preferable that your babies stay in the same room as you, to allow you to bond and breastfeed frequently. Initially, both babies can be nursed simultaneously. Your lactation consultant will suggest several breastfeeding positions, but the most commonly used is the clutch hold, supported by pillows and nursing props.

Breastfeeding after Augmentation

Women who have had breast implants can nurse successfully, provided there was no serious damage to the milk ducts during surgery. In general, breastfeeding is more successful in women who had implants placed under the fold of the breast, as opposed to implants placed near the areola. Some of my patients with implants have expressed concern about leakage contaminating their milk and harming the baby. The research on these types of health risks is inconclusive, though some studies have suggested that leaking from the implant into the breastmilk may contribute to chronic gastrointestinal disorders in children. If you have implants, be sure to consult your pediatrician about breastfeeding, and if you are considering getting implants, make sure to weigh the risk to your ability to nurse in the future. Many of my patients who are now mothers and had implants when they were younger, now question if not regret their earlier decision due to health concerns for themselves and their babies.

When You Should Not Breastfeed

One of the common reasons a woman stops breastfeeding is on the advice of her doctor, often because she is prescribed a standard medication that the practitioner fears will interfere with the milk. The caution, however, is usually not warranted, and more often reflects a doctor's lack of familiarity with or support of breastfeeding. In fact, most drugs prescribed by doctors have little if no influence on milk supply nor do they affect the baby. Chemotherapy and radiation therapy for cancer are the biggest exception to this rule. Mothers with mastitis, thrush, or common illnesses like the cold and flu should be encouraged to continue nursing.

There are, however, some infections that can be passed to baby through breastmilk. If you suffer from any of the following, you should not breastfeed:

- HIV (Although a study in Africa found that mothers who exclusively breastfed for up to six months did not increase the risk of HIV transmission, the virus can be passed to infants through breastmilk.)
- Active untreated tuberculosis
- Classic galactosemia
- Active herpes lesion on the nipple (infant may nurse on the other nipple)
- Cancer chemotherapy or radioactive isotopes

Difficulties with Breastfeeding

Most women experience some minor discomfort in the first few days and weeks after giving birth, most commonly from engorgement, plugged ducts, sore nipples, and, on rare occasions, mastitis. Relief is available in many forms, from homeopathic remedies to breastfeeding techniques. In addition, nipple confusion can be an issue for many babies.

Engorgement

As the new milk begins to come in, it is not uncommon for many women to experience engorgement, or swelling and fullness of the breast from milk accumulation. Though engorgement usually happens the first week following delivery, your breasts can become engorged at any time during breastfeeding if you do not empty your breasts while nursing or if you miss feedings. Engorgement is more common in first-time mothers, and decreases with each baby.

Engorged breasts feel heavy, warm, and tender, and the skin can be tight, shiny, and exquisitely tender. Fullness can also cause nipples to become flattened, which makes it more difficult for your baby to latch on. This can lead to lumps, plugged ducts, and infection, called mastitis. Plugged or blocked ducts will feel like a lump or knot under the skin. When possible, you want to avoid becoming engorged as it takes the pleasure away from breastfeeding and has resulted in mothers wanting to stop breastfeeding altogether. Frequent feedings reduced the incidence of engorgement.

Engorgement is more common in mothers who experience cesarean or premature births because feedings can be delayed or interrupted. Fullness also occurs when feedings are restricted to particular times, rather than nursing as the child demands, or when bottles are used frequently. Nursing frequently, at least 1½ to 2 hours during the day and up to 3 hours at night for at least 15 minutes on each side, can help prevent engorgement. Breast pumps can also be helpful. See the *Mastitis* entry in Part IV for more details on remedies to relieve engorgement.

In addition to engorgement, many new mothers complain of sore nipples. Most of my patients report that there is at least a slight amount of soreness associated with nursing in the first few weeks. This can be aggravated by improper positioning. Sometimes the soreness is limited to the moment your baby latches on, and for some mothers this can be more severe and include cracking, blistering and bleeding of the nipples. In more severe cases, the pain can continue in between feedings.

Mastitis and Thrush

Mastitis is an infection or inflammation of the breast. For any new nursing mother with flu-like complaints, mastitis must be among the first conditions ruled out. Generally due to engorgement or improper nursing, mastitis can be extremely painful and is usually associated with hard, swollen, engorged breasts. There can also be a discharge from the nipple. Treatment includes warm compresses, nursing or pumping to empty the breasts, and rest and medications. In my experience, I have found a well-chosen homeopathic remedy can bring relief within a few hours. The remedies are often the same for plugged ducts or mastitis. If you do not improve, consult your physician immediately.

Thrush is caused by a yeast infection that can be passed between the mother's nipple and the baby's mouth. Thrush takes the form of white patches in the baby's mouth and on the tongue. It can be located in the mouth and on the nipple. Mothers with both mastitis and thrush are encouraged to continue breast feeding while receiving treatment. See *Mastitis* and *Thrush* in Part IV.

Nipple Confusion

Your baby can become confused between your nipple and that of the bottle. This is commonly referred to as nipple confusion. The way your baby latches on and sucks during breastfeeding is different mechanically than during bottle feeding. Breastfeeding requires more work and coordination in order to suck properly, while milk flows out more freely with the bottle, meaning less work for baby. Babies can quickly become accustomed to the easier bottle nipple, making them less inclined to breastfeed. To avoid this, do not give newborns artificial nipples for the first three to four weeks following birth. Artificial nipples, either in the form of a bottle or pacifier, can interfere with both you and your baby learning to breastfeed correctly. The best nipple for your baby is yours.

After several weeks to a month, a bottle of expressed milk can be introduced. Some parents have noted that if they wait too long (several months) to introduce a bottle, it may not be as easily accepted by their baby. We started gradually, once a day, in order to ensure that our son would accept a bottle as well. Parents usually find that baby will take a bottle more willingly when given by another person (for example, dad or a caregiver) when mom is not in the room.

Relactation, Adoptive Nursing, and Donor Milk

Perhaps a mother had not wanted to nurse and then changes her mind. Perhaps she is experiencing difficulty nursing a premature baby, or wants to try to breastfeed her adopted baby. There are innumerable reasons why women would want to nurse, even if it seems like a tremendous if not impossible challenge. With support, dedication, and patience, many mothers (including adoptive mothers) have been able to lactate or simulate breastfeeding. It is also important to consider baby, who may not want to begin taking the breast if a bottle has been given for too long. For more information, contact your nearest La Leche League group.

Women who want to breastfeed their baby and cannot or choose not to try relactation can now work with an alternative supplemental breastfeeding system. The SNS (supplemental nursing system) is a tiny tube filled with supplement that attaches along side breast and nipple. SNS allows mother to experience nursing despite not having enough milk.

When a mother is not able to breastfeed or her baby is not able to tolerate formula, she has a resource in milk banks, which store milk donated by other mothers. Common candidates for the milk bank are preterm infants whose mother has not been able to establish a milk supply, or the infant who cannot tolerate formula and is inconsolable and failing to thrive.

The donor mothers have been carefully screened for infections and must be in good health. At the milk bank, the donor milk is pasteurized, in theory retaining most of its nutrients, and is then tested for bacteria. You need a medical prescription in order to use a milk bank, but you don't need to live near a bank, as the milk can be shipped. Since the banks are nonprofit organizations, they offer a reduced fee for the milk. Some medical insurance policies are covered, and no family is refused if unable to pay.

Breastpumping and Storing Milk

I credit the invention of the breast pump with allowing me to exclusively breastfeed my children, especially when I had to go back to work. The breast pump lets you pump your milk, store it, and use it at a later date. Although nothing replaces breastfeeding, the modern day breast pump has been a gift. Leaving a caretaker with your milk is not the ideal situation, but offers in many cases the best alternative for a working mother. It is not uncommon to feel guilty, as I did, but at the very least I knew that by pumping at work as well as nursing my baby at night, I was able to do the best that I could for both of us.

Designed to imitate the rate of your baby's sucking, which translates to approximately 45 to 55 times a minute, breast pumps come in all shapes and sizes, including manually operated, battery powered, and electric. Modern breast pumps are clean and easy to use, varying in appearance from simple, motorized gadgets to fancy all-in-one machines enclosed in black leather bags resembling briefcases. Electric pumps can be rented or bought and, depending on your needs, you may want to lease one before you buy to make sure you have the right machine for you. For the first month, I chose to rent the pump. Early on, though, my husband and I realized that it was more cost effective to buy a breast pump, and it proved to be an essential item in my household, especially with my schedule as a working mother.

When I was researching pumps, my goal was to find a pump that allowed me to produce the most milk in the shortest amount of time with the greatest degree of comfort. Following are considerations that may prove helpful as you decide on the breast pump that best fits your needs.

Electric pumps: For efficiency, consider the electric pumps, especially those that pump at least 25 cycles per minute. Slower pumps with longer suction time become tiresome, lead to frustration, and can cause breast and nipple pain.

Automatic cycles: Pumps with automatic cycles are superior to the manually self-adjusting cycles. Most women find automatic cycling more comfortable.

Suction strength: Look for a pump that has an adjustable suction strength. This needs to be adequate in order to imitate baby's suck. Strength that is too high can cause pain. Whereas low pressure will not be efficient for milk extraction.

Single or double scoop?: Breast pumps also offer single- or double-pumping action. There are advantages to both. When I was at work and wanted to write, eat, or speak on the phone and needed an extra arm, I found the single pump handy. However, double pumping was more efficient and took nearly half the time to produce twice the milk. Simultaneously pumping both breasts has been shown to increase milk production, which is a good thing when you want to be guaranteed of a lot of extra milk. A single pump is more handy is you are a stay-at-home mom and choose to breastfeed one breast and pump the other for a feeding.

Breast pump shield size: It is best to use a pump that provides various choice of breast shield to accommodate large- and small-breasted women. The one-size-fits-all pumps may not suit every breast.

Manual pumps: Manual pumps are more reasonably priced, but you will want to avoid using one if you have carpal tunnel syndrome or wrist or arm conditions. Some pumps can be done by the foot, offering an alternative to arm and wrist strain.

Additional tips:

1. Pump in the morning, when milk is usually more abundant.
2. If you are at home with baby, simultaneously nurse baby while pumping. This will increase milk supply.
3. If you experience pain while pumping, stop. This may mean the pump is not of good quality or you are not using it correctly.
4. Pump session should not be longer than 20 minutes.

Hand Expression

Referred to as the Marmet Technique and devised by Chele Marmet, Director of the Lactation Institute in Los Angeles, hand expression can be used for breastmilk storage as an alternative to pumping or if you are in a bind. Keep in mind that it takes a little practice, and a live demonstration can be helpful. Some women have found hand expression to be more effective than pumping.

With hand expression, you are using your fingers to empty the milk reservoirs behind the nipple. The technique demands that you employ both proper finger placement and motion to put pressure on the reservoirs. To begin, place your thumb and first two fingers one to one and a half inches beyond the nipple, with the thumb above and fingers directly below at a 12 o'clock and 6 o'clock position. Bear in mind that your fingers may or may not be at touching the areola—you should measure your placement based on the nipple. With your fingers together, push back toward the wall of the chest; for larger breasts, lift before pressing back. To compress and empty the milk reservoirs, roll the thumb and fingers forward. Repeat this motion—positioning the fingers, pushing back, and rolling forward—until you have emptied the reservoirs. To milk the other reservoirs, reposition your fingers, keeping the thumb and fingers on opposite sides of the breast.

Storing Your Liquid Gold

When my son was two years old, I was invited to a wedding in Colorado. My friend Nancy and I attended, though without our families. As breastfeeding mothers, both of us faced the dilemma of what to do with our "liquid gold." Several times a day, including during a lovely hike in the Rockies, we had to pump our milk and then toss it. We were thankful, to say the least, for our handy, battery-operated pump. Throwing away our precious breastmilk was unusual, because we would have otherwise stored it for use at a later date. Fortunately, unless you are facing circumstances like these, you don't have to worry about throwing away excess milk, as it can easily be stored and kept frozen.

Your milk will not look like cow's milk, perfectly white and creamy. Human milk naturally separates, with the fat rising to the top. If this occurs, shake it and it is ready to use. The color of your milk can vary, reflecting your food choices, be they green vegetables, seaweed, fruit drinks, or even food dyes. A pinkish tinge may signify blood, possibly from cracked nipples. If this does not cease, speak to your practitioner.

Your pumped milk can be stored in many different ways. Before pumping, it is best to wash your hands. Always use clean containers that have been washed in hot, soapy water, then rinsed and left to air dry. If you are freezing your milk, you will need to decide whether to use glass, plastic containers, or plastic bags. Research indicates that all are suitable, though my preference is glass, as claims (albeit unsubstantiated) have circulated about possible links between freezing water in plastic bottles and cancer. After glass, the next best choice is clear, hard plastic (polycarbonate) followed by cloudy, hard plastic (polypropylene). For all containers, use a tight lid.

Cooled breastmilk can be added to already cooled or frozen milk. Leave approximately 1 inch space at the top of container if freezing. When you store your milk, be sure to keep it to quantities of 2 to 4 ounces; this will avoid waste.

Most of my pumped milk was conveniently stored in breastmilk freezer bags. These plastic bags are specially designed for the long-term storage of milk. The plastic bags, which you will date, conveniently fit in the freezer, and can be thawed with the least amount of wasted excess milk. Frozen milk stored in a standard, combination refrigerator-freezer can be kept for three to four months. In a deep freezer that is separate from the refrigerator, milk can be stored for six months or longer.

Short-term storage at room temperature shows that milk is still viable up to ten hours after pumping. When I was at work, my breast pump came complete with insulator, in which I placed frozen packs to keep the milk chilled until I came home. Refrigerated milk can be used within eight days after expression.

Use the milk with the earliest date in the freezer to thaw. To thaw your frozen milk, leave it in the refrigerator for at least four hours or under the faucet with cool water. Do not leave it at room temperature to thaw. Once it has thawed, you can use warm water in the faucet. To warm milk, place the container in a bowl of very warm water. Avoid heating the milk on the stove or in the microwave. Always test the temperature of the milk on the wrist before beginning feedings. Once thawed, the milk can be refrigerated for up to 24 hours. Thawed milk should not be refrozen.

Breastfeeding in Public

Breastfeeding mothers face a common dilemma when it comes to nursing in public places. A hungry baby is impatient, and, as every parent will attest, the sooner you meet her needs, the better for everyone. But making sure your baby is comfortable and satiated can often mean nursing in places you wouldn't normally choose. Nursing in public can be uncomfortable for the mother as well as for strangers, yet mom and baby cannot stay home all the time, nor should they have to.

The most common reason women cite for not wanting to nurse in public is apprehension about showing their breasts. If you wear appropriate clothing, though, there is very little to reveal. Many nursing and mother-oriented magazines contain advertisements for blouses and shirts designed with breastfeeding slits, making it possible to nurse without even lifting your shirt. You can also use light blankets, caps, or cover-ups to place over baby while nursing, though you may find this a less popular option with your baby if she does not like her face covered.

Breastfeeding in public is a matter of cultural perception as well as personal comfort. While an increasing number of print ads are beginning to show nursing mothers and babies, our comfort with breastfeeding does not necessarily extend to public places. In his overview of breastfeeding in the media at a La Leche League international conference, Dr. Jack Newman showed that advertisements still depict breastfeeding mothers exclusively in the home environment, while bottle feeding mothers are portrayed with their babies, in public and back to work. What is the underlying message? Breastfeeding is acceptable at home in private, but not in public where it is seen as a kind of improper exposure.

Even in my office, mothers have asked permission to be able to nurse. A doctor's office should always be breastfeeding friendly, as should any other public venue women may frequent with their babies. Fortunately, as more women demand places in which to breastfeed, public facilities, and particularly restrooms, are being designed to accommodate their needs. When I was nursing my babies, I appreciated the lounges available in many public restrooms, and as you spend more time in public with your baby, you will likewise find yourself developing an eye for semi-private places that support breastfeeding. And don't forget about the privacy of your car!

Weaning

Especially at the beginning, you may feel like you are nursing around the clock: your baby is always hungry, whether night or day. An infant's seemingly endless capacity to nurse is not surprising, given how much she is growing, doubling or tripling her weight in the first year. Your milk flow is programmed to respond to your child's changing nutritional demands. As your child begins solids, you will find that the frequency with which she nurses will begin to diminish and, as a result, your milk supply will decrease as well.

Around the world, the average age to wean a child is approximately four years old. Although your toddler has different needs than when she was a baby, many of the same reasons to breastfeed still apply. She receives valuable nutrients, vitamins, and immunity from your breastmilk, even though she is eating solid foods as well. Breastfeeding also offers comfort, security, and warmth.

Different agencies recommend various breastfeeding time frames. The American Academy of Pediatrics currently recommends breastfeeding for a minimum of one year or longer if desired. Canadian Pediatric Society and UNICEF recommend two years or longer. There is a common misconception that nursing longer will make your child dependent. I had the pleasure of breastfeeding my two sons a total of nine years, and both are now independent and mature. As a working mother, one of the ways I was able to meet their needs was through breastfeeding.

Many mothers wean their children early because they report feeling exhausted and moody, and assume breastfeeding to be cause. In my experience, breastfeeding fatigue is a symptom rather than a cause, and responds well to homeopathic remedies, allowing a mother to feel better about breastfeeding and about taking care of her family and responsibilities. But whether you are weaning an infant or a toddler, the process varies from mother to mother and even child to child, and can feel alternately like an important milestone and bittersweet loss. When asked about the weaning process, Diane Bengson, author of the book *How Weaning Happens*, says, "Gradually, with love."

According to Bengson, there are four basic categories of weaning: abrupt, planned or gradual, partial weaning, and natural weaning.

1. Abrupt weaning involves a sudden stop in breastfeeding. Sometimes a baby or toddler has made the decision to stop and weans herself. Often, mothers tell me this is more difficult for them than for their child. In other instances, unavoidable situations, such as a medical condition, requires a mother not breastfeed. A sudden cessation of breastfeeding in a woman who was nursing frequently can lead to engorgement and breast infections, and she should take precautions to avoid this if possible.

2. In the planned or gradual weaning, the mother and baby are gradually nursing less frequently. The feedings are replaced by food and beverages, and the lack of nursing does not necessarily mean there is a lack of attention and comfort. In addition, mother may distract child with playtime and books in lieu of nursing. This method is used successfully and lovingly with a minimum of stress.
3. In partial weaning, the mother eliminates some feedings. In my household, when each child was around two years old, I found myself getting fatigued by having to wake several times a night, and decided to stop my middle-of-the-night nursing. I would keep all other feedings, as I enjoyed nursing. Since our children were in bed with us, I let my sons know in advance that we would soon be discontinuing middle-of-the-night breastfeeding. When the night finally came, I slept in another room while my husband attempted to soothe, calm, and offer replacement drinks. Although I got a good night's sleep, it took several weeks of adjustment before I was back in the family bedroom. I was then able to thoroughly enjoy my breastfeeding when the sun was up for another several years and allowed them to naturally wean.
4. Natural weaning is child led weaning, which allows child to stop nursing according to her own timetable.

Formula Feeding

While a staunch supporter of breastfeeding, I recognize there are mothers who choose to not breastfeed or cannot breastfeed for a variety of reasons. The decision to formula feed your baby is a personal one and does not mean you will be any less bonded with your baby. It does mean you will face complicated decisions about what kind of formula to give her. From your first day at the hospital, you will face a dizzying array of choices, brands, and formulations, each of which will purport to offer the most complete nutrition for your child. None of these are a perfect substitute for breastmilk, but some come closer than others.

In choosing an infant formula, be sure to read the labels: there are several common brands to choose from, and they vary in protein, fat, and carbohydrate content, as well as enrichments. Ultimately, though, the success of the formula depends on how well your baby tolerates it. Vitamins and minerals are similar in most formulas, since they are strictly regulated.

Here's what to look for in a formula:

1. Pay attention to proteins, and particularly the whey to casein ratio. Formulas are made in varying percentages, ranging from 100% to approximately 48% whey. Consider beginning with a whey-based formula that has a similar ratio to breastmilk (approximately 80% whey and 20% casein, the opposite of cow's milk). This proportion should be easier for your baby to digest, with less strain on the kidneys and hence less chance of dehydration. Formulas that are higher in casein may give baby a feeling of fullness, making them more economical, but harder to digest. Because casein causes curds, it can lead to discomfort and constipation.
2. The carbohydrates in many formulas consist of corn syrup, lactose, and other sugars. Corn syrup is a refined carbohydrate along with sugar, white flour, and white rice. The increased amount of consumption of these refined products is linked to rising rates of obesity and diabetes mellitus. Lactose is milk sugar, naturally occurring in human, cow, and goat milk. Some infants may be intolerant of the lactose found in formulas and suffer from tummy pain, gas, and diarrhea. If this is the case, consider formulas that are whey-based and lactose- and casein-free. Lactose-free milk is sweetened with corn syrup and glucose.
3. Iron in breastmilk is absorbed at rate of 50 to 75%, whereas iron in formula is absorbed at 5 to 10%. Because infants take in such a small amount of iron in formula, the companies add iron to compensate. Although iron can be hard to digest and cause intestinal upset, choose an iron-fortified formula; it is best to avoid the low-iron options.

Transitional baby milks (follow-up or follow-on formulas) are also marketed to meet the needs of babies twelve months and older. This milk contains more calcium, phosphorus, iron, and protein compared to standard infant formula.

Other considerations:

1. Formulas come with expiration dates. Pay attention to it.
2. Always follow mixing instructions exactly. Mixing in too much or too little water may cause serious harm to newborns and young infants.
3. Discard bottle if it has been out of the refrigerator for more than two hours.

4. Discard bottle of remaining formula after baby has fed. The germs from baby's mouth could reproduce in the bottle.
5. Any unused formula can be refrigerated and used within 48 hours.
6. Warm milk slightly by holding the container or bottle under warm tap water, or placing in a bowl of warm water. In general, cold drinks are not healthy. Avoid using the microwave to warm baby's milk. Because of heat dispersion, the milk may feel cool to touch, but inside could have hot spots that would burn a baby. In addition, any type of heat source can change the content of the milk. In one study, microwaving altered an amino acid the milk which was then shown to be toxic to the kidneys.
7. I remember my mother testing the temperature of the formula on her wrist. This method is still recommended today.
8. Hold baby in your arms when feeding her. Alternate arms with each feeding.
9. Avoid leaving baby alone with bottle while lying down. She could choke. Also when lying down, formula can travel to the middle ear through the eustachian tube and lead to ear infections.
10. Bottles can be sterilized in the dishwasher, by washing in hot soapy water, or by immersing nipples and open bottle in a pan of boiling water for 10 minutes. Be sure to clean the bottles first with a bottle brush. Let the cleansed equipment air dry.
11. There are many types of nipples to choose depending on the age of the baby. Infants usually require a smaller hole size, while larger nipples with larger holes are appropriate for older babies. For the full-time bottle-feeding baby, experiment with various types of nipples to see which one works best. If baby is both breastfeeding and bottle feeding, use a nipple with a wide base.

Alternatives to Standard Baby Formula

Some babies do not tolerate or are allergic to the standard cow's milk-based formula. Other options for allergic babies include soy-based formulas, hypoallergenic formulas, and even goat milk formulas. If your baby is not tolerating her formula, I recommend that you work with your practitioner on finding the proper alternative. The goat milk formula requires giving baby a vitamin supplement, but it is easier to tolerate and digest and less allergenic than cow's milk based.

Soy-based formulas: It is recommended that a baby starts with a cow's milk-based formula. For families who are concerned about allergies, the research has not proven that a non-cow-based formula, like soy, will lessen tendency to allergies: up to 50% of babies allergic to cow's milk formula can show sensitivity to soy-based formula as well, and due to immature intestines, feeding soy formula to newborns and young infants may make them susceptible to soy allergies. As a plant protein, soy lacks important protein building blocks that your baby needs. Soy also contains a binding protein called phytates that can make it harder for the body to use calcium, iron, and zinc. As a result, soy-based formulas contain extra quantities of these minerals. The American Academy of Pediatrics has expressed concern that soy is also high in aluminum and manganese, which may be toxic to infants. Researchers have speculated that high levels of manganese have been linked to behavior problems and attention deficit disorder later in life. Soy formula is also saltier, which may begin to alter baby's palate choices later in life. Corn syrup (corn is also an allergen) is often used as a sweetener. Soy milk is not recommended in small or preterm babies.

Lactose-free formula: Lactose has been known to produce lactose intolerance in children and adults, but it is an important component in breastmilk. It provides energy and is important for the growth of healthy bacteria in the intestine and for calcium absorption in the gut. Lactose-free formulas may be helpful for babies who have rare metabolic diseases or for babies following a diarrheal illness. Unfortunately, most formulas contain corn syrup or sucrose (refined car-bohydrates) as replacements for lactose. This is not one of the more common formulas, and due to the fact that it is a specialty formula, it may lack the nutrients that are found in standard formulas. It should only be used if advised by your practitioner.

Hypoallergenic formula: For babies who are dairy sensitive or show extreme signs of allergies or a strong response when they drink formula, there is the hypoallergenic formula. Hypoallergenic formula is for babies who have severe digestive problems, and are not able to tolerate cow's milk or soybean-based formulas. The protein in hypoallergenic formulas has been predigested or broken down so that it is easier to digest and causes less reaction. Apparently, the taste is bitter, unpleasant, and is not able to be disguised despite higher amount of sweeteners such as corn syrup. These are also higher in salt, and in price.

How Much Formula Should You Feed Your Baby?

Give small frequent feedings and use the following guidelines:

- Newborns: 2 to 3 ounces per feeding
- 1 to 2 months of age: 3 to 4 ounces per feeding
- 2 to 6 months: 4 to 6 ounces per feeding
- 6 to 12 months: 6 to 8 ounces per feeding

Your baby will require approximately 2 to 3 ounces of formula per pound a day. Contact your practitioner if baby is not gaining weight. Signs of not getting enough or getting too much include:

- Slow weight gain or excessive weight gain.
- Extreme irritability or crying with obvious cramping after feeding.
- Baby's skin is wrinkly, thin, and loose. No healthy "baby fat."
- Abundance of spitting up or projectile vomiting. Try feeding in smaller amount at more frequent intervals.

The Business of Formula

One of my patients who recently delivered in the hospital discovered to her surprise that the nursing staff was very intent in making sure she had appropriate commercial formula materials, packets, and samples. Despite insisting on her choice to breastfeed, she was presented repeatedly with the more expensive, less nutritious alternative.

Infant formula is big business, and companies are devoted to convincing potential customers that formula feeding is just as easy, healthy, and "natural" as breastfeeding. Their public opinion campaign has proved effective—so effective that, in 1981, the World Health Organization (WHO) adopted the International Code of Marketing Breastmilk Substitutes to counteract the powerful formula companies, like Nestle. The policy prohibited public advertising of bottles, nipples, and formula, and discouraged media promotion and offers of free formula samples to mothers as well as health care workers. Although infant formula companies like Nestle have adopted a "breastfeeding is best" attitude, formula companies are still alleged to violate the code.

Formula presents a number of disadvantages, not only nutritionally, but economically and environmentally.

1. In developing countries, the use of contaminated water in formula prepara-

tion leads to more than one million deaths as a result of diarrhea. Many of these deaths could have been prevented by exclusive breastfeeding.

2. Baby formula is more expensive and less cost effective than breastfeeding, a problem that particularly impacts developing nations and economically challenged populations. Breastfed babies are healthier, which means fewer visits to the doctor, and fewer days missed for working parents. Standard formula can cost approximately $1200 per year, and hypoallergenic up to $2500 a year (plus cost of bottles etc.). A breastfeeding mother may use approximately $600 a year for extra food.
3. Most baby formula comes from cow's milk, making it unsuitable for children who are lactose intolerant.

If you find that you are not able to breastfeed or are losing your milk supply too soon, do not distress. If you have to use formula, any guilt, grief, and sadness can be mitigated by six months when wholesome and nutritious solid foods can be introduced into the diet, thereby slowly reducing the need for formula as your baby grows and relies more on solids.

SUMMARY

WHAT IS IN BREASTMILK?

Breastmilk is the perfect food, formulated specifically to meet your baby's needs at various stages of development from newborn to toddler. Following birth, a mother generates her first milk, known as colostrum. Colostrum is antibody-rich and has anti-infective properties that lines and protects baby's throat, lungs, and gut. Colostrum is thicker and more yellow in color than mature breastmilk.

Following the colostrum, the first milk that a mother makes is referred to as transitional milk. It is yellowish in color and contains less fat and lactose and more protein than mature milk. A mixture of colostrum and mature milk, transitional milk appears within a few days to a week postpartum.

Mature breastmilk usually appears a few weeks later but can occur earlier in mothers who have breastfed before. During a nursing session, a mother generates two types of breastmilk: foremilk and hindmilk. The foremilk, which happens at the beginning of a session, is more watery and free flowing, higher in carbohydrates, and lower in fat. Hindmilk comes when you are ending a period of nursing, and is two to three times higher in fat and slightly higher in protein than the foremilk. During feedings, remember to empty your breasts, so baby gets the right amount of hindmilk for energy and growth.

Breastmilk contains essential nutrients for baby, including milk fat, omega-3 fatty acids like DHA, proteins like casein and whey, and vitamins and minerals like calcium and phosphorus.

BENEFITS OF BREASTFEEDING

Breastfeeding confers benefits for both babies and mothers, aiding in babies' development, preventing certain illnesses, controlling weight, and promoting bonding.

THE BEST DIET FOR NURSING MOTHERS

If you are nursing, make sure to eat a healthy varied diet high in calcium (including non-dairy sources) and DHA. Also, you may notice that baby is sensitive to certain foods you eat; eliminate them from your diet while you are nursing.

HOW TO BREASTFEED

Breastfeeding is a learned skill, and there are many resources available to help mothers nurse comfortably. To help you and your baby into the right placement for breastfeeding:

1. Find a position and place in which you can be relaxed and focused.
2. Make sure the baby is comfortable and calm too.
3. To begin, place the breast into baby's mouth. The right amount of breast tissue is key to a proper latch on, but this will only happen if baby's mouth is open wide enough. It is important that baby latches on at least an inch beyond the nipple to ensure she gets the proper amount of milk. The nipple, including most of the areola, goes far into the back of baby's mouth, with her tongue under the breast and forward. Pull your baby to you and use your free hand to hold, support, and offer the breast for proper latch on.
4. If you are not satisfied with the latch on, or there is pain, start again.
5. As you breastfeed, baby's nose should be nestled and pressed against the breast.

BREASTFEEDING POSITIONS

Proper positioning is key to breastfeeding success. If you are experiencing difficulty, a lactation consultant can help you figure out the best position for you and your baby. The most common positions are the cradle hold, clutch hold, cross-cradle position, and side-lying position.

BREASTFEEDING FOR SPECIAL NEEDS: CESAREAN BIRTH, PREMATURE BABY, TWINS, AND AUGMENTATION

If you have had a cesarean birth, a premature birth, twins, or breast augmentation, you can still nurse. However, it is important that you work with practitioners who are knowledgeable about breastfeeding.

WHEN YOU SHOULD NOT BREASTFEED

You should not breastfeed if you have HIV, active untreated tuberculosis, classic galactosemia, active herpes lesion on the nipple, or undergoing chemotherapy.

DIFFICULTIES WITH BREASTFEEDING

Most women experience some minor discomfort in the first few days and weeks after giving birth, most commonly from engorgement, plugged ducts, sore nipples, and, on rare occasions, mastitis. Relief is available in many forms, from homeopathic medicines to breastfeeding techniques. In addition, nipple confusion can be an issue for many babies if they were given a bottle or pacifier as newborns.

RELACTATION, ADOPTIVE NURSING, AND DONOR MILK

Women who were not initially able to nurse (including adoptive mothers) have been able to lactate or simulate breastfeeding. Women who cannot relactate can try an alternative supplemental breastfeeding system. When a mother is not able to breastfeed or her baby is not able to tolerate formula, she has a resource in milk banks, which store milk donated by other mothers.

BREASTPUMPING AND STORING MILK

Designed to imitate the rate of your baby's sucking, breast pumps come in all shapes and sizes, including manually operated, battery powered, and electric. Hand expression, in which you use your fingers to empty the milk reservoirs behind the nipple, is another alternative to pumping.

Always use clean containers (either glass or plastic) to store your pumped milk. Leave approximately a 1 inch space at the top of container if freezing. Refrigerated milk can be used within eight days after expression; frozen milk will keep for three or four months.

BREASTFEEDING IN PUBLIC

Nursing in public is becoming more common; you can use blouses with breastfeeding slits or cover-ups to do so discreetly.

WEANING

Around the world, the average age to wean a child is approximately four years old. The American Academy of Pediatrics currently recommends breastfeeding for a minimum of one year or longer if desired. There are four basic categories of weaning: abrupt, planned or gradual, partial weaning, and natural weaning.

FORMULA FEEDING

If you cannot or choose not to breastfeed, look for a DHA-enriched, iron-fortified, whey-based formula, with a similar ratio to breastmilk (approximately 80% whey and 20% casein).

Some babies do not tolerate or are allergic to the standard cow's milk-based formula. Other options for allergic babies include soy-based formulas, hypoallergenic formulas, and even goat milk formulas.

Give small frequent feedings and use the following guidelines:

- Newborns: 2 to 3 ounces per feeding
- 1 to 2 months of age: 3 to 4 ounces per feeding
- 3 to 6 months: 4 to 6 ounces per feeding
- 6 to 12 months: 6 to 8 ounces per feeding

Your baby will require approximately 2 to 3 ounces of formula per pound per day.

chapter 13

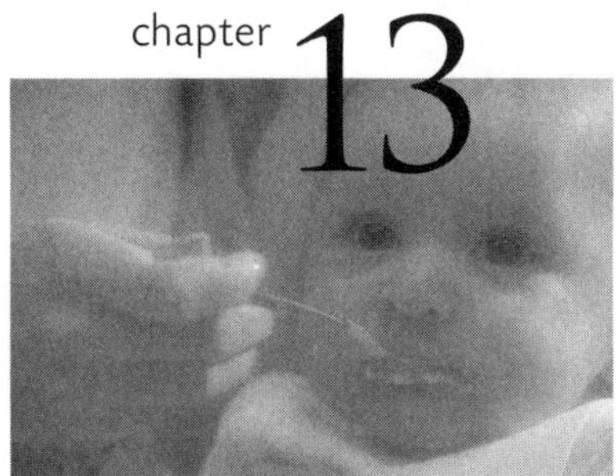

Healthy Nutrition

To our children we can give two things—roots and wings.

—*Chinese proverb*

FROM THEIR BIRTH until they leave home as young adults, our children depend on us to make vital decisions about their diet and nutrition. We are responsible for more than simply feeding them, however; we also model for our children a variety of ways of thinking about, preparing, and consuming food that will impact their eating habits and health throughout their lives. Snack foods, meal times, shopping routines, and cooking techniques are all part of the nutritional education we provide children as they grow up.

Most of us have adopted at least some of the eating routines of our childhood, whether a big family meal on Sunday or eggs with breakfast each morning, but many parents I talk to are also interested in changing the habits they grew up with in favor of diets that are lower in animal fats, higher in organic fruits and vegetables, and more ecologically sustainable. As I tell my patients, there is no one diet suited to all families. Rather, holistic practices teach us about the best available choices for families based on the ages, activity levels, tastes, and medical histories of each member. Even with our busy schedules and hectic lifestyles, we can offer nutritious meals to our families without too much time, preparation, and training.

Food trends seem to change almost as quickly as the seasons. Each year brings a new diet, new marketing gimmicks, and new claims and criticisms about what we eat and how we eat it. The low-fat/high-carb diet of the previous decades has given way to high-protein/low-carb recommendations, while slow foods, raw foods, blood-type diets, and other forms of vegetarianism and veganism offer alternatives to the processed and treated "instant" meals that crowd the grocery shelves. With so many diets claiming to be the healthiest, planning meals for your family is no simple task. Everyone, it seems, wants to tell you what to eat, what to buy, and how to cook it.

This chapter is designed to cut through the competing messages to the basic facts about nutritious and healthy eating, helping you make the choices that correspond with the needs of your family as well as with your time and budget. The common thread is that **your food be as freshly prepared, organic, in season, and varied as possible**. This is important whether you are vegetarian, vegan, or a fan of steak-n-potatoes (the latter hopefully in moderation). Whatever your food preferences, nutritionists concur that the following diet can meet your family's nutritional needs and help lower risks of cancer, heart disease, and diabetes:

- Rich in plant-based foods
- Rich in whole grains, fruit, and vegetables
- Low in animal fat
- Low in animal-based products (including dairy)

The Standard American Diet

The standard American diet is a recipe for risk, consisting of the very ingredients that contribute to the nation's increasing rates of heart disease, stroke, and cancer. It is rich in foods that are harmful to the body—processed, unrefined products, sugars (also known as simple carbohydrates), bad fats (saturated, hydrogenated, partially hydrogenated, and trans fats), as well as dairy and animal-based foods—while low in beneficial plant-based foods and whole grains and fiber (the complex carbohydrates).

Many of these standard foods also seem the most convenient: prepackaged dinners and snacks, sodas and fast food are often tempting precisely because they are easy to prepare, easy to find in the supermarkets, and popular with kids. Eating habits are among the most difficult aspects of our lives to transform, given our emotional, psychological connection to foods we love, remember, or simply rely on for an easy meal.

Perhaps your children are school age, and you have been a little lax on reading the labels. It is not too late to begin making healthy changes—the key is to do it slowly, one box of Frosted Flakes at a time. After the box is used, replace it with a healthier variety. Savvy parents know that abrupt changes to their child's diet will only provoke protest and refusals to eat, so try first looking for organic, low-fat, or fruit juice sweetened versions of foods you already enjoy, as well as for new products that can serve as healthy alternatives. Eating healthfully does require more attention to ingredients, and occasionally more time in preparation: our food culture privileges convenience over health, so eating better will always mean spending more time choosing, cooking, and consuming meals.

At the same time, though, better eating doesn't have to be complicated; it simply means making different choices at the grocery store and adopting different routines in the kitchen. A diet based on a variety of fresh, organic foods provides more of the nutrients that are vital to the health of children and adults alike. When we say that a food is "nutritious," it means that it can be broken down by the body into proteins, carbohydrates, fats, vitamins, minerals and water, all of which are crucial to good health.

The USDA MyPlate

In June 2011, the old USDA food pyramid was replaced with MyPlate (and in Spanish MiPlato), a joint project of the US Department of Agriculture and Health and Human Services. It was designed to visually communicate the five food groups: fruits, vegetables, grains, protein, and dairy. Each group is also sized to reflect proportion. The imagery used is of a place setting with the plate divided into 4 quarters colored to represent fruits, vegetables, grains, and protein. To the right of the plate a circle is given representing a glass of milk. The corresponding government website www.choosemyplate.gov/MyPlate instructs readers on building a healthy eating style based on variety, amount, and nutrition. The website also notes the importance of caloric intake for the individual depending on their age, sex, height, weight, and amount of physical activity. Unlike past projects, the new guidelines do list nutritious food sources that include whole grains, fresh vegetables and fruits in season, nondairy calcium sources, vegetarian protein sources, and healthy oils.

Nutritional Building Blocks 101

Protein and Amino Acids

Protein is essential for nearly all the biological processes in the body, including growth, repair, metabolism, muscular and bone strength, hormonal systems, immune functioning, the nervous system, and skin elasticity and regeneration. Although protein provides the body some energy, it is not our primary source: most energy comes from fats and carbohydrates.

When we consume proteins, our bodies break them down into smaller building blocks called amino acids. Most of them can be manufactured by the body, but nine essential amino acids must be supplied from the diet and hence can come only from the foods we eat.

Protein is derived from both animal and plant sources. Plant sources include beans, soy products, and nuts, while animal sources include meat, poultry, fish, eggs, dairy products, and breast milk. Nutritionists have long urged people to consume "complete proteins," those proteins that contain all nine essential amino acids not manufactured by the body. Animal proteins are complete, while plant sources must be combined to provide all the essential amino acids. Rice and beans, for instance, a staple in many ethnic diets, provide a complete protein. Natural peanut butter on whole grain bread is also a complete protein. Food combining to make a complete protein does not need to happen in the same meal.

Because your baby is growing so rapidly, she needs approximately three times more protein than an adult for each pound of body weight. During the first year of life, your baby needs 1 gram of protein per pound of body weight. From twelve months to fifteen she needs ½ gm of protein per pound of body weight. This is actually a much smaller amount than we think we need. A three year old with a weight of approximately 30 lbs only needs sixteen grams (approximately ½ ounce) of protein a day. A grown adult of 130 lbs needs approximately 2½ ounces (75 grams) of protein a day. For example, 1 tablespoon of peanut butter, ¼ cup of cooked dry beans, or ½ ounce of nuts are equivalent to one ounce of protein. Not very much.

In general, we are overly concerned in the United States with getting enough complete protein in our diets. Despite claims to the contrary, we rarely suffer in this country from a shortage of protein.

Carbohydrates

Along with fat, carbohydrates are the body's primary energy source. The building blocks for carbohydrates are sugar molecules, or saccharides. Sugar, starches, and fiber are all carbohydrates: sugars are known as simple carbohydrates, while starches and fibers are considered complex carbohydrates. Most carbohydrates come from plant sources, with the exception of milk, which contains the simple sugar lactose.

Sugars (Simple Carbohydrates)

Sucrose (table sugar), brown sugar, powdered sugar, fructose (sugar in fruit and in honey), molasses, and lactose (milk sugar) are all simple carbohydrates and are quickly and easily digested. Although these simple sugars are appreciated by most young palates, you should limit your child's consumption. Refined sugar causes tooth decay, is full of empty calories, and causes blood sugar fluctuations that can have a detrimental impact on behavior.

Read the label. You would be surprised how many of our foods, especially the processed and refined ones, contain added sugars. One of the biggest culprits is juice, which many people consider a healthy alternative to soda. Like soda, however, juices are full of simple sugars and should be consumed in moderation. Increased awareness of the sugar has prompted baby food manufacturers to remove sugar from most foods, except for many of the desserts.

Starches and Fibers (Complex Carbohydrates)

Complex carbohydrates are considered more nutritious than simple sugars, as it takes longer for them to be digested and absorbed in the body. Your child feels full for a longer period of time without the up-and-down fluctuation of blood sugar levels. Except for fiber, both sugars and starches are broken down into glucose, a sugar. The glucose is then used for energy or stored for later use. When your child eats more carbohydrates than the body needs, it may be stored as fat. Grains, legumes, nuts, seeds, potatoes, breads, pasta and other vegetables are all starches. The carbohydrates you give your children should be mostly complex, such as unrefined whole grains and brown rice. Minimize processed white foods (white breads, white rice and white flours), which act like simple sugars in the body.

Fiber, also a complex carbohydrate, passes through the intestine undigested. Fiber is plant based, and is also known as roughage. Although it is possible to live without fiber, this complex carbohydrate is vital to your child's health now and later on as an adult. Fiber occurs in insoluble (not dissolvable in water) and soluble forms, and both play important roles in digestion. Insoluble fibers include cellulose and lignin, which work as bulking agents and keep the intestines cleansed, preventing constipation and bowel conditions like diverticulosis and colon cancer later in life. Water-soluble fibers (pectin, psyllium, and gums) act by slowing the digestion of other carbohydrates, helping regulate sugar levels, prevent diabetes, and lower cholesterol.

Good sources of fiber include legumes and beans (kidney beans, lentil beans), nuts, almonds, seeds, grains (oat bran, wheat bran, brown rice), fruits (dried figs, apples, raspberries, pears) and vegetables (broccoli, Brussels sprouts, spinach, cauliflower). Many nutritionists concur that, for children over the age of two, 50 to 60% of her calories should come from carbohydrates, preferably healthy complex carbohydrates. The daily recommendations are approximate: for a two-year-old child, 3 ounces (85 grams); for school-age children, 6 ounces (170 grams); for teens, 8 ounces (240 grams). For example, one cup of brown rice is equivalent to 2 ounces (30 gm).

Fats and Lipids

Although we are inundated with negative information about fats, they are essential to your child's good health. They give your child energy and serve a crucial role in infant and childhood development. The fat in breast milk, for instance, aids your child's developing nervous system and brain function. Fats also cover and protect vital organs, provide insulation to keep your child warm, help the absorption of the fat-soluble vitamins (vitamins A, D, E, K), and are involved with hormonal production. The benefits of fats do not go away as we age, nor do all bodies store fat in the same way. Women generally have a higher body fat percentage than men precisely because fat is so important during the childbearing years.

Saturated Fats

The building blocks of fats are known as fatty acids, but not all fatty acids are created equal. When reading labels, you will want to be familiar with two different types of fat: Saturated fatty acids and unsaturated fatty acids (also called monounsaturated and polyunsaturated fats). Saturated fatty acids are considered the unhealthy fats, and these most often come from animal sources such as meat, poultry, lard, shortening, eggs, and butter. Certain plants also yield saturated fats; palm kernel oil, hydrogenated oils, chocolate, palm oil, cocoa butter, and coconut oil are plant-derived fats you will want to limit in your diet. These fats have been linked to arteriosclerosis and heart disease.

Unsaturated Fats

Unsaturated fats occur in both monounsaturated and polyunsaturated forms and are considered "good" fats, those our bodies need to sustain energy, ward off disease, and regenerate cells. Avocados and vegetable oils (olive, canola, and grapeseed) are excellent sources of monounsaturated fatty acids, while fish, seed, and nut oils (safflower, sunflower, walnut, soy and corn oil) all contain polyunsaturated fatty acids (PUFA). PUFAs are shown to decrease atherosclerosis.

Certain unsaturated fats, known as essential fatty acids (EFAs), are considered crucial because our body cannot make them and we thus must get them from a proper diet. All the body's cells, including brain cells, make use of EFAs. They help lower the risk of heart disease and colon and breast cancer, as well as improve vision, skin integrity, mood, attention span, and learning skills. EFAs are particularly important for children and seniors.

Children typically get more than enough fat in their diet; however, like most of us, they could improve the good fat to bad fat ratio. According to the FDA, a two-year-old child should not have more than 2 teaspoons of fats per day and a four-year-old, 4 teaspoons a day. The recommended amount for school aged children and adolescents is 5 teaspoons.

Two of the most widely known essential fatty acids are linolenic acid (omega 3 fatty acids) and linoleic acid (omega 6 fatty acid), both polyunsaturated fats. Other important fatty acids include gamma linolenic acid (GLA), eicosapentaenoic acid (EPA) and docosahexaenoc acid (DHA). These EFAs are found in plants, seafood, and in small amounts of meat. The best sources for omega 6 fatty acids are warm-weather plants such as nuts, seeds, and corn, sunflower, sesame, and safflower oils. In general, Americans tend to get enough omega 6 fatty acids in their diet but not enough omega 3 fatty acids. Omega 3 fatty acids are found in coldwater fish and cold-weather plants: walnuts, pumpkin seeds, canola oil, wheatgerm, eggs, flaxseed, green leafy vegetables, soybeans, tuna, sardines, cod, mackerel, and salmon all provide omega 3 fatty acids.

If your child is being breastfed, there is no need for either flax or fish oil. If mom does not eat fish on a regular basis, she could add fish oil to her diet. Nursing mothers can also increase the fat content of their breast milk by taking flaxseed. There are, however, some precautions with flaxseed as it may interact or slow down absorption of some medications. Do not take flaxseed at the hour of medications, and consult your physician if you have questions about its usage.

Flaxseed is one of the richest natural sources of omega-3 fatty acids. It also contains lignans, which studies suggest may play an important role in cancer prevention. Flaxseed comes as an oil or as raw seeds. Try adding them to your child's diet, beginning at 8 months, as follows:

- Flaxseeds: Take ½ teaspoon and grind well in blender or grinder just prior to serving. Mix into food. Within a few hours the ground seeds become rancid and you must discard.
- Flaxseed oil (buy from the grocery or health food store): Take one teaspoon and place in baby's bottle or drink daily. Alternatively, it can be rubbed into skin. Oil can be stored in refrigerator for 2 months.

In addition to being excellent sources of omega 3, fish oil and cod liver oil are high in DHA, a compound that works like food for your brain. Touted as a means of improving concentration and mental stamina, fish oils are currently enjoying popularity in health food stores and are even being added to baby formula. Cod liver oil is also a rich source of vitamin D, which is especially advantageous during the colder winter months, when sun exposure (our main source of vitamin D) is low. In the summer months, it is best to switch to fish oil.

When choosing a fish oil, look for brands that are more pure and contain fewer pollutants. Choose a company that tests for mercury, lead, and other harmful ingredients. The oil should be from wild fish, not farm-raised. Fish oils made from sardines and anchovies have fewer contaminants because they are small fish and have a shorter life span, while larger longer-lived fish like mackerel and salmon contain more toxins. You can get this information by directly contacting the company and inquiring about manufacturing processes.

In addition, there are different grades of fish oils. The most basic is the standard cod liver oil (although there are high grade purified versions). Slightly better is the health food-grade fish oil made from fish body oils. These come in capsules. Finally, pharmaceutical-grade fish oils are purer, taste better, and are richer in long-chain omega 3 fatty acids. These oils can be taken in liquid form and are more expensive. In general, liquid form is superior to capsules. Take 1 teaspoon of fish oil for every 50 lbs of body weight daily.

Hydrogenated Fats

Hydrogenated fat is made when a high-pressure hydrogen mixes with an unsaturated fat. This chemically processed fat also contains trans fatty acids, which raise LDL (bad cholesterol) levels and lower HDL (good cholesterol). In addition, the trans fatty acids may be linked to obesity, diabetes, immune system conditions, and sexual dysfunction in men, including low testosterone, abnormal sperm production, and prostate disease.

These unhealthy hydrogenated, partially hydrogenated, and trans fats are found in most processed foods, such as donuts, potato chips, French fries, candy bars, peanut butter (except the natural varieties), salad dressings, cereals, cookies, crackers, shortening, pretzels, and fried foods. Like sugar, the taste of trans fats can be "addictive." Moreover, we often eat trans fatty foods without even knowing it, thinking we have opted for the healthy, "low-fat" option. Be sure to read the fine print on the nutrition label. Don't buy them! They last longer on the store shelf, are less expensive than saturated fat, and to many palates they taste good. But the long-term effects are not worth the short-term gratification.

Vitamins and Minerals

Necessary in small amounts, vitamins and minerals help the body carry out vital metabolic reactions and processes. The thirteen essential vitamins our bodies need occur in either fat-soluble (A, D, E, and K) or water-soluble (C and the eight B-complex vitamins) forms. Fat-soluble vitamins are stored in fat tissue, and hence remain in the body for much longer periods of time. It is rare, for this reason, to have a deficiency in vitamins A, D, E, or K, and toxicity is a possibility if you consume too much of them. The water-soluble vitamins, on the other hand, are eliminated quickly in urine and need to be replenished more frequently. We get all of our vitamins from food with the exceptions of vitamin D, which we get from sun exposure, and, on a smaller level, vitamin K, which the body is able to produce. In general, vitamins and minerals are best taken with food, to help absorption and avoid nausea. Fat-soluble vitamins should be taken with food containing some fat, as it is in this form that they are best absorbed.

In an ideal world, no one would need to take vitamin supplements: we would get all the nutrition we required from organically grown whole foods and would never have to worry about whether to take that multivitamin. Of course, few if any of us are able to get all the vitamins and minerals we need from our diet, and the same holds true for our children. I'm often asked by parents if they should give their child vitamins, and I generally respond, cautiously, yes. Supplements bear important similarities to manufactured drugs, with side effects that often go unstated and variations in quality according the brand. Given the nutritional quality of today's food, though, I believe we do need to offer our children some form of supplementation.

I am not a fan of taking tons of pills, so I try to make it simple and choose the least adulterated and healthiest whole food products in our family. Keep in mind that vitamins are not necessary during the first year while a baby is breastfeeding or taking a fortified baby formula. But after twelve to eighteen months, it is a good idea to consider supplement options for your child. In our home, we use a whole food based nutritional product which is made from 17 different fruits and vegetables, to complement healthy eating and fill in the gaps when we are not able to eat as well. The fruit capsules are made from apples, oranges, pineapples, cranberries, peaches, acerola cherries, and papaya. The vegetables include carrots, spinach, broccoli, kale, cabbage, parsley, beets, and tomato, along with barley and oats. They are gluten- and dairy-free. The fruits and vegetables are juiced and the water is removed at low temperatures to preserve the nutritional quality, vitamins, minerals, fiber, phytonutrients, and antioxidants (and enzymes). Prior to encapsulation, the product is tested for the presence of pesticides, herbicides, and chemicals. They are made into gummies, chewables, and capsules. According to research, whole food nutritional products are better absorbed than processed vitamins. Nowadays, there are many competing products that encapsulate vegetables and fruits. It is always best to have the real thing, so consider these not as replacements for the real thing but available options to fill in the occasional gaps and lapses in the diet.

VITAMINS AND MINERALS

THIAMINE (VITAMIN B1)

Role: Coenzyme that metabolizes carbohydrates into glucose, used by the body for energy and proper brain function, and helpful for chronic hepatitis B infection.

Food sources: Whole-grains, green leafy vegetables, legumes, sweet corn, brown rice, berries, yeast, sunflower seeds, oats, avocado, pasta, tofu, artichoke, tuna, and salmon.

Deficiency: Memory loss and confusion. Alcoholics, otherwise rare. Associated with beriberi (anemia, paralysis, weakness).

Excess: Excreted in the urine.

Recommendation: Children ages 1 to 3: 0.5mg/day
Children ages 4 to 8: 0.6mg/day
Children ages 9 to 13: 0.9mg/day

RIBOFLAVIN (VITAMIN B2)

Role: Coenzyme that helps the breakdown of proteins, fats, and carbohydrates. Maintains the health of the skin, mucous membranes, and eye, and stimulates red blood cell production.

Food sources: Whole grains, fortified breads, cereals, peas, spinach, sweet potato, artichoke, tofu, almonds, milk, meat, eggs, and cheese.

Deficiency: Skin conditions, inflammation of tongue, and light sensitivity. Rare in the United States.

Excess: Excreted.

Recommendation: Children ages 1 to 3: 0.5 mg/day
Children ages 4 to 8: 0.6 mg/day
Children ages 9 to 13: 0.9 mg/day

NIACIN (VITAMIN B3)

Role: Coenzyme, known as nicotinic acid. Metabolizes food, particularly sugars, and helps to maintain a healthy digestive tract, skin, and nerves. Produced in the body from tryptophan, an essential amino acid.

Food sources: Fish (tuna, swordfish, salmon), meat, brewer's yeast, milk, eggs, legumes potatoes, peanuts, wheat germ, wheat bran, barley, rye, buckwheat, wild rice, and mushrooms.

Deficiency: Pellagra, diarrhea, dermatitis, and dementia. Occurs in countries with corn-based diets, rare in developed countries.

Excess: High doses can cause a skin flush (like a hot flash) along with headaches, nausea, and itching.

Recommendation: Children ages 1 to 3: 6 mg/day
Children ages 4 to 8: 8 mg/day
Children ages 9 to 13: 12 mg/day

PANTOTHENIC ACID (VITAMIN B5)

Role: Metabolism of carbohydrates, proteins, and fats. Development and growth. Produced in intestine.

Food Source: Meats, poultry, legumes, soybeans, lentils, split peas, yoghurt, avocado, mushrooms, and sweet potato.

Deficiency: Rare.

Excess: Diarrhea.

Recommendation: This is an unofficial recommendation, as deficiency is rare.
Children ages newborn to 3: 2 to 3 mg/day
Children ages 4 to 7: 3 to 4 mg/day
Children ages 7 to 10: 4 to 5 mg/day

PYRIDOXINE (VITAMIN B6)

Role: Coenzyme, promotes the metabolism of carbohydrates, proteins, and fats.Supports red blood cell production, helpful for PMS symptoms,and the health of the brain and skin.

Food sources: Brewer's yeast, animal products (liver, organ meats, eggs, chicken, tuna, salmon), brown rice, butter, vegetables (carrots, peas, potato, sweet potato), wheat germ, walnuts, whole grain cereals, soybeans, avocado, garbanzo beans, prune juice, sunflower seeds, and artichoke.

Deficiency: Skin conditions, neuropathy, mental confusion, insomnia, and seizures. Alcoholics, otherwise rare.

Excess: Nerve damage after taking megadoses for months.

Recommendation: Children ages 1 to 3: 0.5 mg/day
Children ages 4 to 8: 0.6 mg/day
Children ages 9 to 13: 1 mg/day

BIOTIN (VITAMIN H, VITAMIN B7)

Role: Metbolism of amino acids and carbohydrates. Helps form energy for body. Produced in intestine.

Food Sources: Meat, liver, brewer's yeast, cauliflower, and peanuts.

Deficiency: Brittle fingernails, scaly skin rash, and thinning of the hair. Raw egg white prevents absorption. Rare.

Excess: Excreted in the urine.

Recommendation: This is an unofficial recommendation, as deficiency is rare.
Children ages newborn to 3: 10 to 20 micrograms mcg/day
Children ages 4 to 6: 25 mcg/day
Children ages 7 to 10: 30 mcg/day

FOLIC ACID (VITAMIN B9)

Role: Coenzyme, known as folacin works with vitamin B12 to manufacture DNA as well as red blood cells. Important for pregnant women in preventing spina bifida in the fetus.

Food sources: Orange juice, yeast, liver, leafy green vegetables, asparagus, pinto beans, lentils, whole grain cereals, artichokes, spinach, kidney, avocado, papaya, wheat germ and fortified breakfast cereal.

Deficiency: Anemia, poor growth and spina bifida (in utero). Alcoholics, the under-nourished, and people with certain absorption diseases.

Excess: Convulsions.

Recommendation: Women who are pregnant or trying to get pregnant should take 400 to 800 mcg of folic acid daily.
Children ages 1 to 3: 150 µg/day
Children ages 4 to 8: 200 µg/day
Children ages 9 to 13: 300 µg/day

CYANOCOBALAMIN (VITAMIN B12)

Role: Helps in metabolism of carbohydrates, proteins, and fats. Vital for blood cells, nerve sheaths and absorption of nutrients during digestion. Vegetarians receive vitamin B12 from fortified foods or may need a supplement.

Food sources: Meat, seafood, yoghurt, cheese, poultry, milk, and egg yolk. It is not found in plants, which is a concern for strict vegetarians and vegans. Potential sources for vegans include foods fortified with vitamin B12 (increasingly common in breakfast cereals, soy products, and plant milks).

Deficiency: Weakness, anemia, numbness, and nerve damage. Can occur in strict vegetarians

Excess: No adverse effects noted in healthy individuals.

Recommendation: Children ages 1 to 3: 0.9 µg/day
Children ages 4 to 8: 1.2 µg/day
Children ages 9 to 13: 1.8 µg/day

VITAMIN C (ASCORBIC ACID)

Role: Helps maintain healthy skin, bone, teeth, ligaments and tendons, aids in red blood cell production. Stimulates wound healing, strengthens the immune system, and has antioxidant properties to protect cell membranes.

Food sources: Citrus fruits (lemon, orange, limes, grapefruit), vegetables (chili peppers, broccoli, green pepper, potato), and fruit (kiwi, strawberry, guava, papaya).
Deficiency: Bleeding, poor wound healing, easy bruising and inflamed gums known as scurvy. Alcoholics, otherwise rare.
Excess: Diarrhea.
Recommendation: Children ages 1 to 3: 40 mg/day
Children ages 4 to 6: 45 mg/day
Children ages 7 to 10: 45 mg/day

VITAMIN A
Role: Important for eye and vision, especially the retina. Stimulates bone growth, regulates the immune system, and helps maintain the skin and teeth.
Food sources: Whole milk, eggs, liver, carrots, red pepper, sweet potato, pumpkin, green leafy vegetables (spinach, kale), fruit (mango, cantaloupe, apricots, papaya) tuna, and fortified foods (usually processed).
Deficiency: Night blindness, xeropthalmia (leading to blindness), dry eyes, and poor resistance to infections. May occur in strict vegetarians, but otherwise rare in the United States.
Excess: Yellow-orange skin on the palms and soles of the feet. Only vitamin on which you can overdose from food—from eating too many carrots!
Recommendation: Children ages 1 to 3: 300 mcg (1,000 IU)/day
Children ages 4 to 8: 400 mcg (1,320 IU)/day
Children ages 9 to 13: 600 mcg (2,000 IU)/day

VITAMIN D
Role: Sunlight triggers its production by the body. Increases absorption of calcium and phosphorus, helps maintain strong bones. Intake of vitamin D through food (and supplementation if needed) important during the cloudy, dark winter months and for those who are unable to go outside.
Food sources: Cod liver oil, egg yolk, fortified cow and soy milks.
Deficiency: Rickets with weak bones and fractures. Only vitamin not found in breast milk, but Mother Nature compensates with sunlight.
Excess: Kidney stones, weight loss, and loss of appetite. May occur from too much cod liver oil.
Recommendation: Children ages newborn to 13: 5 µg (~200 IU)/day

---

VITAMIN E
Role: Known for antioxidant properties to protect cells from free radicals. Plays a role in the immune system, metabolism in the body, cancer and Alzheimer's prevention

and heart function. Natural form is labeled as "D." The synthetic form, known as dl-alpha-tocopherol, is half as active and not recommended.
Food sources: Polyunsaturated vegetable oils and seeds (safflower, sunflower, canola, corn), grains (wheat germ oil, oat bran, fortified cereals), dark green leafy vegetables almonds, peanuts, avocado, blackberries, rolled oats, peaches.
Deficiency: Hemorrhage, anemia, and swelling (in infants). Rare.
Excess: Excessive bleeding.
Recommendation: Children ages 1 to 3: 6 mg (9 IU)/day
Children ages 4 to 8: 7 mg (10.5 IU)/day
Children ages 9 to 13: 11 mg (16.5 IU)/day

VITAMIN K

Role: Role in blood clotting and the maintenance of strong bones, and prevention of heart disease.
Food sources: Dark green leafy vegetables (spinach, kale), vegetables (broccoli, onions, lettuce, cabbage), soybeans, and cereals. Manufactured in the body by friendly bacteria in the digestive system.
Deficiency: Bruising and easy bleeding. Deficiency rare, though possible after prolonged use of antibiotics (see "Test and Procedures Following Birth" in Chapter 4).
Excess: Blood clots. Rare.
Recommendation: Children ages 1 to 3: 30 mcg/day
Children ages 4 to 8: 55 mcg/day
Children ages 9 to 13: 60 mcg/day

CALCIUM

Role: Vital for healthy bones, teeth, nerves, and muscles. Absorption of calcium requires vitamin D, silicone, and fluoride.
Food sources: Traditionally dairy is considered an important calcium source. Pasteurized milk changes nutrients and makes it difficult for the body to properly use the calcium. Nondairy sources include broccoli, dark leafy green vegetables (kales, collard green, turnip greens, Chinese greens, okra), hummus, figs, sesame, blackstrap molasses, fortified soy milk, flaxseed, almonds, soy, beans (navy, white, Great Northern), and almond butter.
Deficiency: Cramps, numbness, palpitation, dental cavities, and stunted growth. Phosphorus interferes with absorption (includes sodium phosphate in sodas), smoking, and excess caffeine cause depletion.
Excess: Impairs kidney, interferes with absorption of other minerals in body. Most cases from malignancy in elderly.

Recommendation: Children ages 1 to 3: 500 mg/day
Children ages 4 to 8: 800 mg/day
Children ages 9 to 13: 1,300 mg/day

IRON

Role: Major component of hemoglobin (red blood cells) which carries oxygen throughout the body. Boosts immune system and good for the brain.

Food sources: Plant sources less absorbed than animal sources. Foods high in vitamin C improve absorption. Vegetables (peas, spinach), beans (lentils, navy beans,white beans, kidney beans, soybeans, garbanzo beans), firm tofu, soymilk, tahini, gains (fortified cereal, oatmeal, cream of wheat, pasta) molasses, fruit (dried apricot, prune juice, raisins), pumpkin seeds, avocado, meat, poultry, and seafood (tuna, shrimp, clams, oysters).

Deficiency: Anemia, fatigue, chilliness, poor concentration, brittle fingernails, and frequent sicknesses. Can occur in women due to menstrual blood loss. Lack of iron causes cravings for non-digestibles such as clay, sand, and ice, known as pica.

Excess: Overdose from supplementation. Keep bottle out of reach of children.

Recommendation: Children ages 1 to 3: 7 mg/day
Children ages 4 to 8: 10 mg/day
Children ages 9 to 13: 8 mg/day

How to Prepare Natural Food for Kids

If your idea of making baby food involves endlessly boiling and mashing vegetables, you may want to think again. You'll be glad to know that cooking for infants can be as varied and creative as you want it be, or as quick and simple as you need it to be. Many of the cooking techniques you use in adult meals—steaming, grilling, stir-frying—translate to infant meals as well, particularly after one year of age. The important difference is that you must plan your meals so that they meet the evolving nutritional and developmental needs of your child. This section will guide you through menu planning, food preparation, and kitchen know-how for infants through toddlers, offering advice that will ideally have you saving the jarred baby food only for emergencies.

The Healthy Kitchen

Food preparation for babies and toddlers does not have to be hard work. In fact, once you get in the rhythm of preparing your baby's food, including having the necessary cookware, utensils, and ingredients, you will be amazed how simple it can be to come up with healthy meals on a regular basis. In addition to requiring the standard pots, pans, and containers that make up the average kitchen, preparing your baby's first meals will go more easily if you have a few additional cookware pieces on hand, including a double boiler or Bain Marie, a blender or food processor, a pressure cooker, and a steamer. These items all offer a useful alternative to boiling, which tends to leach vitamins and other nutrients from the food you are cooking. To retain vitamins in fruit and vegetables, you will want to keep heating, water, and cooking time to a minimum. My preferred methods of cooking for babies are thus steaming, baking, and pressure cooking, all of which cook food thoroughly without losing nutritional content.

Iron cookware: There is still something to be said for tradition when it comes to iron cookware. Used for generations before us, iron pots offer something even our fanciest cookware lines have yet to perfect: nutritive value. Cooking in iron adds iron to your food, making even your pots and pans "nutritious." Iron cookware is especially good for preparing grains and soups. Iron content of foods, especially acidic foods, can be dramatically increased by preparation in iron cookware.

The blender or food processor: Particularly during the first year, you will be pureeing, blending, mashing, and otherwise liquefying much of your baby's food. Especially at the beginning, infant "solids" more closely resemble liquids: food should be smooth and lump-free. For this reason, you will likely want to invest in a good blender or food processor, one that lets you control the consistency of the food, is easy to clean, and safe to use.

The hand grinder: If you would rather spend your money on something other than an expensive blender or food processor, the hand grinder is the perfect alternative for you. Place steamed vegetables, grains, or fruit in this inexpensive hand gadget, and you soon have pureed baby food, ready to serve. Hand grinders also allow you greater control of the texture of food, which has made it one of husband's favorite kitchen tools.

The double-boiler or Bain Marie: Doubling boiling is a favorite method among chefs because it allows for indirect heating—perfect for preparing foods for delicate palates, be they gourmand or infant. A double boiler consists of a pot within a pot, with water boiled in the lower. The food portion placed in the upper pot is heated evenly and quickly, making double boiling a perfect way of preparing infant dishes.

The pressure cooker: One of the favorite kitchen items in our house is the pressure cooker. We found it an invaluable asset for preparing baby food, since it steams quickly with little loss of nutrients. Place a sweet potato, carrot, or other vegetable with a small amount of water and *voila*: delicious steamed vegetables in a matter of minutes. As with any kitchen utensil, however, be sure not to leave the pressure cooker unattended while children are around.

Steamers: Steaming rather than boiling your vegetables results in minimal loss of nutrients. Simply place the vegetable-filled steamer in pan with an inch or so of boiling water and cover. Depending on the vegetable, steaming can take as little as five to ten minutes.

A note on microwaves: Despite their convenience, microwaves remain one of my least favorite methods of preparing baby food. An unnatural heat source—and potentially a harmful one, too—microwaving alters your food in ways that conventional heating does not. Also, because microwaves heat unevenly, they can be dangerous for young mouths. One section can feel cold and another piping hot. If you do use a microwave, completely stir food after heating, and check the temperature throughout.

In the kitchen, clean utensils, grinders and cookware thoroughly with dishwashing soap and hot water or in a dishwasher. Let air dry. I prefer to use natural cleaning products when possible. Avoid any additional harmful chemicals that may come in contact with baby. Wash your hands frequently, not only before you handle food, but throughout the day.

The Healthy Grocery Shopping Trip

As you stroll down the aisle of your supermarket—or better yet, your weekly local farmer's market—you will encounter more and more food labeled "organic." Organic food implies both a method and a philosophy: it represents an agricultural process free of chemicals, herbicides, or pesticides, as well as a way of understanding the relationship between our bodies, our land, and our buying power. In the past, organic food was limited to a few health food stores and was prohibitively expensive. However, as the demand has increased, organic food has become both more plentiful and affordable.

The difference between conventional and organic farming begins at ground level. In an effort to reap the largest and most profitable harvest, conventional farmers use pesticides and chemical fertilizers to treat the land and plant, increasing yield at the expense of nutritional value, taste, and healthfulness. The chemicals sprayed on crops seep into the soil and remain in residue form on the plant itself. These residues are known to be toxic to the immune system, nervous system (brain), and hormonal system, and can cause cancer. In other words, conventionally grown food can pose a serious health threat. In addition, the soil suffers from these farming methods, left polluted with chemical and depleted of precious nutrients.

Food that is good for you comes from healthy soil, and organic farming employs methods that are beneficial for the both the soil and consumer. Compared to conventionally grown food, certified organic produce is also more nutritious and flavorful, and is never genetically modified.

Recently, the Environmental Working Group listed the twelve most contaminated conventionally grown foods, known as the *Dirty Dozen*. Use organic for the following when possible:

Apples
Celery
Cherries
Grapes (imported)
Nectarines
Peaches
Pears
Potatoes
Red Raspberries
Spinach
Strawberries
Sweet Bell Peppers

These fruits and vegetables were tested and found to be cleaner, with less likelihood of pesticide residue. Conventional products can be eaten if organic is not available:

Asparagus
Avocado
Bananas
Broccoli
Cauliflower
Kiwi
Mangoes
Onions
Papaya
Peas
Pineapples
Sweet corn

For my vegetarian and vegan colleagues, the phrase *healthier meat, poultry, and fish* may seem like an oxymoron. Not all meat is the same, however, and if you and your family are meat-eaters, make sure it is the healthier version. Look for the following qualities when shopping for meat, poultry, fish, or eggs.

- Free-range (the animal is able to move instead of being cramped in close proximity)
- Cage-free
- Hormones free
- Antibiotic free
- Organically fed
- Free of growth hormones

Currently, most of the fish sold in American markets is farm-raised. This means that fish like trout, catfish, and salmon, which used to be caught in their natural habitat, are farmed in a controlled environment—and not necessarily a healthy one! A study by the U.S. Environmental Protection Agency concluded that it was safe to eat farmed salmon no more than once a month, while wild salmon could be eaten eight times a month. Not surprisingly, wild fish is considered more flavorful than farmed fish. The following are some reasons why it is best to eat wild fish, and avoid farm-raised fish:

- The waters in which they are raised have been found to be unhygienic.
- The fish receive vaccines and antibiotics.
- They are given substances to enhance their pink color (this is particularly true of salmon).
- Farmed fish contains high levels of contaminants and cancer-causing chemicals.

Food Temperature

Just like breast milk, food should be served slightly warmer than room temperature. Be careful to monitor food temperature, as a baby's mouth is more sensitive to temperature than yours. My mom always did her temperature test by placing a little bit of food on her wrist. In our home, we also tested the spoonful of food by touching it to our upper lips.

According to practitioners of Chinese medicine, cold foods and drinks are not healthy for anyone, but especially babies. Particularly in the cold weather and right after vigorous exercise, room temperature or slightly warmer foods and liquids are easiest to digest; the body has to work harder to warm cold substances in the stomach. There is no reason to serve your baby very cold or very hot food, so aim for Goldilock's rule: not too hot, not too cold, but just right.

Food Storage

One of the best ways to avoid kitchen burnout—that moment when the thought of cooking leaves you so exhausted you'll turn to the first baby food jar you see—is to make enough food to last you several meals. Anyone who cooks is familiar with the concept of leftovers, but storing food for babies involves special considerations, since infants are far more sensitive to bacteria than adults. Below are some simple guidelines on storing quantities of baby food. You want to be able to do preserve food with as little loss of nutrients as possible and no harmful bacterial growth, so err on the side of freshness and caution. If you are not sure, discard.

- Use a clean spoon or utensil when taking a small portion out of a larger container. Never double dip once spoon is used.
- Discard any leftover food that has come in contact with baby's saliva.
- Discard leftover baby food that has been mixed with breast milk or formula.
- Discard leftover cereal that has been mixed with any liquid.
- Opened baby food (either homemade or commercial) can be left in the refrigerator for 1 to 2 days. When possible use glass containers instead of plastic, the latter having been in the news lately regarding toxins. Chemicals found in plastics, such as phthalates, have been found to affect the hormonal system, especially in children.
- When freezing leftovers, abide by the frozen rule: only freeze once. Frozen food that has been thawed should not be refrozen. This includes baby food that was originally made from frozen vegetables or fruit.
- Most foods, including vegetables, fruit, grains, dairy, eggs, beans, tofu, and pasta can be kept frozen in small portions to be used as needed. One of my favorite methods of storing frozen food is in ice cube trays or, alternatively, small muffin tins. The portions are baby-size (two tablespoons are ideal), which means less waste. In addition, the frozen food portions can be removed one by one. Fill cubes halfway initially,

as baby may only consume approximately one tablespoon of food, then increase the portion size as baby's appetite increases. Once the food cubes have solidified (this can take 8 to 12 hours), transfer them to plastic freezer bags. Be sure when storing frozen baby food to use freezer bags, not storage bags, and to always label and date the package. Homemade baby food can be kept in the freezer for up to three months.

- To thaw frozen food, place it in the refrigerator overnight, defrost it in the microwave (checking thoroughly for temperature variations), or heat it on the stove top or in a double boiler.

Choking Hazards

When my boys were young, my husband, their caretaker, and I took a CPR course in our area. We found the information invaluable and empowering, and if you have not yet done so, sign up for a class. Knowing what to do in case of a choking incident could mean everything to your child.

Cooking hazards for infants and toddlers (up to three years of age) include:

- Grapes (cut in quarters and give only after one year)
- Any chunky or hard food
- Hard or chewy candy, gum, jelly beans (another good reason to not have it around)
- Meat, hot dogs
- Tree nuts (after one to two years)
- Popcorn, pretzels
- Dried fruit, raisins, cherry with pits, raw apples slices, pears slices, berries
- Vegetables like raw carrot sticks
- Olives, whole

Meal Planning

Birth to Six Months

For the first six months, your baby should need only breastmilk or, alternatively, formula. At this stage of development, a baby's ability to suck is well developed, as is his or her rooting reflex, in which the baby automatically turns the head to locate a breast to suck from. The rooting reflex can be triggered by stroking the cheek, a technique recommended to help newborns learn to breastfeed. Infants at this age also possess a strong tongue-thrust reflex, preventing solids from entering the esophagus.

Six Months

As you introduce your baby's first solid food, keep in mind that portion sizes will be small: first meals may consist of no more than one to two tablespoons of solid food. At this age, your child's primary source of nutrition is still breast milk or formula, so aim for a gradual transition into solids. You may find it easier to introduce new foods at the end of the day, when the supply breast milk is generally lower. When we started our boys on solids, however, I preferred that our nanny give the boys their solid food while I was away at work. That way, I could do the breastfeeding when I came home. Avoid eating sessions after breastfeeding as the food may hinder proper absorption of nutrients in mom's milk.

Feeding your baby is a project from beginning, middle to end. It is not fast food. Between the eating, playing, and clean-up, it can take some time. Enjoy it.

First foods should be easily digested, non-allergenic, and as similar as possible to breast milk. Consider the following guidelines for introducing first foods, and be sure to discuss them with your practitioner as well. When selecting fruits, vegetables, and cereals, always buy the healthiest available version—fresh, organically grown without preservatives. Avoid canned jars and the commercially processed or refined cereals. All the foods listed below are cooked except for the bananas and avocados which can be eaten raw.

Fruits and sweet vegetables: Bananas, apples, pears, carrots, and sweet potatoes are all excellent starter foods. Their sweet taste makes them similar to breast milk, and, when mashed, they are easily digested. It is not uncommon to hear that it is better to introduce vegetables before fruit, as fruit could foster a sweet tooth later on. But in fact, the sweeter vegetables like carrots and sweet potatoes may be the preferred vegetables in the beginning: like breast milk, they are palatable and healthy, making them an ideal way of transitioning from liquid to solid nutrition. Be sure to use organic fruits and vegetables when possible.

- Mashed bananas: Bananas are easy to prepare and can be mixed with a few drops of breast milk or formula for a smooth consistency.

- Avocado: High in vitamins and nutrients, avocado is an excellent first food. Like bananas, you will want to introduce this food first in mashed form.
- Sweet potatoes and carrots: These classic starter foods should be cooked and mashed, either by hand or in a blender.
- Apple (cooked applesauce): Apples or pears can be sliced or cooked (steamed or pressure-cooked) with 2 tablespoons of water. When tender, blend into a smooth sauce.

Cereals: Rice cereal is the most common cereal to start with, since it is easy to digest and generally not allergenic. Other kinds of cereal and organic whole grains (brown rice, barley, whole grain oats, or millet) can be given after six months old. The healthiest and most economical way to prepare grains is at your home, and as your infant grows and can eat more varied grains and cereals, you may find it convenient to cook batches for the whole family. When possible, use an iron pot. When the grain is cooked, transfer to a grinder or processor, using water, breast milk, or formula to liquefy. To begin, dilute ¼ teaspoon of the cereal with breast milk or formula.

Once you have ascertained that your baby has done well with other fruits or vegetables, they can be mixed in for a tastier treat.

Seven to Nine Months

At this stage, you can slowly introduce finger foods. Your baby is becoming a more curious, interested eater, and can pick up food and morsels. However, this means that many things go in the mouth, so watch for small bits of food and objects that could be hazardous. While food should still be mashed and pureed, you can progress to slightly thicker, chunkier substances. Possibilities include:

- Rice, brown rice, oat, barley, millet, pasta
- Cooked vegetables, including zucchini, yellow squash, carrots, peas, asparagus, green bean, and mashed potatoes
- Cooked and strained fruits such as peaches, apricots, nectarines, plums, pear, and prunes
- Tofu
- Teething biscuits

Nine to Twelve Months

As your baby approaches her first year, foods can be increasingly solid in consistency. She can now hold cups and bottles and is beginning to use utensils (but still makes a mess!). She can also eat finger food and bite-sized vegetables. While your child should ideally still be on a vegetarian diet, your options are expanding significantly.

- Cereals/whole grains (can be mixed), healthy crackers, healthy cereal (O's), bagels, rice cakes, pasta
- Vegetables can include asparagus, broccoli, cauliflower, eggplant, smashed potatoes, artichoke, beets, corn, cucumber, spinach, brussels sprouts, and turnips
- Fruits such as cantaloupe, kiwi, mangos, papaya, pitted cherries, dates, and grapes (quartered)
- Protein sources include beans, legumes, tofu, tahini, creamy nut butters

Avoid giving your baby honey, both raw and in baked goods, in the entire first year. Honey may contain botulism spores which may cause botulism, a potentially fatal illness.

Twelve to Eighteen Months

After a year of carefully preparing healthy meals for our children, we typically inaugurate their first birthdays with big, sugary, frosting-coated cakes. From now on, "forbidden foods" often become a way of celebrating, rewarding, or distracting our children. It doesn't have to be this way, though. I encourage you to still be mindful of what you are preparing for your child, particularly as she becomes a more active participant in the world. Although many healthcare providers argue that you can now introduce foods like cow's milk, beef, fish, and ice cream, I encourage you to keep them to a minimum, if you use them at all. A semi-vegetarian diet can meet all of your child's needs and there is no reason to rush into "grown-up" substances like meat and sugar, since they are often also the least healthy components of our diet.

By one year old, nearly half of your child's nutrition will be coming from solid foods. She can now feed herself with a spoon and fork, but may be apt to walk around and graze throughout the day instead of sitting down for a formal meal, and her appetite may vary from day to day. Portion sizes should be gradually increasing, though: until age five, a toddler needs one tablespoon of the major food groups for each year old. A four-year-old needs four tablespoons of vegetables three to five times a day. Additional foods you can now include:

- Tomatoes
- Citrus
- Fruit juice
- Wheat
- Honey
- Strawberries, berries

For a child with family history of allergies, consider waiting to introduce the following:

- Eggs until age two
- Peanut butter and shellfish until age three
- Whole nuts until four years old (these are also choking hazards, so always monitor your children if they are eating nuts)

I often hear parents complaining about their toddlers, "As a baby, she used to eat everything, and now she is so picky!" I reassure parents that it has nothing to do with them. As a toddler, your baby is becoming more independent, and so are her food choices. Toddlers are known to be finicky eaters and to boycott eating if things are not done their way (for instance, if foods touch each other).

Toddlers love to be involved in projects, so why not let them help you prepare some simple fare? Give her a job to do: pull celery strings, pour and stir ingredients. Sometimes I would even give my son a job of tearing discarded lettuce leaves, just to keep him busy. And he loved it! Now that my children are school aged, they still enjoy cooking with us.

One and a Half to Two Years

Hopefully at this stage you are still offering your toddler nutritious grains, fruit, vegetables, and nondairy, vegetarian proteins. Her diet, however, is expanding all the time and so are her abilities to coordinate utensils and eat more complicated meals like small sandwiches. Your toddler is likely restless at the table, making it a challenge to keep "standard" meal times. It is at this age that you might want to consider snacks as a way of providing nutrition throughout the day.

I use the word snack advisedly, since our associations with snacking often involve sugary, salty, or fatty foods that offer a quick burst of energy. For toddlers and young children, however, healthy snacking can become a primary source of nutrition. If you find your toddler has difficulty sitting still, consider keeping out a grazing tray. On a plate, tray or muffin tin, place two or more healthy foods cut to bite-sized morsels for them to graze on. Keep this at their level. Avoid offering fresh food that has browned or been out more than two hours, and always be in the same room as your child when food is concerned. Arranging the food in interesting ways, making it pleasing to look at, and giving it fun names are all ways to encourage a finicky toddler to try it. Good grazing foods include:

- Fruit slices
- Cooked, diced vegetable chunks
- Avocado slivers
- Tofu chunks
- Brown rice balls
- Nut butter on apple slice, banana, or cracker
- Sweet potato morsels
- Dollop of mashed beans on a cracker or vegetable
- Dips such as tofu, guacamole, hummus, and smooth natural peanut butter

Kids tend to fill up on whole grain and rice crackers and cereals, so use these sparingly. Many of my families come to my office with plastic containers full of easy and healthy finger food. Obviously, certain foods travel better than others, but you may want to keep snacks on hand for "emergencies."

Food Allergies and Sensitivities

Allergy symptoms occur when the immune system reacts to food as if it were a foreign invader in need of annihilation. True food allergies affect approximately 2% of children.

The more common form of sensitivity is known as food intolerance, and it typically affects digestion, causing distension, gas, and diarrhea. Lactose (milk) intolerance is a common example. Technically speaking, intolerances are not true allergies because the immune system is not affected, but whether an allergy or intolerance, food sensitivities can be annoying and uncomfortable.

Food allergies are more severe than intolerances because they involve more organs, involving whole systems in the body. Signs of food allergy can include the following:

Digestive System

- Spitting up
- Vomiting
- Diarrhea
- Bloating
- Rumbling noises
- Gas
- Constipation
- Mucus in the stools
- Diaper rash
- Redness around anus

Respiratory System

- Watery eyes
- Runny nose
- Sneezing
- Cough
- Wheezing/asthma (can be life threatening)
- Swelling in the throat and choking (can be life threatening)
- Dark circles under the eyes
- Recurrent ear and respiratory infections

Skin

- Rash
- Hives
- Puffiness and swelling

Behavior

- Crankiness
- Irritability
- Fatigue

Reactions can begin the moment food touches the lips or they can take several hours. They can happen the first time your child eats a particular food, or they can develop over time. Symptoms vary from very mild to severe and life threatening, and may also be dose related, i.e. affected by the amount consumed.

Preventing and Discovering Food Allergies

Parents who have allergies have a chance of passing allergic reactions on to their children, although it may be to a different food or not to food at all; a family history of allergies such as asthma, hay fever, and eczema also increases your child's risk. Mothers who are allergic to specific foods should thus avoid them during pregnancy and while breastfeeding. In addition, mothers should avoid highly allergenic foods, even if they do not typically react to them.

Starting solids too early has also been linked to food allergies. Many families with allergies are reluctant to introduce solids, and prefer to wait as late as possible. If allergies run in your family, delay solid food until closer to six to seven months. When introducing foods, avoid giving your baby any foods to which other family member are allergic. If your older child reacts to carrots, for example, delay introducing carrots.

Avoid common allergenic foods for at least the first eighteen months. Begin introducing new foods slowly. When offering and introducing a new food, give it individually, rather than as part of a mixture. Also, wait at least four to six days between introducing new foods. This will give you an opportunity to see whether baby is tolerating the new addition. One easy rule of allergenic foods is to avoid the "hairy fruits." such as kiwi, peach, apricot, strawberry, and mango (hair is on the inside).

Introduce new foods in the morning. In this case, if your child has a poor reaction to it, you have the rest of the day to treat it. If your child reacts to a food, avoid giving it to her. Sensitivity to one food may mean your child will be sensitive to other foods in the same group. Vary your child's food choices.

Breastfeed and avoid formula. Mother's milk has been shown to decrease the likelihood of allergies, so continue to breastfeed as long as you can, ideally into the toddler years. If you are obliged to use formula, consider the hypoallergenic formulas: often children who are allergic to cow's milk formula will have similar reactions to soy and goat milk formula.

The Elimination Diet

If you suspect that your child may have an allergy to a particular food, eliminate the food and keep track of her progress. Initially, parents are going to assume it is a new food causing the reaction. However, your child may become more sensitive to a food over a period of time—weeks, months, or even years. If you are not sure which food she may be sensitive to, start with a food diary. On a piece of paper, list the foods that your child has been consuming for several days. Perhaps you can come up with a few possible suspect foods. Consider first the foods in the high allergenic list on the following page first that are known suspects and remember that the more processed and refined foods you buy, the more likely your child is consuming hidden ingredients.

Avoid all high allergen foods in general during this time period, whether or not they are on your list, and give your child organic, unprocessed, low allergy foods instead. It is easier if the whole family is able to eat the same foods together. This diet includes avoiding dairy, wheat, soy, sugar, refined processed food, food with additives, preservatives or dyes, corn, chocolate, and eggs.

Stay on the diet for three weeks. After three weeks, begin re-introducing foods on the suspect list, and note if there are any symptoms. Once you have tracked down the particular food, eliminate it from the diet for awhile. Be sure to stay in contact with your practitioner as this can be very difficult if there are more than a few foods that your child is allergic to. At this point, I also find it helpful to give a child a homeopathic remedy, selected based on her total symptoms. If five children come to my office with allergy symptoms, they may all leave with a different remedy choice, because they all have different complaints and different dispositions.

Some patients come to me with extensive skin tests performed by an allergist, a doctor who specializes in treating allergies. Skin testing is usually reserved for a child with severe allergy symptoms. In addition to the skin test is a blood test that can check for antibodies to determine specific allergies; ImmunoCAP® tests for IgE. I find the day-to-day perceptions of parents to be the more reliable indicator of allergies. Skin tests can present with a false positive reading (which I also see with the TB skin test), and in fact tend to offer a more accurate picture of what a child is not sensitive to, as a negative reading can be more dependable. Conventional medicine does not recognize IgG as a true "allergy" which is why insurances do not pay for testing; they will, however, pay for IgE testing. In fact, allergists who give "allergy shots" over weeks and months are trying to convert the allergic patient who reacts with IgE to get them to change it to IgG (which insurances pay for, which means it is conventionally accepted). It is very difficult to tell a family that has made dramatic dietary changes based on IgG testing that there may be other aggravating factors in the allergic patient's immune system imbalance.

If you are breastfeeding and your baby is colicky and fussy after feedings, your baby may be reacting to the food you are eating. Begin an elimination diet for yourself. In each food group, eat only organic, low-allergenic foods. For the first two weeks, eat only the following foods:

- Grains: rice or millet, rice drink
- Protein: lamb, turkey
- Vegetables: green and yellow squash, boiled potato, sweet potato
- Fruit: pears

After two weeks, slowly begin introducing foods on the low-allergy list. Avoid the foods on the high allergy list.

This diet is extremely limiting and most women find it difficult to maintain. Refer to Chapter 5 and Part IV as well to find remedies for colic and instructions for swaddling that will complement this elimination diet. This can help baby's fussiness, which means that mom can begin to add food back into her diet, albeit slowly.

Common Allergenic Foods

Ironically, we desire the very foods that we are sensitive to and that our bodies have the most difficult time digesting and incorporating.

Nearly 90% of food allergies are caused by these foods:

- Dairy (especially cow's milk)
- Eggs (especially egg whites)
- Peanut and tree nuts (walnuts, pecans, almonds, macadamia, hazelnuts)

- Shellfish and fish
- Soybean and soy products (tofu)
- Wheat

Additional high-risk allergenic foods:

- Chocolate
- Corn
- Dairy products (cheese, milk, yoghurt)
- Fruit (citrus, strawberries, berries, coconut, mango, melons, papaya)
- Grains (buckwheat)
- Legumes (beans)
- Preservatives and chemical additives in food (food colorings, blue dye, red dye, and yellow dye #5)
- Protein (fish, shellfish, pork)
- Spices (cinnamon, mustard)
- Sugar
- Vegetables (tomatoes, onion, peas)
- Yeast

Low allergenic foods:

- Fruit (apples, applesauce, apricots, bananas, cranberries, dates, grapes, mangoes, peaches, pears, plums, raisins)
- Grains (barley, rice, oats, rye)
- Protein (chicken, lamb, salmon, turkey, veal)
- Vegetables (asparagus, beets, broccoli, carrots, cauliflower, lettuce, squash, sweet potato)

If your child is allergic to one or more foods, you will need to be an especially close reader of food labels. Learning what products to eliminate means knowing the many forms in which an allergic substance can appear in foods—not an easy task considering the different names substances like wheat and soy can masquerade under in the foods we consume everyday. Common food allergies and ingredients to avoid are listed below.

Cow's milk: Avoid soy milk, goat milk, buttermilk, cheese, ice cream, yogurt, margarine, sour cream, cocoa mixes, creamy foods, gravies, baked goods, breads, whey, casein, and sodium caseinate, a common ingredient in hot dogs, desserts, and other products.

Wheat: Avoid gluten, cornstarch, durum, semolina, pasta, bread baked goods, flour, and farina. Increasingly, stores are stocking wheat-free products: look for labels that advertise themselves as wheat- or gluten-free.

Corn: Avoid corn syrup, caramel, and many baked goods with corn flour.

Soybean: Avoid tofu, edamame, miso soup, soy sauce, veggie burgers, textured vegetable protein, hamburgers, sausage, and hot dogs.

Nuts (peanuts and tree nuts): Peanuts are legumes from both the pea and bean family which is why a child with a peanut allergy may be able to tolerate the tree nuts. Peanuts can be found in the ingredients lists of many products, including mixed nuts, cookies, candy, and cakes, as well as in dishes in Asian restaurants. Tree nuts (hazelnuts, almonds, walnuts, pecans, and cashews) are found in baked goods, candy, and oils.

Eggs: Avoid egg substitutes, albumin, globulin, ovalbumin, and vitellin. Many commercially prepared foods contain egg such as cakes, cookies, pancakes, ice cream, pasta, salad dressing, and custards. Egg whites should not be given to children under one year of age.

The Dairy Dilemma

As we become more educated about dairy products—about the additives and antibiotics common to most and the difficulties our bodies have digesting them—many parents are increasingly looking for alternatives to milk, cheese, yogurt, and their dairy-based derivatives. I am often asked by both new and experienced parents what I recommend on the subject of diary. Is it safe to include in their child's diet? Is it safe to leave it out? These questions came up in my household when our children were toddler age. My husband is from a small, picturesque village in Switzerland, a country where milk, chocolate, and cheese fondue are nothing short of the national identity. Having grown up around dairy farms, my husband naturally wanted our kids to have dairy in their diet. As our children were breastfed till nearly school age, I argued the only milk they needed was mine. We were in the middle of a dairy dilemma. As a final compromise, our children's main beverage is water, but they enjoy their milk and Swiss cheese sparingly.

For years, the National Dairy Council has been telling us on billboards, "Milk Does a Body Good!" But does it really do a body good? Humans are, after all, the only animal that drinks another species' milk. Across the animal kingdom, milk is made for babies and is species specific: its nutrients are designed to support young life until it is able to digest adult foods. Evidence is mounting against milk as a healthy part of the diet, for either child or adult. Among the many reasons milk is falling out of favor are the following:

- 75% of people worldwide are lactose intolerant, symptoms of which include stomach cramps, bloating, gas, distension, and diarrhea after drinking milk.
- Milk is high in fat.
- Once considered the primary means of obtaining calcium, dairy is less popular with nutritionists and health advocates. Instead of milk, they recommend any of the numerous non-dairy calcium sources, including vegetables like broccoli and kale and a wide variety of legumes. These sources are healthier for your child and just as full of bone-strengthening calcium.
- Milk consumption has been linked to breast cancer, colon cancer, prostate cancer, diabetes, allergies, heart disease, and more.
- Unhealthy milk comes from unhealthy cows, and nowadays, our cows are certainly sicklier: hardly surprising since they are regularly given drugs, antibiotics, and hormones all meant to increase productivity. In addition, many dairy cows are on forced feeding plans, which can lead to breast infections that require even more antibiotics. Most conventionally produced milk also contains recombinant Bovine Growth Hormone (rBGH), a genetically engineered drug that helps increase milk production. rBGH may be associated with breast, colon, and prostate cancer. Not surprisingly, this conventional milk is substantively different than natural milk, contaminated with growth hormone, antibiotics, and pus from infections.

- Breastmilk or formula should be the only milk for your baby during the first year. Avoid cow's milk and other diary products before her first birthday, and the later the better, if possible. Cow's milk is one of the most common allergies in young children, so if you want to include dairy in his or her diet, try other sources, such as yogurt (look for the Live and Active Culture seal), kefir, and goat milk.

Many of my patients are using goat's milk as an alternative to cow's milk. Research indicates that human bodies better tolerate goat's milk, since the protein and fat in goat's milk are more easily digested and less allergenic than cow's milk. This is primarily because goat's milk does not contain agglutinins, which in cow's milk causes fat globules to cluster. As a result, goat's milk is more easily broken down by the body, so much so that people who are lactose intolerant can often tolerate goat's milk. The mineral content is slightly different, too. Goat's milk contains more calcium, but less vitamin B12 and folic acid than cow's milk. For this reason, you can now find some goat's milk supplemented with folic acid. Goat's milk also contains no antibiotics or hormones, and does not stimulate an immune response—that is to say, there is no mucus formation from goat's milk.

The benefits of goat's milk are not only limited to the body. It is little wonder, given its versatility, that the goat occupies a central role in economies and food practices around the world. Ecologically, it uses less grazing space and offers an easy supply of milk, making it an ideal livestock choice for people in a variety of regions. Here, following the custom throughout the world, some families are beginning to keep a goat in their backyard for goat's milk.

Other alternatives include non-dairy milk drinks made from soy, rice (horchata is a Mexican rice milk), oats, nuts and seeds. In the past, these milks had to be prepared at home, but now health and grocery stores stock a number of commercial brands. Pay attention to nutritional labels, however, as even these alternatives can contain additives, and are sometimes quite sweet. Use organic when possible.

To make a quick nut milk, use ½ cup organic nuts (raw cashews, blanched almonds, or sesame seeds). Almond and sesame are the highest in calcium. Grind to a fine powder in blender and add 1 cup of cold water. Sweeten if needed. Milk can also be strained if desired. Be sure to use the high nutrient pulp!

Cage-Free Eggs

Until recently, we have been encouraged to avoid eggs due to their high cholesterol content. Current nutritional trends are revising the conventional wisdom on eggs, however, and they are now considered acceptable choices in non-vegetarian circles. After human milk, eggs rank second in terms of providing high-quality protein, though as with any food, it is important to consider the source. Better quality eggs come from healthier hens. I prefer the cage-free, hormone-free, organically raised eggs over those from commercial hens that are caged and conventionally fed. Hens that are allowed to roam (free-range) produce eggs that are lower in cholesterol.

Egg whites are common allergens, so be cautious in including eggs in your baby's diet. Although I prefer babies remain on a predominantly vegetarian diet, many doctors allow infants to begin egg yolks as early as 8 months. Egg whites should be avoided until after one year old. Due to their tendency to harbor salmonella, it is best to avoid raw eggs.

Foods and Additives to Avoid

Genetically Modified Organisms

You may already be seeing food labeled "non-GMO" at your local grocery store. But what is a GMO? Even if you did not know that GMO stands for Genetically Modified Organisms, chances are good that you have been eating these foods since they entered the marketplace in 1996. A GMO is created when a gene or DNA from one organism is inserted into another organism, fundamentally changing its structure and creating a new breed of plant. Supporters of GMOs argue that these altered foods offer a number of advantages, including increased resistance to pests, improve ripening and shelf life, and enhanced nutrient values.

Consumer advocates, however, are worried about the lack of labeling: many times, we simply do not know if a product has been modified or not. As concerns mount about the health consequences of GMOs, more people are demanding clear identification of products as either modified or unmodified. By definition, organic foods have not been genetically altered, one reason many people find organic foods desirable. While the long-term effects of GMOs on the body remain to a large extent unknown, definitive problems include:

- Food allergies: According to the FDA, GMOs may trigger allergic reactions. The York Nutritional Laboratory reported a 50% increase in soy allergies in 1999-2000. Significantly, soy is the most genetically modified crop.

- Danger to plants and animals: GMO crops designed to resist weed killers may be propagating a whole generation of superweeds that will be difficult to eradicate.
- Harm to immune system: Rats fed with genetically engineered potatoes suffered immune system damage.
- Possible increased antibiotic resistance.

Chemicals, Additives, and Preservatives

Whether your child has an allergy or not, it is important to familiarize yourself with food labels, as many of the most unfamiliar substances in processed foods are sulfites, preservatives, and dyes, known to cause sensitivities.

The nutrition facts listed on packages of food give you information regarding the product's nutritional values (or lack of). Be sure to pay attention to portion size, or amount per serving, listed at the top. Often, foods are packaged to look like single servings, while their nutritional information, calories, and fat content are based on multiple, smaller servings. The amount of fat, carbohydrates, sodium, and vitamins and minerals all appear in boxes below the serving size. Below these will be a list of ingredients, with the most predominant ingredient listed first. Once you begin reading labels regularly, you may be surprised to see how high on the list sugar often appears, generally in the form of corn syrup. Sugar is also disguised under the names sucrose, dextrose, fructose, and maltose. Salt (sodium) is another additive to avoid. Used as a flavor enhancer and preservative, salt causes the body to retain water, increases blood pressure, and is linked to a number of health problems. Foods high in salt include soy sauce, chips, cheese, hot dogs, cold cuts, and pizza. Retrain your family's taste buds—put away the salt shaker. As an alternative, try using more lemon and unsalted herbs.

As a rule, fewer ingredients on the label mean a healthier product. Long ingredient lists often indicate a number of additives and preservatives, which you will recognize by their long chemical names.

Nitrates

When I was growing up, my mother was not an avid reader of food labels—that is, until she met my stepfather, at which point our diets all changed for the healthier. One of the things my mom refused to buy was food laden with nitrates, the preservatives used in cold cuts, ham, bacon, hot dogs, and charbroiled burgers.

Studies suggest a possible connection between these chemical preservatives and cancer, including leukemia in children. In the body, nitrates become nitrosamines, which are linked to cancer and type-2 diabetes. Minimize or avoid smoked, grilled, or charbroiled foods, as they have potentially carcinogenic qualities.

Nitrates are naturally occurring in our soil, but even these natural forms can pose health risks. Because conventional farming often adds too much nitrogen-based fertilizer to the soil, you may want to buy organic versions of the following vegetables: root vegetables and green vegetables such as spinach, beets, cabbage, lettuce, broccoli, celery, radish, and to a lesser extent, carrots, cauliflower, French beans, parsnips, peas, and potatoes.

If you want to eat cured meats, buy the variety without hormones, preservatives, or chemicals.

Monosodium glutamate (MSG)

The controversial flavor enhancer MSG is known to cause adverse reactions. Common complaints include headache, stomach upset, nausea, vomiting, diarrhea, shortness of breath, anxiety attacks, and more. For years a staple in Chinese restaurants, MSG is also found in a wide array of products, and as the FDA does not require that MSG be listed, it can often go unrecognized in our food.

Definite sources of MSG:

- Autolyzed yeast
- Calcium caseinate
- Gelatin
- Hydrolyzed protein
- Sodium caseinate
- Yeast extract

Possible sources of MSG:

- Textured protein
- Carrageenan
- Vegetable gum
- Seasonings and spices
- Flavorings (natural, chicken, beef, pork, smoke)
- Bouillon, broth, stock

- Barley malt
- Malt extract and flavoring
- Whey protein, whey protein isolate, whey protein concentrate
- Soy protein, soy protein isolate, soy protein concentrate, soy sauce, soy extract

Allergenic Preservatives

Humans have always relied on preservatives to make food last longer. In centuries past, common preservatives were sugar, salt, and vinegar; now however, we rely on a wide array of chemicals and additives to ensure our food keeps for long periods of time. Sulphur dioxide, sodium benzoate, nitrates, tartrazine, sorbic acid and pimaricin are just a few of the preservatives commonly used in our food, and many of these have been known to cause allergic reactions, including life-threatening shortness of breath.

One of the most popular preservatives is sulphur dioxide, or sulphites. Sulphites can be found in wine, dried fruits, salad bars, certain brands of juices, dried sausage, pickles, and hamburger patties. Other common preservatives include sodium benzoate, found in soft drinks, fruit juices, cake mixes, and commercial puddings, and tartrazine, known as FD&C Yellow Number 5, used to color foods and cosmetics. It is derived from coal-tar and is found in cheese, snacks, medications, macaroni and cheese, candy, soda, pasta, and more.

Sugar

Anyone who has seen a child's face light up at dessert time knows the almost universal appeal of sugar for young palates. Candy and other sweets are the stuff of childhood fantasy: from holidays to birthdays, from movies to songs to games like Candyland, sugar figures prominently in young imaginations. Even our terms of endearment like "honey" and "sweetie" link love and affection to the pleasures of sugar.

At the same time, many of us are unaware of sugar's negative impact on children's health and behavior. Quickly and easily digested, simple sugars cause blood sugar fluctuations dramatically, as anyone who has watched their children after a night of trick-or-treating can attest. Sugar consumption is linked to diseases such as diabetes, obesity, and heart disease, and is known to suppress the immune system for several hours following ingestion, making your child more vulnerable to illness.

Moreover, sugar works like a drug. I have observed with my youngest son that the more sweets he eats, the more he craves them. For children with hyperactivity and attention deficit, the addictive quality of sugar poses a particular problem. These children frequently test positive for abnormal glucose intolerance, indicating that they may be more sensitive to sugar after ingesting it. When sugar is taken out of the diets of children with hyperactivity, studies suggest that their behavior improves.

Not all sweets work in the body in the same way. How your child reacts to sugar is influenced by a food's *glycemic index* (GI), which measures the rate at which the food affects blood sugar levels. Sweets with a high GI indicate that glucose enters the bloodstream more quickly, in turn stimulating a rapid insulin response which causes broad swings in blood sugar levels: hence, the irritability and mood changes your child experiences after eating a food with a high index. Carbohydrates are ranked according to their glycemic index. Foods with a lower glycemic index like legumes or vegetables are digested more gradually and release sugar more slowly into the bloodstream, while candy, soda, and other sugary foods release high amounts of glucose almost immediately upon ingestion. In general, foods with a lower glycemic index are more helpful in weight management, better for insulin levels, and keep you satiated for a longer period of time.

Foods with a low glycemic index include whole grains, brown rice, oatmeal, most types of pasta, non-starchy vegetables (yams, beets, celery, green beans, broccoli), fruit (grapefruit, grapes, peach, cherries, apples), legumes (lentils, split peas, garbanzo beans, lima beans, navy beans, pinto beans, kidney beans, baked beans), and dairy (yogurt, milk).

Refined and processed sweets and grains usually have a high glycemic index and should be avoided. Eating an orange has a lower GI than drinking orange juice due to the fiber in the fruit. Juice is almost always high in sugar content will raise blood sugar more quickly if consumed on an empty stomach. Rather than relying on juice, give your child fresh fruit instead. Be sure to read the label as well: in many processed and refined foods—breakfast cereals are a prime example—sugar is often one of the main ingredients.

I allow my children to have sweets in moderation, almost always substituting refined sugar for a natural sweetener, of which there are a number available for baking and cooking:

- Maple syrup
- Sucanat
- Fruit juice
- Raisins
- Honey
- Brown rice syrup
- Molasses
- Barley malt

As a mother of school-aged children, I find it nearly impossible to avoid refined sugar in my children's diet. My kids go to school, have play dates, and attend birthday parties—they are exposed to sugar, processed food, and junk food regularly. While I cannot regulate my children's diets constantly, I also realize the strongest foundation for establishing healthy eating habits is the home. At the very least, I know that my husband (who does all the meal preparation) packs them well-balanced, nutritious lunches for school.

Stevia

Stevia is an herb used as a sweetener in place of sugar. While the whole leaf is not FDA approved as a sweetener, stevia is sold in the US as a dietary supplement and is widely used around the world with no serious side effects reported. In this country, though, it remains controversial, with speculation that the FDA has kept stevia on its list of unsafe food additives in order to avoid competition with the synthetic chemical sweetener, aspartame. Studies of rats fed excessive doses of stevia have yielded few conclusive findings on potential health consequences. By 2008, the FDA designated highly refined products from the stevia leaf as "GRAS," or "generally regarded as safe".

Xylitol

Known as the natural sweetener, xylitol is made from wood sugar and also found in plums, strawberries, and raspberries. It is considered to be as sweet-tasting as sugar and is commonly used because it doesn't cause tooth decay or affect blood sugar levels. Although it is advertised as not having the side effects of sugar or artificial sweeteners, overuse of xylitol has been linked to diarrhea and some studies have linked it to weight gain and liver, brain, and kidney conditions. A recent study found that xylitol decreased the rate of ear infections in children.

Artificial Sweeteners

Artificial sweeteners touted for sweetening foods without calories have gained popularity over the years. Sucralose (Splenda) and aspartame (Nutrasweet and Equal) which are found in thousands of food and beverage products have been linked to serious side effects. Sucralose, a sugar derivative, is still considered an artificial chemical once it enters the body. Adverse reactions exists and have been shown to affect growth, thymus gland, kidney, liver, and red blood cells. Aspartame, which comes from the chemicals aspartic acid, phenylalanine, and methanol has been linked to a long list of serious problems effecting the heart, brain, immune system, and causing birth defects. Most reactions to food additives reported to the FDA come from aspartame. I do not recommend that children or adults use any of these products.

Vegetarian Diet

Other than the importance of preparing food for you and your family that is fresh, unrefined, organic, varied and in season, I have found that not one specific diet is best for everyone. In my office, I meet many families who have varied dietary preferences. Many families have chosen vegetarian diets based on moral and health reasons.

The history of the vegetarian diet spans back through the millennia. In the East, Hindus and Buddhists refrained from eating meat as they deemed animal life to be sacred. In the West, philosophers in Ancient Greece, Leonardo da Vinci, Trappist monks and Seventh Day Adventists led various degrees of vegetarian lives. The term is loosely used today; however, it usually is defined as a diet that is exclusively plant based and abstinence from animal food. Some people consider themselves vegetarians, but also include fish, chicken or eggs in their diet.

A vegetarian diet is adequate as long the diet is balanced and high in nutrients. Often it is healthier than the standard American diet. Because it is a plant based diet, healthy vegetarian food is high in fiber, vitamins and low in saturated fats. Research shows that vegetarians tend to have lower rates of heart disease, obesity, diabetes, and cancer. Vegetarians are also able to get enough calcium, protein and iron from non-animal sources. Strict vegetarians or vegans, who completely abstain from animal foods including dairy and eggs, need to be careful about their vitamin B12 intake (see "Vitamins and Minerals" in Chapter 13).

Common varieties of vegetarian diets include:

Vegan Diet: A vegan diet is a plant based diet. Vegans abstain from animal food (including dairy, eggs and honey) and using animal products (clothes such as silk, wool, leather, and lanolin, gelatin).

Lacto-vegetarian: Vegetarians who include dairy products in their diet.

Lacto-ovo-vegetarian: Vegetarians who include dairy and eggs.

SUMMARY

The common thread when planning meals for yourself and your children is that **your food be as freshly prepared, organic, in season, and varied as possible**. Whatever your food preferences, nutritionists concur that the following diet can meet your family's nutritional needs and help lower risks of cancer, heart disease, and diabetes:

- Rich in plant-based foods
- Rich in whole grains, fruit, and vegetables
- Low in animal fat
- Low in animal-based products (including dairy)

THE STANDARD AMERICAN DIET

The standard American diet, which includes a lot of prepackaged foods, is rich in foods that are harmful to the body—processed sugars, hydrogenated and trans fats, dairy, and animal-based foods. The new USDA MyPlate divides foods into five food groups that include grains, vegetables, fruit, milk, meat, and beans and gives recommended portion sizes and healthy eating tips for each.

NUTRITIONAL BUILDING BLOCKS 101

Protein and Amino Acids: Protein is essential for nearly all the biological processes in the body, including growth, metabolism, muscular and bone strength, immune functioning, and the nervous system. During the first year of life, your baby needs 1 gram of protein per pound of body weight. From twelve to fifteen months she needs 0.5 gm of protein per pound of body weight.

Carbohydrates: Carbohydrates are the body's main source of energy. Minimize your child's consumption of sugars and simple carbs and emphasize fiber and complex carbs. A two-year-old child should have 3 ounces (85 grams) of carbs; school-age children, 6 ounces (170 grams); teens, 8 ounces (240 grams).

Fats and Lipids: Fats give your child energy, aid your child's developing nervous system and brain function, protect vital organs, help the absorption of fat-soluble vitamins, and are involved with hormonal production. Limit saturated, hydrogenated, and trans fats; emphasize monounsaturated and polyunsaturated fats, especially omega-3 fatty acids and DHA found in flaxseed, fish oils, and many other foods.

Vitamins and Minerals: Necessary in small amounts, vitamins and minerals help the body carry out vital metabolic reactions and processes. The thirteen essential vitamins our bodies need occur in either fat-soluble (A, D, E, and K) or water-soluble (C and the eight B-complex vitamins) forms. Ideally, we would get all the nutrition we need from foods but we may need to offer our children some supplementation.

HOW TO PREPARE NATURAL FOODS FOR KIDS

Many of the cooking techniques you use in adult meals—steaming, grilling, stir-frying—translate to infant meals as well, particularly after one year of age. The important difference is that you must plan your meals so that they meet the evolving nutritional and developmental needs of your child. Preparing your baby's first meals will go more easily if you have a few additional cookware pieces on hand, including a double boiler or Bain Marie, a blender or food processor, a pressure cooker, and a steamer, which cook food thoroughly without losing nutritional content.

Compared to conventionally grown food, certified organic produce is more nutritious and flavorful, and is never genetically modified. When shopping for meat, poultry, fish, or eggs, look for free-range, hormone- and antibiotic-free, and organically fed. Wild fish is preferable to farm-raised fish.

Baby food should be served slightly warmer than room temperature. Leftovers should be stored in glass containers. It can be refrigerated for up to two days or frozen for up to three months.

MEAL PLANNING

As you introduce your baby's first solid food, around six months of age, keep portion sizes small—no more than one to two tablespoons of solid food. First foods, mostly fruits, vegetables, and cereals, should be easily digested, non-allergenic, and as similar as possible to breast milk.

By seven to nine months, slowly introduce finger foods. As your baby approaches her first year, foods can be increasingly solid in consistency but should still be mostly vegetarian. Avoid honey in the first year.

By one year old, nearly half of your child's nutrition will be coming from solid foods and portion sizes should be gradually increasing. By two years old, her diet is expanding all the time and so are her abilities to coordinate utensils and eat more complicated meals like small sandwiches. At this age you might want to consider healthy snacks as a way of providing nutrition throughout the day.

FOOD ALLERGIES AND SENSITIVITIES

Allergy symptoms, such as spitting up, vomiting, sneezing, swelling in the throat, rash, or hives, occur when the immune system reacts to food as if it were a foreign invader in need of annihilation. True food allergies affect approximately 2% of children. The more common form of sensitivity is known as food intolerance, and it typically affects digestion, causing distension, gas, and diarrhea.

If the parents are allergic to specific foods, avoid those foods for the first eighteen months. Also, avoid common allergenic foods like eggs, nuts, and shellfish. If you suspect that your child may have an allergy to a particular food, eliminate the food and keep track of her progress.

FOODS AND ADDITIVES TO AVOID

Avoid genetically modified organisms (GMOs), chemicals, additives, and preservatives (such as nitrates, monosodium glutamate, and sulphites), sugar, and artificial sweeteners.

VEGETARIAN DIET

A vegetarian diet is adequate as long the diet is balanced and high in nutrients.

chapter 14

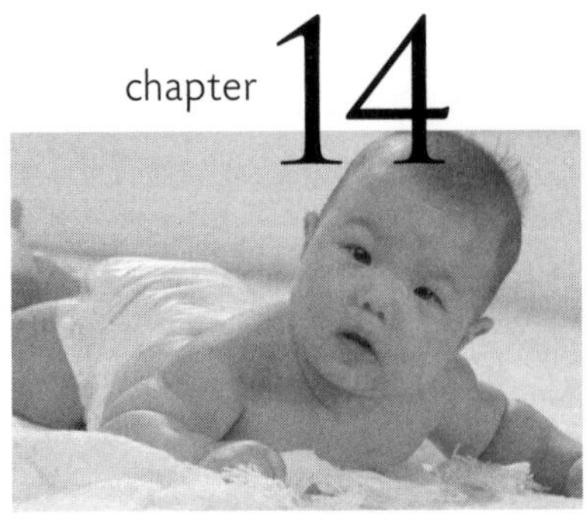

Vaccines

We should quietly hear both sides.

–Goethe

ONE OF THE FIRST MAJOR HEALTH DECISIONS facing new parents is whether or not to vaccinate. Often, the first vaccination is the hepatitis B shot given to newborns. At two months of age, babies are given hepatitis B again, DTaP (diphtheria, tetanus, pertussis), Hib (meningitis), polio, and pneumococcal vaccines. The vaccination schedule continues from there. Vaccinations are recommended by our healthcare system for every child, and are often required before he or she begins school. No vaccination is 100% safe, however, and sometimes a child can experience a reaction after a shot—discomfort, allergic reactions, and even death have occurred. As a result, a growing number of parents have begun to question the safety and effectiveness of vaccines. The information in this book is designed for parents who have chosen to vaccinate their children as well as for parents who have chosen not to. This chapter will guide you in making an informed choice regarding your child's vaccination schedule, and will offer alternatives to those parents seeking options other than full vaccination. For more information on vaccinations I recommend the resource list at the back of the book.

Many of us do not even regard vaccinations as a decision: for medical, legal, and personal reasons, we assume vaccinations to be compulsory rather than voluntary, and we hesitate to question the consequences or even necessity of infant and childhood inoculations. But vaccinations—for decades the proud standard of medical advancement—are no longer immune to controversy. In recent years, concerns about vaccine injuries, autism, and mercury in flu vaccines have increased as professional journals and newspapers report with increasing frequency on possible links between vaccinations and chronic diseases. In my office, the most common question I hear from concerned parents is, "What should I do about the shots?"

My response is multi-faceted. The fact that I am both an M.D. and a holistic practitioner places me in a unique position. As an M.D., I am well aware that the standard of care is to vaccinate; as a holistic practitioner, I recognize that vaccinations can present short-term and sometimes long-term risks for patients. Although the goals of conventional and holistic medicine are the same—to raise happy and healthy children—the differences in approaches can be vastly different, and the choices offered can be confusing and even frustrating for parents. After careful consideration, my husband and I decided not to vaccinate our children. In my office practice and in my lectures, however, I am careful to emphasize that our decision to not vaccinate was a personal family decision, and as a caretaker to many families, I do not impose this course of action on my patients. I recognize that vaccinations prevent many severe and life threatening illnesses, and it would be naïve to trust that healthy lifestyles and natural parenting approaches are always going to provide us with adequate solutions. Although homeopaths have been treating infectious diseases successfully for several centuries, I would not hesitate to rely on medicine and technical advancements of the 21st century when needed.

As I was writing this chapter, both of my children came down with chickenpox. I was humbled by the extremity of the illness and the suffering my older son in particular endured. While I wished I could alleviate his discomfort, I also had to acknowledge that vaccines can have side effects just as harmful—and sometimes more harmful—than the illnesses they prevent. I have witnessed the tragedies that have occurred following a shot, and provided care to many children who have responded poorly to vaccination. In accordance with the law and the various exemptions that each state permits, I strongly support a "pro-informed-choice" attitude—one that encourages parents to make educated, informed decisions regarding vaccinations and every other aspect of parenting. My experiences as a parent and a doctor indicate that the decision to vaccinate is no longer black or white. There are many shades in between that will set a tone that is right for your family. Some of my patients fully vaccinate to schedule, some not at all, and others vaccinate selectively. The goal of this chapter is to provide you with an overview of vaccines, including the pros, cons, illness information, risks, and benefits, as well as advice on how to avoid vaccine side effects.

The Immune System

Holistic medicine maintains that the immune system is our best ally in fighting illness. We all know something about the immune system, but few people could explain exactly how it works to ward off disease. What is the immune system? And what part does it play in health, disease and inoculation? This section offers an overview of our bodies' natural system of protection—how it works, why it works, and how your children can benefit from a healthy immune response.

Germ Theory

How do we get sick? Louis Pasteur, the controversial 19th century scientist, taught us about the germ theory, which remains an integral component of mainstream medicine. His theory is founded on a warfare model of disease: like invading armies, germs attack us from outside the body, and if we succumb, the result is illness. Vaccines developed from this logic; they are meant to "fight" invading illnesses by first mimicking that illness in the body, causing temporary immunization.

Holistic medicine, on the other hand, acknowledges that children get sick, especially in the early ages, and that sickness is vital in assuring your child's health in the future. But children do not become sick because of the strength of the germs, but due to their own vulnerability. If they are already in a weakened state, they stand a higher chance of contracting whatever illness they are exposed to. This thinking helps to explain why only some children become sick if exposed to a sick person. During the cold and flu season, I see hundreds of sick children and adults, at close range. Yet it does not mean that I become sick all the time. If the host is resistant to becoming infected, she will not; it is only when we are susceptible to illness that we become sick. In contrast to mainstream medicine, which combats illness, the holistic approach focuses on factors that can naturally strengthen the body's constitution, such as nutrition, exercise, balanced relationships, and preventive forms of natural medicine.

When your child gets sick, she experiences a natural progression of symptoms. Let's say your daughter has been playing with her friend Claire, who has a bad cough and runny nose. If your child is vulnerable to infection, she can get sick from her exposure to Claire. Typically, the bacteria or virus enters through the mouth or nose. The immune system becomes activated at the level of the tonsils. Once your child becomes "infected," the inflammatory process begins. She can come down with fever, runny nose, sore throat, cough, and even rash which can last from a few days to over a week. This is followed by a healing phase. This cycle—exposure, infection, inflammation, and healing—will occur over and over throughout childhood and adulthood, and does not mean that you or your child is unhealthy. Generally, illness strengthens the immune system, making it better able to respond to bacteria or viruses in the future. If your child is chronically sick, however, you will want to talk to your practitioner about possible reasons for a low immune response.

Innate and Adaptive Immunity

In the course of a day, we are exposed to countless potentially harmful organisms and substances. But the body has remarkable ways of protecting itself, and many of these disease-causing agents do not affect our health. The reason is the immune system, an advanced, complex system that defends the body against foreign invasion of microorganisms and infectious germs like bacteria, viruses, parasites, and fungi. Among the immune system's most important features is its ability to recognize its own cells and to differentiate cells that do not belong, especially ones that can cause harm. It is, in this way, a "smart" system, capable of evolving and strengthening according to changing environments and conditions. Although there are many types of microorganisms, this book addresses the most common bacterial and viral infections and the vaccines designed to combat them.

Over thousands of years, the immune system has evolved to help protect the body. When germs encounter the body, the immune system responds in multiple ways to protect it. The initial barriers are skin and mucous membrane in the mouth and gut. This immediate first line of defense is called the *innate immune system*. Innate immunity offers general protection and responds with fast acting cellular defense against foreign microorganisms and germs. Symptoms such as fever, swollen glands, and runny nose are signs of an immune response.

Once activated, the first line of defense then stimulates the *humoral* or *adaptive immune system* to produces antibodies and other specialized immune cells such as T-cells to aid and assist in the healing process. The adaptive immune system (also known as acquired immune system) develops over the course of your child's lifetime, responding to different diseases naturally or through vaccinations. This adaptive defense is able to remember, recognize, and mount an attack against specific organisms. When it detects germs that the body has never encountered before, within days or weeks it can begin to remember pathogens, so that it can be more effective in responding to them in the future and protecting the body in the event of re-infection. As far back as ancient Greece, physicians observed that if someone had been infected with the plague, they would not get it again. Now we know that this is due to acquired immunity.

Although your baby is born with a weaker immune response compared to you, nature gives her protection through her mother. Antibodies passed from mother to baby through the placenta and in breast milk are part of what is called passive immunity. Your baby is given a temporary immunity to diseases during early childhood that can last from six to twelve months or even longer. Following this period in early infancy, your child will become sick on a periodic basis, but as she gets older, the immune system will adapt to prevent frequent illness.

How Vaccines Work

With a vaccination, a bacteria or virus is injected into the body and the body responds by producing antibodies with the goal of defending the person from attacks of the same bacterium or virus in the future. The bacteria and viruses in a vaccine exist in killed, weakened, or altered live state, and trigger an immune response without causing the disease. Vaccine-induced immunity is known as artificial immunity.

After a shot, the body responds with an increased resistance and an immunological memory. With several exposures, the body begins to remember, respond, and protect the body from the disease. This immunity builds over time and is referred to as acquired immunity. Your child can acquire immunity to a disease in a multitude of ways, and not simply through vaccination: exposure to an illness, actual infection by that illness, and antibodies passed from mother to child are all important means of building immunological memory.

Pros and Cons of Vaccinations

As I noted earlier, our healthcare system is overwhelmingly pro-vaccination, but critics of the program have become more outspoken in recent years. Here is a summary of the arguments.

Pros of Vaccination

Many of my patients have told me that they have been unable to broach the subject of selective or non-vaccination without serious repercussions and threats from their practitioners. Many physicians are, in fact, pro-vaccine, and believe that based on decades of declines in illnesses like whooping cough, diphtheria, polio, measles, mumps, and rubella. Vaccines are effective in preventing these illnesses, and supporters point to many of the following arguments as evidence that the benefits of vaccination outweigh the risks.

1. **The vaccination program in the 20th century is hailed as one of the most considerable achievements in public health**. National vaccination programs are responsible for eradicating some of the most devastating illnesses of the past centuries, including polio, diphtheria, and smallpox.
2. **Supporters of vaccines acknowledge that shots have potential side effects and risks, but maintain that they are rare occurrences.** Media reports on possible vaccine side effects such as autism have not been adequately proven, and vaccination supporters argue that they provoke unnecessary fear among the public.
3. **Children who are not immunized can raise the risk of infection for everyone else.** The potential for an epidemic decreases when adequate numbers of children (at least 75%) are vaccinated. This phenomenon is called herd immunity, and can protect the children who are not immunized. A low herd immunity increases risk.

Cons of Vaccination

Supporters of vaccination argue that possible reactions to vaccinations do not overshadow the program's larger public benefits. Side effects, they contend, are an unfortunate and minor consequence to positive medical advancement. But like many parents, I have heard numerous reports and personal stories that would suggest vaccinations pose serious risks to children and are by no means wholly safe. Listed below are the three major criticisms of the vaccination program in its current form.

1. **Like any medication, every vaccine has the risk of injury or death.** Vaccines exist in both live and killed forms, though, in general, live vaccines are more potent and thus result in longer immunity as well as potentially stronger adverse reactions. The live oral polio vaccine, for instance, was

discontinued when it was discovered that it caused more cases of paralytic polio than the actual disease. Currently, measles, mumps, rubella, and chickenpox are live virus vaccines. It is also difficult to prepare vaccines in such a way that they are similar to the illness but not dangerous. If your child has experienced a bad reaction to a prior shot, she may respond poorly to another vaccine.

In addition, pharmaceutical companies add antibiotics, preservatives, and toxic disinfectants to vaccines. A few of the most common vaccine additives include aluminum, formaldehyde, egg products, and mercury. All of these additives can pose known health risks, though mercury has received the most scrutiny by medical professionals, parents, and the media alike. Toxic to the neurological system and the kidneys, high levels of mercury can cause neuro-developmental conditions such as tics, speech delay, sleep disorders, attention deficit disorder, and autism. Few vaccines still contain mercury, often in the form of an antibacterial compound called thimerosal (trade name: Rithialate), which contains 50% ethyl mercury and has been in use since the 1930s. The younger the age that the infant or fetus is exposed to mercury, the greater the possibility for health risks, and studies have shown the mercury levels increase according to the number of shots a child has received containing mercury. Diptheria, tetanus, pertussis, *Haemophilus influenzae* type b (Hib), and Hepatitis B contained thimerosal as a preservative in the past. The flu vaccine still does. Polio, MMR, chickenpox vaccines do not contain mercury.

2. **Vaccination is different than natural immunity .** Because vaccines grant an artificial immunity that is often temporary, many critics will not refer to them as immunizations at all. Unlike natural immunity, vaccines work by tricking the body into thinking it has been exposed to the real illness, which generates an immune response that is supposed to protect the child. Yet the natural routes of exposure (through the mouth, nose and intestine) via the innate immune system are bypassed and the bacteria or virus are injected directly into the bloodstream, triggering the adaptive immune system. The injections thus circumvent the body's natural defense mechanism and may cause a chronic imbalance in the immune system. Common childhood illnesses help the immune system to mature and become stronger, making it

more effective in dealing with challenges from viruses and bacteria later in life. Vaccinations don't offer lifetime immunity, and instead shift the illness to vulnerable adults who are susceptible to a more dangerous version of the disease. Chickenpox during adulthood, for instance, is a risky disease, presenting far more complications than the childhood version. In addition, naturally-acquired illnesses usually occur one at a time. By giving shots that may contain 4 to 6 bacteria and viruses at once, we could be overstimulating the immune system. Could you imagine your child having diphtheria, tetanus and whooping cough at the same time?

3. **Increased use of vaccines corresponds to a rise in chronic diseases among children.** With the number of available vaccines increasing in the last decades from eight to thirty, there is little doubt that our children are immunized with greater frequency and for a wider array of diseases. Critics to the vaccine program point out that as nutrition, hygiene and literacy improved, the severity and frequency of many of the devastating illnesses from the 19th century were on the decline, even before the vaccinations were introduced. Nowadays, the childhood illnesses of a bygone era like chickenpox and measles have given way to a host of chronic diseases and disabilities, which are increasing at epidemic proportions. Since the mid twentieth century, conditions affecting the brain and neurological diseases have quadrupled, learning disorders are up 1000 times, and allergies, asthma, and ear infections are now chronic childhood conditions. While studies have yet to definitively link vaccines to these more unusual illnesses, researchers are beginning to question the role of vaccines in neurocognitive disorders like autism, Asperger's, and attention deficit disorder, chronic conditions like asthma, and diseases like SIDS and leukemia. Researchers suspect that the link between vaccines and some of these conditions may be due to the effects of the vaccines on infants whose immune systems and organs are immature and developing. Critics to mass vaccination point out there are no long term studies to determine the effects of vaccinations.

Standard Vaccinations

Vaccines are compulsory in the United States, and follow a protocol established by the Centers for Disease Control. However, exemptions do exist. When a child is school age (including pre-school), you will be asked about your child's medical history, including dates of vaccinations. For the families in my office practice who have opted to either vaccinate selectively or not at all, they will need to justify a reason for their action or lack of action. After explaining to schools that the law allows exemptions, most families have found the school administrators work smoothly with the family. Most parents reported they simply signed a waiver provided by the school. Each state has different requirements regarding exemptions. The following types may be available in your state:

- Philosophical: Some states allow the vaccines to be waived based on one's personal beliefs.
- Medical: Most states permit medical exemptions. The patient's doctor must write why the child is medically unable to receive a vaccination. As of 2017, California, Mississippi, and West Virginia only allow for medical exemptions.
- Religious: Most states allow one to file a religious exemption based on beliefs that oppose vaccination. Families usually are obliged to offer proof of affiliation with their organization.

The standard vaccination schedule, with recommended ages for each vaccine, set by the Centers for Disease Control is as follows:

- **Hepatitis B:** birth, 1 to 2 months, 4 months, 6 to 18 months
- **Polio:** 2 months, 4 months, 6 to 18 months, 4 to 6 years
- **Diphtheria, tetanus, and pertussis (DTaP):** 2 months, 4 months, 6 months, 15 to 18 months, 4 to 6 years old,
- **Haemophilus influenzae type b (Hib):** 2 months, 4 months, 6 months, 12 to 15months
- **Pneumococcus:** 2 months, 4 months, 6 months,12 to 15 months
- **Measles, mumps, and rubella (MMR):** 12 to 15 months, 4 to 6 years old
- **Chickenpox (Varicella):** 12 to 18 months
- **Influenza:** every autumn 6 months and older

COMMON CHILDHOOD DISEASES AND VACCINES

HEPATITIS B

Hepatitis B (HBV) is a virus that affects the liver. It is most common in adults from ages 20 to 39. The demographics of this illness make it an unusual choice for a mandated vaccine. It is typically seen in those who are sexually promiscuous or use IV drugs (60 to 80% of drug users have evidence of exposure). It is possible for an infected mother to transmit HBV to her baby during birth; it is for this reason that pregnant women are routinely screened for hepatitis B. Amongst children, it is those born to infected mothers who are at highest risk for developing chronic hepatitis B infections.

Symptoms: Often the initial infection has no symptoms. In fact, 30% of people show no signs or symptoms of the disease, and symptoms in children are less common than in adults. When symptoms do manifest, they may resemble a general flu-like feeling, including weakness, loss of appetite, nausea, headache, fatigue, diarrhea, joint pain, and pain in the right upper abdomen. Jaundice, including yellowing of the eyes, dark urine, and light-colored stools are also possible signs of HBV.

Complications: 5 to 10% of cases in adults become chronic and cause liver damage, liver cancer, and liver failure. Babies born to mothers with hepatitis B are at risk for contracting the disease at birth with a 90% risk of chronic infection. Otherwise, hepatitis B is not considered a childhood disease.

Vaccine: The CDC recommends that all infants be injected with the first dose of hepatitis B vaccine at birth before being discharged from the hospital. Hepatitis B is given at birth, 1 to 2 months, 4 months and 6 to 18 months old. The hepatitis B vaccine may be given together with Hib meningitis, called the Comvax.

Risks of Vaccine: Risks to the vaccine include Guillain-Barre, multiple sclerosis, diabetes, arthritis, and auto-immune diseases. Antibody levels from the vaccine probably decrease by the time a vaccinated child has reached the teen years when exposure is more likely. In addition, the hepatitis B vaccine has been known to contain mercury.

POLIO (PARALYTIC POLIO)

Poliomyelitis (polio) is caused by a virus that enters through the mouth and implants in the throat and intestines. The virus attacks the brain and spinal cord, and can cause paralysis in different muscle groups. Only 1% of polio cases become the classic paralytic polio.

Symptoms: Surprisingly, most cases of polio go unnoticed. Ninety-five percent of symptoms include minor complaints such as sore throat, stomachache, nausea, and headache. The incubation period for polio is commonly 6 to 20 days.

Complications: Complications of paralytic polio is paralysis which is more common in the legs. In severe cases there can be paralysis of the muscles used for breathing and swallowing, which can be fatal.

Vaccine: Up until recently, there were two polio vaccines: the inactivated polio virus or killed virus (IPV) given as a shot, or the oral polio virus (OPV) taken by mouth. The OPV was discontinued in 2000 due to its links to cases of paralytic polio (known as VAPP, or vaccine-associated paralytic polio). Children now receive four doses of IPV (inactivated polio virus) at 2 months, 4 months, 6 to 18 months, and 4 to 6 years of age.

Risks of Vaccine: One of the more debilitating reactions associated with the oral polio vaccine is Guillain-Barre syndrome (GBS), a condition that presents symptoms similar to polio. Some polio vaccines were found to be contaminated with monkey virus (known as simian virus 40 or SV40), contracted from the monkey tissue used to grow the polio virus. SV40 is now linked to cancer (lung, brain, bone, lymphatic), including non-hodgkins lymphoma.

DIPHTHERIA

Diphtheria is a highly contagious disease, most common in poor and densely populated areas. There are only about five cases a year in the United States; the overall mortality rate is 5 to 10%.

Symptoms: Diptheria begins with the general symptoms of fever, chills, headache, cough, runny nose and sore throat. A characteristic thick membrane forms in the throat, making it difficult to breath. Although diphtheria can affect the skin, it most often attacks the respiratory tract. The incubation period for diphtheria is two to five days.

Complications: Complications from diphtheria include breathing problems, infection of the heart (myocarditis), kidney damage, and temporary paralysis of limbs and muscles.

Vaccine: Diphtheria is given with tetanus and pertussis (DTaP) at 2, 4, 6, 15 to 18 months, and 4 to 6 years old, and later on as the Td. The CDC recommends that adults get the boosters of tetanus-diptheria (Td) vaccine every 10 years.

Risks of Vaccine: Since the diphtheria vaccination is given either in combination with pertussis and tetanus, or with the tetanus, side effects cannot be isolated. There have been reports of outbreaks of diphtheria following vaccination.

TETANUS

Tetanus (*Clostridium tetani*) bacteria exist in soil as spores. Tetanus is not a contagious disease, but enters the body through a break in the skin, such as a puncture wound, burn, or major injury, where it then affects the nervous system. According to an article in the Journal of the American Medical Association in the 1960s, "Good wound care is probably the single most important factor in the prevention of tetanus in fresh wounds." Tetanus is more common in adults, with about 30 cases a year.

Symptoms: The incubation period can last from three days to several months, but averages eight days and is followed by early symptoms that include difficulty swallowing, painful spasms, and tightening in the jaw (also called lockjaw) as well as in the neck and abdomen. These symptoms can progress to severe muscle spasms and contractions in the neck, chest, belly, and back.

Complications: Complications associated with tetanus include pneumonia, fractures (from severe muscle spasms), and brain damage. The death rate is 11%, especially in people over sixty years old due to spasms in the respiratory muscles.

Vaccine: The tetanus toxoid is given in a trivalent injection known as the DTaP, which is given at at 2, 4, 6, 15 to 18 months, and 4 to 6 years old. Later on it is given as the Tdap (diphtheria, tetanus, and acellular pertussis) or alone as tetanus. An alternative to the vaccine booster series is the Tetanus-Immune globulin (TIG) shot which can be given following a serious injury (within the first 72 hours). This shot provides protection for the injury via passive immunization: the body does not develop its own antibodies.

Risks of Vaccine: The tetanus toxoid vaccine, TT, contains mercury; the Td and Tdap vaccines do not contain mercury. The adverse effects of the tetanus vaccine include incidence of tetanus, Guillain-Barre syndrome, and arthritis.

PERTUSSIS (WHOOPING COUGH)

In the days of our great-grandmothers, the 100-day cough, now known as whooping cough or pertussis, was considered a common childhood illness in the United States. It is a contagious disease, caused by the Bordetella pertussis bacterium, and spreads from contact with an infected person who coughs or sneezes. Pertussis can be difficult to diagnose by laboratory exam as the test, which analyzes a culture taken from a swab inside the nose, will most likely be negative if a child has been vaccinated, has started antibiotics, or has been sick for more than two weeks. There are approximately 10,000 reported cases (and 10 deaths) a year, though this is considered underreported.

Symptoms: Like many illnesses, pertussis starts with those familiar common cold symptoms—runny nose, fever, and mild cough. Within two weeks, the cough becomes more severe with fits of many rapid coughs followed by the characteristic long inspiration with a crowing sound or high-pitched whoop. Thick mucus builds up in the lungs, which triggers coughing fits severe enough to cause choking, gagging, vomiting, and, less often, blueness in the face, also known as cyanosis. In between attacks, the child looks normal. Older children, adolescents, and adults may have whooping cough without the characteristic cough, and may be diagnosed with bronchitis or a simple cough. From beginning to end, the stages of whooping cough can last 2 to 3 months earning the name the 100-day cough. The incubation period is commonly 7 to 10 days, with a range from 4 to 21 days.

Complications: Complications associated with whooping cough may include pneumonia, ear infections, dehydration, convulsions, and, in rare instances, brain damage or death. It poses a greater danger to children less than 1 year in age due to the small size of the air passages, and infants are thus at the highest risk for pertussis and its complications. Pneumonia is the most common complication and cause of death. Though complications are less severe in older children and adults, pertussis can account for nearly 7% of all adult coughs.

Vaccine: The pertussis vaccine is given as a part of the DTaP (diphtheria, tetanus, and acellular pertussis) series which is given at 2, 4, 6, 15 to 18 months, and 4 to 6 years old.

Risks of Vaccine: The severe complications caused by the original whole-cell pertussis vaccine, including local swelling, fever, high-pitched screaming, convulsions, mental retardation, disabilities, and death, led to the development of acellular vaccines (acellular pertussis 'aP'). Reactions to acellular form of the pertussis vaccine are milder compared to the whole-cell vaccine; however, severe reactions to the acellular vaccine also occur, including encephalitis and death. The pertussis vaccine is only given to children less than seven years of age as it can cause severe reactions over the age of seven. The pertussis vaccine should not be given to children who have a history of convulsions, brain disorder, or abnormal development. Some of my patients have refused the pertussis shot if there is a family history of seizures.

HAEMOPHILUS INFLUENZA TYPE B (HIB)

Haemophilus influenzae type b (not related to the flu) is a bacterium that lives in the mucous membrane in the mouth and nose in 90% of healthy people. Sometimes the haemophilus type B strain (HiB) can cause pneumonia and meningitis. Hib is contagious and spreads through person-to-person contact. Hib infections occur most often during the late winter and spring. Some cases of sinus and ear infections are also caused by Hib. The peak incidence is at 6 to 7 months. Children less than 6 months old are protected by maternal antibodies, as breastfeeding offers protection for children from meningitis. The longer a child is breastfed, the less risk of meningitis. This protection has been documented by researchers to last up to 5 to 10 years.

Symptoms: Hib meningitis starts with vague symptoms such as high fever, headache, nausea, and vomiting. Symptoms specific for meningitis include neck and back stiffness, sensitivity to light, sleepiness, and a severe headache. Babies may be cranky, drowsy, or refuse to eat. Approximately 25% of children who have Hib develop seizures. Other serious signs are mental confusion, shock, and coma. In severe cases of Hib, a child can die within several hours. The incubation period is not known.
Complications: In general, meningitis is a serious illness that can affect both children and adults in viral and bacterial forms. While viral meningitis is less severe and often requires no treatment, bacterial meningitis constitutes a serious health threat. Hib is the most common cause of bacterial meningitis; other common causes are *Neisseria meningitidis* (meningococcus) and *Streptococcus pneumoniae* (pneumococcus). Nearly all cases occur in children under 6 years of age. Complications from bacterial meningitis can include pneumonia, arthritis, pericarditis (infection around the heart), hearing loss, and learning disabilities. The death rate is 5 to 10% in patients without adequate medical treatment.
Vaccine: An earlier Hib vaccine was introduced in 1985, but was discontinued when discovered to result in increased susceptibility to the illness for children over 18 months in the first week following the vaccine. Currently, a newer and more effective conjugate Hib vaccine is in wide use. The schedule for the Hib vaccine is 2,4,6, and 12 months. The Hib vaccine may be given together with Hepatitis B, called the Comvax.
Risks of Vaccine: Reactions to Hib vaccine include fever, irritability, prolonged crying, diarrhea, vomiting convulsions, shock, collapse, Hib meningitis, and Guillain-Barre syndrome. It is difficult to determine the reactions because the Hib vaccine is usually given with the DTaP.

PNEUMOCOCCUS (PCV)

Streptococcus pneumonia (pneumococcus) is a bacterium that can lead to meningitis, pneumonia, blood infection and ear infections. There are 90 types of Pneumococcal bacterium known, and 30% are already resistant to antibiotics. Most children and adults live with pneumococcal organisms in their nose and throat. Those at high risk of developing an infection include children with weakened immune systems, those with spleen and kidney diseases, children of Native American descent, African American children, and children who spend a minimum of four hours a week in a daycare setting.
Symptoms: Pneumococcus can cause a variety of illnesses that include ear infections, pneumonia and meningitis. If a child has meningitis symptoms to look for irritability, listlessness, poor feeding, vomiting, rash, stiff neck and seizures.

Complications: Complications of pneumococcus include pneumonia and meningitis.
Vaccine: The 13-valent pneumococcal conjugate vaccine (PCV13), also known by the name Prevnar13, is given at 2, 4, 6 and 12 to 15 months of age with a minimum of 6 weeks between doses.
Risks of Vaccine: Many researchers question the effectiveness of this vaccine based on several factors:

- Prevnar13 may reduce the effectiveness of other vaccines (Hib, Pertussis, and polio) if it is given as the same time. Children in a clinical study who received the pneumococcal vaccine suffered high fevers, seizures, and other reactions, including twelve deaths.
- Although the vaccine was marketed as a way of decreasing ear infections, no research indicates that it is effective in this regard. Some research has provided evidence that this vaccine may be the most reactive vaccine, with a high incidence of fever and local reactions.

MMR

Measles, mumps, and rubella (MMR) vaccines are given as a single shot of live viruses beginning at 12 months, with a second dose given at 4 to 6 years old. In 1998, Dr. Andrew Wakefield of the London Royal Free Hospital and his colleagues suggested the MMR vaccine (especially the measles and mumps vaccines given together) may be the cause of an inflammatory bowel condition in children which may be linked to autism.

MEASLES (RUBEOLA)

Measles used to be a common childhood virus before the vaccine. It occurred primarily in children aged 2 to 6 years, and almost every child had measles by the age of 15. It is quite contagious with an incubation period of approximately 10 to 20 days. A cyclical disease, measles outbreaks happen around the world every two to three years and more often in the late winter and early spring.
Symptoms: Most cases are mild, and begin with a cold, a high fever, red sensitive eyes, and a hacking cough. On the fourth to fifth day, a rash appears. Characteristically, Koplik spots, small white spots in the insides of the cheek, appear before the rash. The rash begins faintly behind the ears and within 24 hours becomes darker as it spreads to the face, neck and arms. In two to three days the rash reaches the legs, while the rash on the face correspondingly fades. With the onset of the rash, the child begins to feel better.
Complications: Rare complications of measles include severely high fevers, deafness, blindness, ear infections, pneumonia, and encephalitis.

Vaccine: Measles, mumps, and rubella (MMR) vaccines are given as a single shot of live viruses beginning at 12 months, with a second dose given at 4 to 6 years old. The vaccine is contraindicated in children who are allergic to eggs.
Risks of Vaccine: Side effects of the vaccine include encephalitis, meningitis, seizures, deafness, Guillain-Barre syndrome, and autism.

MUMPS

Mumps is a mild viral infection with an incubation period of fourteen to twenty-five days. It is contagious and spreads by person-to-person contact. Mumps is considered a mild viral illness in children, and more severe in teenagers and adults. 20% of mumps cases have no symptoms.
Symptoms: Mumps begins with the common symptoms of fever, headache, and fatigue. Within 24 hours, it leads to the characteristic swelling of the cheek (one or both sides) caused by inflammation of the salivary gland. The illness is finished within a week.
Complications: Complications from mumps are rare and may include inflammation of the ovaries, testicles (more common in adults), and pancreas, deafness, encephalitis, and meningitis. Inflammation of the testicles occurs in 20 to 30% of male adolescents and adults, though sterility is rare. Most of the cases of deafness (80%) are one-sided and occur in 1 out of 20,000 cases.
Vaccine: Measles, mumps, and rubella (MMR) vaccines are given as a single shot of live viruses beginning at 12 months, with a second dose given at 4 to 6 years old. The vaccine is contraindicated in children who are allergic to eggs.
Risks of Vaccine: The risks of the vaccine include meningitis and diabetes mellitus, as it affects the pancreatic gland.

GERMAN MEASLES (RUBELLA)

German measles is a mild viral illness, also known as the *three-day measles*. It occurs cyclically around the world every six to nine years. Most often it strikes in the winter and spring and is spread by coughing and sneezing. There is an incubation period of 14 to 21 days. The vaccine can be given alone or as part of the MMR shot.
Symptoms: Rubella is a mild rash and fever that lasts for two to three days. Common symptoms include a low-grade fever, swollen glands, rash, and fatigue for a few days. A rash appears on the face and then spreads downward, fading by day three to five. Infection usually gives lifelong immunity.
Complications: Complications are rare, although women who contract rubella suffer from arthritis in 70% of cases. The purpose of the vaccination is to prevent

Congenital Rubella Syndrome in babies. Congenital Rubella Syndrome occurs when a mother contracts rubella in her first trimester. If she is not immune to rubella (either through having the illness or through vaccine), her fetus is at risk for birth defects. In addition, she may suffer a miscarriage. Twenty percent of babies exposed to this virus in utero are at risk for deafness, birth defects, and eye and neurological defects including mental retardation.

Vaccine: Measles, mumps, and rubella (MMR) vaccines are given as a single shot of live viruses beginning at 12 months, with a second dose given at 4 to 6 years old. The vaccine is contraindicated in children who are allergic to eggs.

Risks of Vaccine: Risks of the rubella vaccine include arthritis, Guillain-Barre syndrome, and thrombocytopenia, a low level of blood platelets, which help blood to clot.

CHICKENPOX (VARICELLA)

The chickenpox virus is part of the herpes family, and is similar to shingles (herpes zoster). It is considered a mild disease in childhood, but becomes more severe in adults. Chickenpox is highly contagious and, in the past, the United States saw an average of 4 million cases a year (nearly 90% of the population). These numbers have decreased greatly since the vaccine was introduced.

Symptoms: Half of the cases of chickenpox occur in children from ages five to nine. Symptoms of chickenpox include fever and runny nose, followed by an intensely itchy rash that crusts over within 2 to 3 days. The rash appears in crops on the body and sometimes in the mouth. It is usually extremely itchy and uncomfortable. The disease lasts 2 to 3 weeks. In adults, the disease is more severe and may last several months.

Complications: The most common complications include a secondary bacterial skin infection in children, and pneumonia in adults. More severe problems include encephalitis (1:4000 to 10,000 cases), septicemia, and osteomyelitis. Less than 1% of children who get chickenpox suffer rare complications, though for both children and adults, severe complications are most likely to develop in those who have compromised immune systems due to other health problems.

Vaccine: The chickenpox vaccine is given once between 12 to 18 months old.

Risks of Vaccine: Widespread use of vaccine may shift disease susceptibility to older populations. Side effects may include Guillain-Barre syndrome, shingles, shock, encephalitis, blood disorders, and, in rare instances, death.

INFLUENZA

The flu is caused by the influenza viruses and usually occurs in epidemics from

November to March. Up to 20% of the population can be affected during the flu season.

Symptoms: Symptoms of the flu are high fever, fatigue, headache, body aches, and can include cold symptoms with cough. Children can also have nausea, vomiting and diarrhea.

Complications: Complications of the flu include secondary infections such as ear infections, sinus infections and more seriously, pneumonia. Children who have serious illnesses with compromised immune systems, as well as the elderly and sickly are more susceptible to complications from the flu. There are over 30,000 deaths per year from the flu, mostly affecting people in high risk groups.

Vaccine: Every year the vaccine is reformulated with the flu strains that are predicted to most likely cause the flu epidemic. Children 6 months and older, are encouraged to get a flu shot every autumn. The flu shot is recommended for women during pregnancy, even though it contains mercury.

Risks of Vaccine: Reactions to the flu shot include flu-like symptoms such as fever, aches, and fatigue. More serious reactions include Guillain-Barre Syndrome, an autoimmune illness.

HEPATITIS A

Like Hepatitis B, Hepatitis A (HAV) affects the liver. Most commonly, HAV is spread by person-to-person contact (fecal-oral route) through eating and drinking contaminated food and water. The HAV is found in the stool of infected persons. For this reason, frequent hand washing is imperative after diaper changes, using the toilet, and before eating. If you or your child has come into contact with HAV, an immune globulin shot can be given within 2 weeks to prevent prolonged symptoms.

Symptoms: Hepatitis A is not considered a long-term chronic infection. Once you have had Hepatitis A, you maintain a lifelong immunity. Hepatitis A usually lasts approximately two months and includes fever, fatigue, loss of appetite, nausea, diarrhea, abdominal pain, dark urine, and jaundice. Up to 70% of children who contract Hepatitis A have no symptoms and it usually goes undetected.

Complications: Adults have more serious symptoms and 15% will have prolonged or relapsing symptoms over a 6 to 9 month period. Death is rare.

Vaccine: The Hepatitis A vaccine is recommended for children in selected areas only and is currently used in a few states. While some argue for a mandatory hepatitis A vaccine, critics stress that HAV does not cause chronic infection, has a low mortality rate, especially among children, and is often asymptomatic in the young.

Risks of Vaccine: Hepatitis A vaccines carry the risk of side effects, including severe illnesses like Guillain-Barre syndrome, convulsions, multiple sclerosis, and jaundice.

ANTHRAX

September 11, 2001 and the events immediately following placed biological and germ warfare, especially of anthrax and smallpox, at the forefront of national consciousness. Anthrax is an infectious disease caused by the bacterium *Bacillus anthracis*. It mostly occurs in wild and domestic animals such as cattle, sheep, goats, camels, and antelopes. There are three forms of the disease: cutaneous (skin), inhaled (lungs), and ingested (gastrointestinal). Humans can contract anthrax by coming in contact with infected animals via an open skin wound, by inhaling anthrax airborne spores, or by eating undercooked meat from infected animals. The inhalation form of the disease is most severe, and is usually fatal.

Symptoms: Anthrax symptoms vary depending on how the disease was contracted, but symptoms usually occur within 7 days. Skin infection begins as a raised itchy bump that resembles an insect bite but within one to two days progresses into a painless ulcer, with a characteristic black area in the center. Nearby lymph glands may swell. With inhalation anthrax, an exposed individual develops flu-like symptoms (which can include fatigue, muscle and body aches, fever, and cough) which can last 2 to 3 days. Following these initial symptoms, the exposed person improves and begins to feel better. After several days, new symptoms appear, including severe breathing problems with bloody, frothy mucous, chest pain, sweating, and shock. The intestinal form of anthrax includes symptoms of nausea, loss of appetite, vomiting, and fever. Subsequently abdominal pain, vomiting of blood, and severe diarrhea occur.

Vaccine: An anthrax vaccine has been licensed for use in humans, and is reported to be 93% effective in protecting against anthrax. The Department of Defense has begun mandatory vaccination of all active duty military personnel who might be involved in a conflict.

Risks of Vaccine: The anthrax vaccine is considered experimental, and American troops were forced to take it beginning in 1998. According to the Military Vaccine Education Center, an organization that aids soldiers who have been injured following vaccines, symptoms from the anthrax vaccination include severe fatigue, weakness, migraines, tremors, tumors, seizures, heart conditions, and death.

SMALLPOX

Once believed to be completely eradicated, smallpox outbreaks are a rare, though still possible, occurrence. A viral disease unique to humans, smallpox can only be propagated through person-to-person contact. The infection is spread by the inhalation of air droplets or aerosols. The disease can lead to death.

Symptoms: The incubation period from time of exposure until symptoms develop is

12 to 14 days. After the incubation period, the person experiences a fever, severe aching, and weakness. Severe abdominal pain and delirium are also possible. Two to three days later, a papular rash (pimples) develops over the face, then spreads to the extremities, turning into a vesicular rash (clear fluid-filled blisters), and finally to a pustular rash (yellowish pus-filled blisters) deeply imbedded in the skin. Eventually scabs form leaving deep, pitting scars. Chickenpox is very similar looking and can be mistaken in the first 2 to 3 days of the rash. However, chickenpox lesions generally develop in crops over several days and are much more superficial.

Vaccine: The Center for Disease Control recommends routine vaccinations only for laboratory staff who may be exposed to the virus. The vaccination poses risks and complications, and the overall stock is low, as the facilities that made it were dismantled after 1980 when smallpox was considered eradicated.

Risks of Vaccine: The smallpox (vaccinia) vaccine is a live virus that has a high rate of side effects. For months following the vaccine, children may suffer with fever, irritability, rash, lack of energy and swollen glands. The site of the vaccine is contagious with live virus and a person who is recently vaccinated can transmit the virus to other areas of the body, which causes lesions to form. Severe side effects are high and include neurological reactions such as encephalitis.

Alternatives to the Standard Vaccination Schedule

Practitioners are increasingly confronted with patients who diverge from the standard vaccine protocol, preferring to vaccinate selectively or not at all.

No Vaccinations

There are many families who have decided to not vaccinate their children at all. Most have seriously considered the risks and benefits of no vaccines. For most, the benefit of not vaccinating is the simple fact that their child will avoid having a vaccine reaction. On the other hand, their children are more susceptible to getting these diseases, and it would be naïve to take the "it won't happen to us" attitude. The truth is, it is possible for any child, even vaccinated ones, to succumb to a serious infectious illness. If you are considering not vaccinating your child, it is important to familiarize yourself ahead of time with the symptoms of the illnesses and options for treatment.

Selective Vaccination

If you are considering selective vaccination, you have multiple options available for delaying or reducing the number of shots your child receives.

- Begin the shot later. Many parents are choosing to start vaccinating at a later age, often at six months or, for some, after one year when the baby's immune system is stronger.
- Choose shots carefully. Inform yourself about which illnesses your child is at risk for, and at what ages. This helps you decide which vaccines are higher on your list. Often families at low risk for hepatitis B will often postpone the hepatitis B vaccine during infancy. The Hib meningitis and pertussis (which comes as DTaP) is often recommended at least during the first year by many pediatricians.
- Allow time in between the shots, stagger the shots, and give one at a time. This avoids overloading the body at one time. By waiting, it also allows the body to recover in between the shots, and may minimize vaccine reactions. This is especially important with the MMR vaccine.

The National Vaccine Information Center also offers guideline questions for determining the timing and type of vaccination schedule best for your family:

- Is my child sick right now? If she is ill, defer the shot until she is better.
- Has my child had a bad reaction to a vaccination before?
- Does my child have a personal or family history of:
    1. vaccine reactions
    2. convulsions or neurological disorders
    3. severe allergies
    4. immune system disorders
- Do I know if my child is at high risk of reacting?
- Do I have full information on the vaccine's side effects?
- Do I know how to identify a vaccine reaction?
- Do I know how to report a vaccine reaction?
- Do I know the vaccine manufacturer's name and lot number?

Homeopathic Vaccines (Nosodes)

With increased public attention to vaccine safety, many of my patients express interest in homeopathic vaccines, called *nosodes*. Nosodes are homeopathic remedies made from the same bacteria and viruses as the vaccines. They are taken by mouth, and have no preservatives, chemicals, or mercury. We as yet have no concrete research or data suggesting that homeopathic microdoses of diphtheria, tetanus, or measles will protect your child.

Travel Vaccinations

In addition to the standard vaccination schedule for children, many shots are recommended for travel in exotic places. Travel is beyond the scope of this book. However, many people come to my office in search of homeopathic and natural alternatives to these shots for the family. We have, as of yet, no formal studies or data suggesting that homeopathic microdoses of hepatitis A, typhoid, malaria, yellow fever, salmonella typhi, and others can prevent these conditions. Most people still prefer to try these preventive remedies in lieu of not doing any form of prevention. Most report excellent success on their voyages.

The Safe Shot Strategy

As physicians, most of my colleagues and I take very seriously our oath to "first do no harm." Most physicians, however, also firmly believe in the success of the vaccine program, making them less likely to acknowledge that their routine shots could do harm. While vaccine reactions cause concern in the medical community, vaccine-related symptoms often go underreported, since they can occur not only immediately following shot but also days and weeks afterward. The longer the time that passes between vaccine and reaction, the less likely your doctor will connect the cause with the effect.

In my own practice, I find I am more cognizant of the variety of ways vaccine reactions can manifest and less tolerant of the pain and discomfort they cause infants and children. Since becoming a holistic physician, my standards have changed as well as the tools I use to treat vaccine-related problems. For instance, I received a phone call from a distraught mother who complained that her nine-month-old boy had been crying constantly for seven days and nights since he received his round of shots. Her pediatrician had gently reassured her that the discomfort would pass and told her to give him ibuprofen in the interim. I saw them in the office, where he was given homeopathic *Chamomilla* 200C for extreme fussiness and irritability. By the next day, the extreme state lifted, and both mother and baby were able to resume their usual daily activities.

Reactions can occur following a vaccination. Those that happen immediately after a shot can include:

- Allergic Reactions (hives, shock)
- Shock, collapse
- High-pitched screaming (persistent crying)
- High temperature
- Excessive sleepiness
- Convulsions
- Inflammation at the site of the shot

Certain conditions may be tied to vaccines, and these may be delayed by days to weeks. The longer the time between a reaction and a shot, the more unlikely your doctor will make the association. In general, most doctors will not consider cause and effect when it comes to vaccines. Taylor, a healthy school aged boy received a set of vaccinations while he had a slight cold. Within two days he was hospitalized in the intensive care unit for pneumonia and a serious blood infection. During the hospital stay, the group of specialists never once mentioned the possibility of a vaccine reaction to the parents. The parents were convinced that their son's serious illness was the result of the vaccines several days prior and tried to discuss this with the boy's doctors, who immediately dismissed the possibility. Delayed side effects could include:

- Blood conditions (hemorrhaging, idiopathic thrombocytopenic purpura)
- Encephalitis (inflammation of the brain)
- Attention deficit disorder
- Learning disorders
- Developmental delays
- Multiple sclerosis
- Arthritis
- Neurological conditions

- Guillain-Barre syndrome (a probable autoimmune disease that attacks healthy tissue. It presents with progressive muscle weakness and can cause paralysis of the legs, arms, breathing muscles, and face. The paralysis can be temporary. GBS can occur following infections, surgery, and immunizations.
- Convulsions
- Diabetes mellitus
- Spastic colon
- Pharyngitis
- Otitis media (ear infections)
- SIDS (for more information, see the SIDS section in Chapter 5)
- Upper respiratory tract infection

To help prevent reactions like these, I recommend parents adopt a safe shot strategy, which means educating themselves on the vaccine, the disease it immunizes against, and the possible side effects of the shot. The safe shot strategy involves four steps:

1. Know your child's vaccination schedule. Identify the shot(s) that are coming up.
2. Familiarize yourself with the disease the vaccination is designed for. What is the disease? What are its complications? How common is it? What is the chance of your child contracting it?
3. Inform yourself about the vaccine. What are the risks associated with it?
4. Monitor your child's health closely both before and after the shot. Contact your physician if your child shows signs of agitation, discomfort, or serious illness. If your child has chronic conditions that might affect his or her immune response, talk to your practitioner before the vaccination.

If you decide to vaccinate, you will want to be sure your child is in good health. For scheduling any vaccination, I encourage the "wait until better" approach. If your child is currently sick or has been recently (in the past two weeks), wait until better. If your child is cranky, fussy or not herself, this may mean that she could be getting sick: wait until better. If your child has been on antibiotics, wait at least six weeks until getting a shot. Antibiotics weaken the immune system and it is not uncommon that children become sick soon after. Wait until better.

For children who suffer from chronic conditions such as allergies, skin conditions like eczema, or recurrent ear infections, I believe it is best to treat these underlying conditions with holistic medicine before vaccinating. Holistic medicine such as homeopathy, will help strengthen your child's constitution prior to getting a shot, lessening the chance that the vaccine could exacerbate the preexisting condition. Unfortunately, so many children live with chronic problems now that we also need to consider the possibility that the condition has been caused by or connected to previous shots.

Typically, your doctor will recommend acetaminophen before the vaccine. Because medications like acetaminophen suppress symptoms, however, they make it difficult to choose a proper remedy if there is any type of reaction. There are several alternative remedies you can use to prevent reactions, which are discussed in detail in *Vaccine Safety* in Part IV.

SUMMARY

Vaccinations—for decades the proud standard of medical advancement—are no longer immune to controversy. In recent years, concerns about vaccine injuries, mercury toxicity, and autism have increased. In accordance with the law and the various exemptions that each state permits, I strongly support a "pro-informed-choice" attitude about vaccinations. Some of my patients fully vaccinate to schedule, some not at all, and others vaccinate selectively, depending upon the risks and benefits of each vaccine.

THE IMMUNE SYSTEM

Over thousands of years, the immune system has evolved to help protect the body. When germs encounter the body, the immune system responds in multiple ways to protect it. The strength of your child's immune system determines whether or not she will get sick when exposed to germs. With a vaccination, a bacteria or virus is injected into the body and the body responds by producing antibodies with the goal of defending the person from attacks of the same bacterium or virus in the future.

PROS AND CONS OF VACCINATIONS

Among the benefits of vaccinations:

1. National vaccination programs are responsible for eradicating some of the most devastating illnesses of the past centuries, including polio, diphtheria, and smallpox.
2. Side effects and risks of vaccinations are rare.
3. Children who are not immunized can raise the risk of infection for everyone else.

Among the criticisms of vaccinations:

1. Like any medication, every vaccine has the risk of injury or death. In addition, pharmaceutical companies add antibiotics, preservatives, and toxic disinfectants to vaccines.
2. Vaccination is different than natural immunity, thus circumventing the body's natural defense mechanism, and may cause a chronic imbalance in the immune system.
3. Increased use of vaccines corresponds to a rise in chronic diseases among children.

STANDARD VACCINATIONS

Vaccines are compulsory in the United States, and follow a protocol established by the Centers for Disease Control. However, exemptions do exist for philosophical, medical, and religious reasons. The standard vaccination schedule, with recommended ages for each vaccine, is as follows:

Hepatitis B: birth, 1 to 2 months, 4 months, 6 to 18 months
Polio: 2 months, 4 months, 6 to 18 months, 4 to 6 years
Diphtheria, Tetanus , and Pertussis (DTaP): 2 months, 4 months, 6 months, 15 to 18 months, 4 to 6 years old
Haemophilus influenzae type b (Hib): 2 months, 4 months, 6 months, 12 to 15 months
Pneumococcal: 2 months, 4 months, 6 months,12 to 15 months
Measles, Mumps, and Rubella (MMR): 12 to 15 months, 4 to 6 years old
Chickenpox (Varicella): 12 to 15 months
Influenza: Every autumn 6 months and older

ALTERNATIVES TO THE STANDARD VACCINATION SCHEDULE

No Vaccinations: If you are considering not vaccinating your child, it is important to familiarize yourself ahead of time with the symptoms of the illnesses and options for treatment.

Selective Vaccinations: You may want to begin shots later than recommended, stagger shots, or choose only shots for those illnesses for which your child is most at risk.

Homeopathic Vaccines: Homeopathic vaccines, called *nosodes*, are made from the same bacteria and viruses as the vaccines, and have no preservatives, chemicals, or mercury. However, we as yet have no concrete research or data suggesting that they are effective.

THE SAFE SHOT STRATEGY

To help prevent bad reactions to vaccines, I recommend a safe shot strategy, which involves four steps:

1. Know your child's vaccination schedule.
2. Familiarize yourself with the disease the vaccination is designed for.
3. Inform yourself about the vaccine and its possible risks.
4. Monitor your child's health closely both before and after the shot.

Before scheduling any vaccination, I encourage the "wait until better" approach. If your child is currently sick or has been recently (in the past two weeks), wait until better. If your child has been on antibiotics, wait at least six weeks until getting a shot. If your child suffers from a chronic condition like allergies or recurrent ear infections, treat these conditions with holistic medicine before vaccinating. Also, keep remedies close at hand to prevent and treat any vaccine reactions.

chapter 15

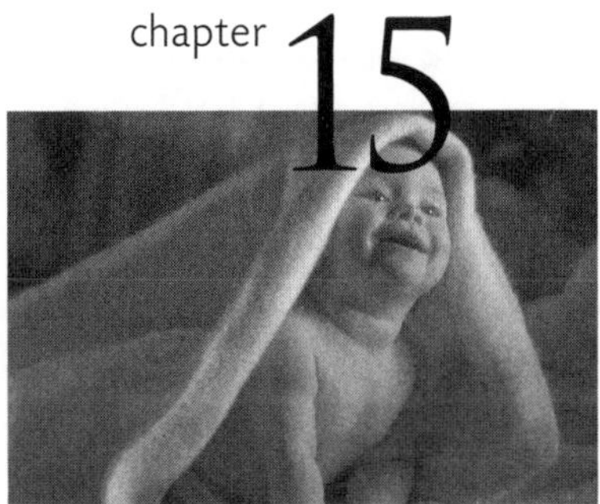

Bonding, Mind, and Spirit

Since philosophy shows us how to live, and since children need the art as well as adults, why don't we teach it to them at an early hour?

The Spiritual Life of Children: The Philosophy of Childhood

Other sections of this book have focused primarily on health of the physical body, on treating and preventing various aches and ailments and nurturing all the innumerable parts that make up your child's corporeal self. No comprehensive understanding of health, however, can exclude the intangible realms of the spirit—the emotions, imagination, curiosity, and wonder. This chapter addresses your child's inner world or soul, which need no less nourishment than the physical body. For my thoughts on the inner lives of children I am eternally grateful to the philosopher Mervyn Brady—the depth of his knowledge and understanding has taught me to be a better human being, physician, and mother. In his workshops, he instructs parents how to tend and cultivate the inner world of their children and I draw from his wisdom throughout this chapter.

Many religions and spiritual practices conceive of the soul as the divine aspect of the self; permanent and insubstantial, the soul is often imagined dwelling in the temple of the body, housed and protected by the physical self. Just as the body takes in food, air, and water in order to subsist, so the soul is fed by impressions from the surrounding world—from those sensory elements that prompt us to marvel, enjoy, and explore. Our physical selves feed and nurture our spiritual selves, just as spirit can inspire, heal, and protect the body. The scent of a perfume, the melody of a lullaby, or a memorable sunset all feed your child's inner word, and suggest that the body, the five senses, and soul are all connected.

Many adults despair about being consumed by life's responsibilities and not taking the time to "smell the roses." Ben Franklin once wrote about a friend who died when he was twenty-five, and was buried fifty years later. He was referring to this friend's inner world, whose flame had gone out at a young age, yet the body did not die until years later. How do we assure that our children's souls remain richly satisfied? Is the soul something that can be remembered or forgotten in the tasks of day-to-day living? Spiritual practices teach adults to appreciate their "child-like" inner selves, and we can also help ensure that our children stay in touch with the moments of wonder, excitement, and newness that nurture their imaginations and feed their souls. At birth, a baby is born with little distinction between body and soul. She is filled with a curiosity, intrigue, and enthusiasm at once spiritual and physical—everything is open to discovery; everything is new. These are exciting years, which also render her vulnerable to the elements and she must be supervised closely. By age three, your child experiences her world in increasingly physical ways, testing the limits of her body—and often the limits of her parents' patience, too. At this age the roots of personality begin to grow and the body starts to occupy a more prominent place than the soul. As your child gains in agility and mental and emotional maturity, her personality has blossomed. By the age of seven, much of the foundation is established.

As the first caretakers to our children, we can begin to plant seeds to help ensure their healthy inner lives as well as outer bodies. Childhood is the time when these seeds can find fertile soil, flourishing in ways that will profoundly impact one's life path. A great deal is possible in early childhood, since the span of time we spend as children is, relatively speaking, much longer than the number of years would suggest. Instead of looking at lifespan as a chronological succession of years, we might view it logarithmically, divided in three equal parts: 10 months (gestation), 100 months (childhood), and 1000 months (maturity). Gestation, which lasts ten lunar months, represents the phenomenal period of growth that occurs in the womb after the egg and sperm unite and begin to rapidly divide, eventually forming a human being. The second period, childhood, spans the 100 months following conception, and corresponds to approximately age seven when the personality is formed. The period of maturity begins at around age seven and lasts until death. It represents a time to develop and establish one's talents, vocations, and spiritual viewpoint.

According to this scale, life is divided into thirds. Although childhood here is seen as approximately seven years' duration, it encompasses one third of a human being's life. These are the years when reason and conceptual thinking are activated; from approximately four to seven years old, your child's intellect will grow by leaps and bounds as she learns to read, write, and use numbers for measuring abstract concepts like time and distance. During this period, many cultures also place emphasis on rituals of initiation; for Catholic children, this is the time when they take their First Holy Communion. Both modern psychology and many ancient schools believe that the years prior to age seven form the basic building blocks of your child's emotional life, prompting the truism, "If you give us a child before he is seven, we have him for life."

Many of us recognize that time seemed to move more slowly when we were children; once we become adults, the years "fly by," as the saying goes. The philosopher Rodney Collin explains this phenomenon by comparing the logarithmic scale of development with a spinning top. If the top spins for thirty seconds, it initially spins quickly, gradually slowing down until it finally falls over still. The thirty seconds represent one's life in years, while the revolutions symbolize the amount of work and energy accomplished by most individuals—more occurs developmentally in the first half of life than the second. To a child, life goes by a relatively slow pace, and the days are filled by new information and impression. While many of us adults are fixed in our habits, children possess a seemingly endless capacity to absorb life lessons, soaking up knowledge like sponges and remembering this information often for a lifetime.

What a Parent Can Do

Childhood imaginations are fed by attention, and it is essential to become intentional in creating "soul moments" for your children. Special time with your child assures her that her inner life is just as important as her other accomplishments, and that she is wonderful just being herself. Personally, I remember waking up early with my dad before he went to work as a medical resident in the hospital. While he was shaving, I would sit up on the bathroom counter looking in the mirror as we both applied Old Spice aftershave to our faces. Memories like these remind me of the magic bond shared by parents and children, especially when we are present and open to each other.

Take some special time every day to be with your child, away from life's hustle and bustle. Allow your child to glimpse your inner world, and invite her to share hers. Apart from all of our errands and chores, it is vital to spend quality time with your child—no matter the age. During these moments, try looking into your child's left eye; tradition maintains that the left eye is where the soul is situated, and by making a conscious effort to connect with your child, you can maximize the time you spend together. Many of these moments can be created when there is change, an unusual occurrence or shift in routine that allows for a creative venture or new activity. It is important to break patterns periodically, as routine tends to put both children and adult souls to sleep. This past New Year's Eve while my husband was working, my boys and I went to their first Korean barbeque restaurant. They enjoyed using the grill at the table and tasting all the special sauces. Instead of racing to get home as midnight approached, I pulled over and we rung in the New Year in the car, all shouting the twenty-second countdown with loads of giggles. Be creative. By giving your children simple, special times that break from the norm, you are feeding their soul and yours. Being around children gives an adult an opportunity to experience a bit of childhood, although from a different vantage point. Many parents cherish special moments of inspiration they receive from their children. One day, when I was driving my then-eight-year-old son Étienne to school, he turned to me and said, "Stars are the homes of angels. The Sun is the home of God."

In teaching children about values, ethics and respect, many families choose various paths. Through religion, families attend church, synagogue or other organized settings together while others prefer a more individual approach that inspires children through nature, cultural traditions and personal beliefs. Celebrations with rituals that mark the rite of passage, such as the Jewish Bar Mitzvah, as well as seasonal festivals, and holidays, both secular and religious, provide yearly familiar images that are meant to instruct and warm the spirit. Blessings, often adopted from American Indian traditions, which celebrate a girl's passage into womanhood (or other milestones) are becoming popular. Family participation helps mark these special occasions for children. I have fond memories of celebrating Thanksgiving at my grandparents' home which was commemorated by the lighting of a beautiful candle in the shape of a turkey.

The Arts: Fairy Tales, Music, and Math

Throughout school, our children are rigorously trained to separate fact from fiction, privilege reason over intuition, and achieve logically rather than imaginatively. While this education prepares them for the responsibilities of adolescence and adulthood, it often fails to fully nurture their capacities for creativity and wonder. Reading, and particularly reading fairy tales, offers an important means of cultivating imagination and "magical" thinking in children. Fairy tales are meant to entertain and also instruct by tapping into a child's deepest desires and fears about the world around her. They are a child's version of myth, helping to explain a phenomenon, experience, or event, and to educate them about themes of life, death, conflict and renewal. These stories are not meant to be read literally or to be interpreted by the intellect. Instead, they are intended for the inner world.

Originally oral forms, fairy tales have been passed down through generations, preserved by Hans Christian Andersen, the Brothers Grimm, and, yes, even Disney. Before the television and video generation, children's inner worlds relied on biblical, folk, and fairy stories for entertainment. The philosopher Plato recommended that children begin their education by reciting fairy tales and myths rather than pure facts. Tales, Plato recognized, are a form of learning particularly suited to a child's mind. Many fairy tales begin with "Once upon a time, long long ago . . . ," a phrase which invites your child to leave the ordinary world of concrete thinking and enter another reality—the world that speaks to the soul. Fairy tales achieve their magic by making use of several important narrative techniques: allegory, fable, parable, and metaphor.

- An allegory is a story that offers a deeper meaning beyond the literal narrative on the surface. Fables and parables are considered simple allegories.
- In a fable, the main characters are typically animals depicted with human qualities and engaged in difficult or improbable conflicts. Fables usually end with a moral lesson meant to teach, for example, about the shortcomings of vanity, the value of hard work, or a similarly communal message. The stories of the ancient Greek writer Aesop are

still some of our most well-known fables. Examples of his tales passed down from oral traditions include the *Fox and the Crow* and the *Tortoise and the Hare.*

- A parable is similar to a fable in that both are allegories; however, a parable narrates events that are possible. Parables are short stories that instruct us by presenting parallels; we are meant to draw connections between the actions of the characters and those of ourselves. In the New Testament, Jesus often taught in parables.
- Metaphors are a crucial element in storytelling, and allow us to draw comparisons between two unlike objects. "All the world's a stage," a popular line of Shakespeare's, demonstrates how metaphor works: the mind is required to forge a connection between the concepts of world and stage, to understand how they relate not concretely, but suggestively. This cognitive skill is crucial for children's abstract thinking and cognitive development.

Over the centuries such writers as Charles Perrault (Mother Goose), the Grimm Brothers, Hans Christian Andersen, and Lewis Carroll compiled fairy tales from oral tradition, or wrote classic stories of their own. They have largely defined the European fairy tale tradition, but children's stories also come from all around the world and all different cultures. Two of my favorites are the African tale called *The Lion Whiskers* and the French story of *Reynard the Fox.*

In addition to children's literature, art forms such as music, dance, drama, painting, sculpture, and crafts can play an important role in your child's emotional health and cognitive growth. Sadly, the arts in many schools suffer from lack of funding, meaning fewer available programs and a greater responsibility on parents to expose their children to music, drawing, and other activities. Cuts to school arts programs are short-sighted, since creative tasks are not a "break" from real education, but fundamental to a child's developing intellect. Studies have shown that children who play a musical instrument have improved reading, math, and standardized (SAT) scores, and studying music and playing an instrument also teaches children about focus, concentration, coordination, and working closely with others. As the ancients demonstrated centuries ago, music is also closely connected to math. The philosopher and mathematician Pythagoras showed that musical intervals can be expressed mathematically, and many philosophers since have looked for the larger harmonies between the planets and the stars, "the music of the spheres." In the Middle Ages, music was studied along with arithmetic, geometry, and astronomy as part of the *quadrivium.* Realistically, however, not all children respond well to music. It may be not be the right timing, type of class, or teacher. As a toddler, my son Étienne was sensitive to noise and did not enjoy going to music class. After several years' hiatus, I encouraged him to try piano lessons and he has enjoyed playing piano ever since.

Popular Culture, Recreation, and Creative Play

Playtime and Toys

Playtime is not simply free time for children; it constitutes an important means of learning social dynamics, solving problems, stretching the imagination, and developing cognitive skills. Playing is a "job" for children, though fortunately one most of them love and can work at for hours. One of the tools of playtime are toys—those objects that are transformed almost magically from inanimate wood, plastic, or fabric into something living and vital. But while a child can turn almost anything into a toy, most are drawn to the gadgets they see on television and at their friends' houses: toys are often more interesting when they belong to someone else.

The trick for any parent is to choose toys that appeal to your child, but which are also safe, stimulating, and long-lasting. Considerations in selecting toys include factors such as safety, enjoyment, interest, durability, noise, and ease in operation, and whether they encourage solo versus interactive play, educational opportunities, challenging thought, and creativity. For safety purposes, avoid sharp edges, small chokeable parts, and strings longer than eight inches. In general, I find handmade wooden toys last and keep their interest longer than the plastic, electronic "toys of the moment." These I call the junk toys: like their junk food counterparts, they are often more gimmick than substance, with battery-operated parts, bright plastic casings, and immense marketing campaigns. After the initial excitement wears off, junk toys quickly end up collecting dust; no one can convince a child that a toy from last year is "cool" once a more interesting one has come along.

Many of these commercial toys are backed by millions of dollars in marketing, as manufacturers make use of our children's increasing consumer savvy. Often, junk toys and junk food are marketed together on billboards, print ads, and television commercials, and grouped in order to encourage multiple purchases—a single character can be seen in the movie, star in a book, be included as a McDonald's play toy (with the kids' meal), and appear on clothing. So what's wrong with these toys? Isn't a toy simply a toy? Like foods that are low in nutritional substance, certain toys are low in education and intellectual substance. They may look good and seem exciting, but they offer very little challenge to your child's imagination. Particularly for boys, toys also frequently glamorize violence, going beyond fake guns and action figures to high-tech video games, paintball games, and elaborate war-oriented toy sets, complete with blood-stained playhouses.

But while parents can try to shield their children as much as possible from these overtly violent games, children tend to naturally gravitate toward certain activities, sometimes to their parents' dismay. One couple recently complained that their three-year-old son goes around "shooting" a stick as if it were a toy gun, an object that has never entered the house. You may never be able to change what your child is fascinated by, but you can change the ways they work through and explore those fascinations. Junk toys also come with a hefty price tag that exceeds their actual cost in dollars and cents. Most are manufactured by children and adults laboring in sweatshops overseas, and the excess packaging and the petroleum-based plastics add to environmental pollution.

Often, the most simple toys or objects are the most interesting. One of my two-year-old patients adores his mother's soup ladle and takes it with him on outings, including to the doctor. Encourage your child to similarly "make" toys for herself from safe household objects; you would be surprised what she comes up with left to her own imagination. When buying a toy, consider its appropriateness and whether it matches the age, temperament, and skill of the child. High-energy children benefit from physically demanding toys like balls and bikes. Other children respond to art projects, books, and puzzles. Likewise it is important to encourage your child to try all sorts of activities, physical and sedentary, social and solitary. A child who is more timid may learn to interact more comfortably with others by playing a game that requires participation, while a social child will benefit from spending time on his own, working on a project that requires greater concentration. But be assured that your child will let you know what is enjoyable and appropriate for her. I thought my boys would enjoy a play kitchen so they could "cook" alongside dad while he prepared our meals. I soon learned that the real thing was of more interest, and our kitchen now resides in my office.

Around age two, most children go through a phase where they are unwilling to share toys; any attempt to play with, take, or restrict a child from her favorites can result in quick tears. Fortunately, children outgrow this phase, but while it goes on, you will want to plan ahead for guests, playmates, and other company. If you anticipate a toy tantrum, you and your child may select a toy that she is willing to share, while putting away treasured objects before the guest arrives. Children will also undoubtedly be given toys you wouldn't normally buy for them. When my son was three, well-meaning friends brought him a plastic fire truck equipped with lights and a siren—his first battery-operated toy. Within minutes it was out of the package and rolling around much to my son's joy. What could I say? Childhood is a receiving period—and kids love to get gifts as much as adults enjoy giving them.

Television and Video Games

As I mentioned earlier, just as the body needs to be nourished, so does your child's inner world. Her soul is fed on impressions which is taken in from the five senses and is important for emotional health and intellectual development. We spend much time and care in an effort to provide healthy nutritious meals for our children. Why not do the same for their inner world? I have seen that as my children get older, they are more exposed to junk food as well as junk impressions—such as certain programs on television, movies and on video games. I realize that some of this is inevitable, but as much as I can, I like to provide them with healthier impressions such as reading a good book, playing a game, or being out in nature. For additional information, see "Television and Video Games" in Chapter 8.

Nature-Deficit Disorder

The astronomic rise in attention deficit disorder, hyperactivity, autism, learning disabilities, and similar conditions in children presents one the greatest health concerns of the new century. While parents and health professionals are beginning to look to environment degradation, vaccines, and toxins as potential causes, others suggest a broader cultural source to the problem. The journalist Richard Louv published *Last Child in the Woods: Saving Our Children from Nature-Deficit Disorder* (2008) in which he coins the term *nature-deficit disorder* to describe the myriad of ways modern life and entertainment alienates and isolates children from the natural environment.

As children spend more time in front of the television or playing video games, they spend less time in outside exploring the world. Wonder at the complexity of nature is replaced by technology, which is impersonal and can negatively affect motivation, social integration, and compassion. Louv believes that nature-deficit disorder is linked to a plethora of ADD-like illnesses as well as the rise in obesity in our children, and recommends that parents encourage imaginary play in a natural environment instead of the latest video game distraction. Many child experts are starting to agree with Louv regarding the inundation of technology and the ramifications for our children. Even if you live in a large city, you can heed his advice by finding the nearest park, walking path, or community garden, by planning a picnic or hike, or by simply planting seeds in pots and watching them grow. As we have become more unrbanized, we are less in touch with the natural environment. Many programs in schools and throughout cities are encouraging children and their families to become involved in recycling, clean-ups, and volunteer efforts meant to raise the awareness about the environment in which we live locally and globally. Growing plants and gardening teaches children vital lessons about ecology, communal responsibility, and environmental sustainability.

Extracurricular Activities

Due to the financial crises our schools are experiencing, many art and sports programs are among the first cut from school programs. In an effort to compensate, parents enroll their children in all types of after-school programs that include sports, music, and arts and crafts. Many children also participate in the scout programs that begin early in grammar school and goes up through high school. It is a wonderful opportunity for children to have a broad education. However, sometimes children are so over-scheduled, and begin to experience the same feelings an adult would who is stressed out and overwhelmed with having too much to do. As parents, it is important for us to monitor our children's commitments, and achieve a healthy balance.

Family Activities

As a working mother, I make it a priority to carve out extra time with my children and to make that time count. Spending time together promotes family values which is important in nurturing a child's intellectual and emotional health. Although not always practical with everyone's busy schedules, eating a meal together is a wonderful way to spend time together. Without too much extra planning, many quality moments can also include physical activity which is healthy for everyone—they might be as simple as taking a walk, playing Frisbee, or visiting the zoo. The canyons by Los Angeles, for instance, are full of lovely trails where kids can feed the ducks. From urban to rural living, every place holds the opportunity for families to explore together. Having a family pet can also play a special role in a child's life. In addition to providing companionship, having a pet can teach a child about responsibility, respect, and care.

Adoption, Assisted Reproduction Technology, and the Changing Family

As reproductive technology continues to advance and adoption becomes an increasingly mainstream choice, more couples are choosing less traditional paths to parenthood. Older couples and same-sex couples are finding success with fertility assisted reproduction, including the use of donor eggs and sperm and surrogate mothers, while the notion of adoption has broadened to include assisted reproduction technology (ART)—the adoption of eggs and embryos. Mixed-race households are more commonplace, as are children who are not genetically related to either parent. The make-up of the American family is changing, but neither adoption nor fertility assistance means that bonding will be any less intense between child and parent. The hormonal and physiological transformations that occur during pregnancy promote bonding, but even more vital is the parenting that follows.

As more people make use of ART, questions about identity and heredity become more central to family life. Parents face the decision of how and when to tell their child about his or her genetic background, and children, particularly of adoption, may or may not want to eventually locate their birth parents. Feelings of abandonment, separation, or anxiety are not uncommon feelings in children who have been adopted, whether they have been informed or not. It is important to have resources available for parents and child to help cope. Homeopaths and other practitioners of alternative medicine have had success easing children and parents through this difficult transition period. Keep in mind that while heredity and family history play an important role in one's health, personality, and development, so, too, does good parenting. I once heard a parent tell her adopted child, "You came from my heart, not my tummy." The reminder is a vital one for all parents: our love for our children encompasses more than biology; it is the most basic expression of our hearts.

The advancements in reproductive technology are astounding, but not without side effects and risks, including the enlargement of the ovaries, thinning of the uterine lining, and more. I encourage couples to try a holistic medicinal and nutritional approach prior to fertility treatments; many parents have had success becoming pregnant through Chinese medicine, homeopathy, and naturopathy, and in this way avoid the invasive and at times risky new medical procedures.

SUMMARY

THE SPIRITUAL LIFE OF CHILDREN: THE PHILOSOPHY OF CHILDHOOD

Many religions and spiritual practices conceive of the soul as the divine aspect of the self. Just as the body takes in food, air, and water in order to subsist, so the soul is fed by impressions from the surrounding world. As the first caretakers to our children, we can begin to plant seeds to help ensure their healthy inner lives as well as outer bodies.

Childhood imaginations are fed by attention, and it is essential to become intentional in creating "soul moments" for your children. Special time and rituals with your child assures her that her inner life is just as important as her other accomplishments.

In teaching children about values, ethics and respect, many families choose various paths. Through religion, families attend church, synagogue or other organized settings together while others prefer a more individual approach that inspires children through nature, cultural traditions and personal beliefs.

THE ARTS: FAIRY TALES, MUSIC, AND MATH

Fairy tales are meant to entertain and also instruct by tapping into a child's deepest desires and fears about the world around her. In addition to children's literature, art forms such as music, dance, drama, painting, sculpture, and crafts can play an important role in your child's emotional health and cognitive growth. Studies have shown that children who play a musical instrument have improved reading, math, and standardized (SAT) scores, and studying music and playing an instrument also teaches children about focus, concentration, coordination, and working closely with others.

POPULAR CULTURE, RECREATION, AND CREATIVE PLAY

Playtime is not simply free time for children; it constitutes an important means of learning social dynamics, solving problems, stretching the imagination, and developing cognitive skills. Considerations in selecting toys include factors such as safety, enjoyment, interest, durability, noise, and ease in operation. When buying a toy, consider its appropriateness and whether it matches the age, temperament, and skill of the child. Likewise it is important to encourage your child to try all sorts of activities, physical and sedentary, social and solitary.

As children spend more time in front of the television or playing video games, they spend less time outside exploring the world. You cannot and should not ban the TV or video games, but monitor what your children are watching and playing and encourage them also to play in a natural environment. Even if you live in a large city, you can find the nearest park, walking path, or community garden, plan a picnic or hike, or grow plants. In addition, you may want to enroll your child in extracurricular programs including sports, music, and arts and crafts or schedule family activities like walks with the pets, visits to the zoo, or making dinner. However, be careful not to overschedule your child.

ADOPTION, ASSISTED REPRODUCTION TECHNOLOGY, AND THE CHANGING FAMILY

Adoption and assisted reproduction technology is becoming increasingly mainstream. This does not mean that bonding will be any less intense between child and parent.

Feelings of abandonment, separation, or anxiety are not uncommon feelings in children who have been adopted. It is important to have resources available for parents and child to help cope.

Advancements in reproductive technology are astounding, but not without side effects and risks. I encourage couples to try a holistic medicinal and nutritional approach prior to fertility treatments; many parents have had success becoming pregnant through Chinese medicine, homeopathy, osteopathy, and naturopathy and in this way avoid the invasive and at times risky new medical procedures.

PART IV

A to Z Guide to Common Childhood Conditions

> The secret of health for both mind and body is not to mourn for the past, not to worry about the future, or not to anticipate troubles, but to live the present moment wisely and earnestly.
>
> *–Buddha*

IN THIS SECTION, YOU'LL FIND A LIST OF COMMON childhood conditions, from the common cold to ear infections to nosebleeds. These are minor self-limiting illnesses that usually do not require a practitioner's attention. The natural treatment of severe illnesses or chronic diseases like eczema, chronic allergies, attention deficit disorder , and asthma requires the expertise of a professional.

Each entry describes conventional treatments for the condition, and gives some suggestions for homeopathic and other natural remedies that may work either as alternatives or complements to the standard treatment. In order to prescribe the correct treatment for your child, don't forget to go through the "case-taking" process described in Chapter 9 to review your child's symptoms methodically (including both subjective and objective observations), assess the situation logically, and take appropriate action. This will help you (and your child) stay composed during a stressful time, and will also help your practitioner if you need to call on one. I am reminded of the quote by Teresa of Avila who wrote, "To worry over our health will not increase our health. This I know." Parents have commented to me that being able to use remedies at home and offer relief to their sick children was very satisfying compared to the alternative of waiting and worrying until the child is sick enough to go to the doctor. I encourage you to start to use remedies if you have not already, and bring this book and remedies with you if you travel, even overnight! One day someone will be glad that you did.

Unless otherwise noted, the dosing and application information for each remedy follows the guidelines outlined in Chapter 9:

Homeopathic Medicine: Homeopathic medicines for home use are available in a variety of potencies from 6 (6X or 6C) to 30 (30X or 30C); 30C is my preference as it does not need to be repeated as frequently. For children and adults take three pellets (or quick dissolve tablets) up to three times a day dissolved under the tongue. In acute cases, take every hour until relieved, or as directed by your practitioner. If you see no improvement after three doses, discontinue the remedy. For infants, place three pellets in ½ glass of water. Let stand for five minutes. Stir ten times. If you are using the hard pellets, they will not dissolve, but the water becomes medicated. Give ¼ teaspoon (can be placed in a dropper) of the medicated liquid to equal one dose. Avoid eating or drinking 10 minutes before or after taking the remedy. When possible avoid touching the medicine. See "Administering Homeopathic Medicines" in Chapter 9 for more details.

Gemmotherapy: The dosage for infants is 5 to 8 drops. Give children ages 2 to 8 years old 12 to 15 drops, and older children and adults, 25 drops. The remedies can be used as often as 2 to 3 times per day during acute illness. Give the drops mixed in water or juice. When possible, avoid eating for five minutes before and after.

ACNE

Adolescence can be a trying period as our children move into young adulthood. To compound the self-esteem issues, many suffer with blemishes on the face. Cystic acne in teenagers is caused by inflammation and clogging of the oil ducts. Common acne is not as deep, but can nevertheless be bothersome to teens. Unfortunately, both commonly occur on the face, but can occur on other places including the chest, back, and neck.

Care and Treatment

Conventional Treatment

Standard medical treatments for acne includes topical medications, antibiotics, and Accutane. Many parents are concerned about the host of side effects especially with Accutane that include birth defects (if taken during pregnancy), depression, anxiety, and irritability.

Homeopathic Medicine

Acne can be treated successfully with homeopathy, nutrition and other forms of alternative medicine. Please see a practitioner who can prescribe an individualized form of treatment.

Gemmotherapy

Oriental Plane Tree is a good general remedy known for its treatment of acne.

European Walnut can also be given if there are deep cysts and pustules.

ALLERGIES AND ALLERGIC REACTIONS

See *Hay Fever and Seasonal Allergies, Hives and Allergic Reactions, Poison Ivy, Poison Oak, and Poison Sumac, Stuffed Nose,* and *Stomachache.*

ANXIETY

While acute episodes of anxiety are common to both adults and children, the condition seems to be on the rise, especially among kids. Recent research indicates that chronic anxiety can affect as many as ten percent of children, and studies comparing schoolchildren in the 1950s to the 1980s report that anxiety levels have substantially increased. Anxiety is defined as an overwhelming sense of apprehension, uneasiness of mind, and fear. From agoraphobia to claustrophobia and panic, anxieties vary in both cause and symptoms, and may be accompanied by sweating, a rapid pulse, restlessness, or feelings of paralysis. If your child is suffering from severe anxiety or panic attacks, see a practitioner for a complete exam.

Causes and Types of Anxiety

According to the National Mental Health Association, the most common anxiety conditions in children are:

Generalized anxiety is typified by the child who worries about everything, including events that occurred in the past, present and future. This can include such worries as health (personal or family), anticipation of upcoming events, and competence.

Separation anxiety comes on when the child is away from home or parents.

Social phobia is more common in teens and revolves around performance and social situations.

Obsessive-Compulsive Disorder (OCD) characterizes a child who has uncontrollable obsessions and compulsions. A common behavior is frequent hand-washing accompanied by a fear of germs.

Post-Traumatic Stress Disorder (PTSD) can result from traumatic events such as an earthquake, abuse, or disaster.

Care and Treatment

Emotionally supporting your child during an anxious period is of utmost importance. Remember that while you may not understand the cause or dimensions of your child's anxiety, the emotion is intense and real for her and she will want you to listen and respond compassionately. When the complaints begin to interrupt sleep or daily activities, consider additional measures for relief.

Conventional Treatment

Standard treatment usually begins with counseling. More severe cases of anxiety are treated with psychotherapy, behavior modification and even medications, such as antianxiety and antidepressants. Many parents resist giving their children medications that have side effects, and prefer to begin with a more natural approach. Homeopathic remedies work well for alleviating acute anxiety, as well as offering long-term relief for chronic suffering and emotional distress.

Homeopathic Medicines

Aconitum napellus is useful for relieving feelings of anxiety and panic stemming from an accident, a fright, or a shocking event. Indications for *Aconite* are nervousness, agitation, a fast heartbeat, and sudden onset of symptoms. In Los Angeles during the 1994 earthquake, it is said that all the local homeopathic pharmacies sold out of *Aconite.*

Argentum nitricum is recommended for anxiety before a test, performance, or event, and is thus a good remedy for stage fright. Other indications for this remedy include fear of heights as well as a sense of claustrophobia that is relieved in cool open air away from crowds. Anxieties about arriving late also respond well to *Argentum nitricum*. The child may feel rushed, warm all the time, bloated in the tummy, and have a desire for sweets.

Arsenicum album is indicated for anxiety accompanied by restlessness and the desire for company. Worries can vary, from the fear of getting into an accident in the car to a fixation with locking the doors in the home at night to prevent intruders, and may include a tendency to obsessive compulsive reactions. The child tends to be chilly and is worse at midnight.

Gelsemium is recommended for fear that manifests as trembling, fright, and anticipatory anxiety. Along with anxiety may be fatigue, diarrhea, and dizziness. *Gelsemium* is also good for stage fright and is well known as a remedy for flu symptoms.

Ignatia amara is the main remedy for loss, sorrow and grief. Indications include a nervous headache, a sensation of a lump in the throat, numbness, intermittent sighing, and uncontrollable weeping.

Kali phosphoricum helps alleviate feelings of nervousness, stress, and exhaustion after hearing about bad news or world catastrophe. Indications for *Kali phosphoricum* are oversensitivity, inability to sleep, and lack of inclination to work or finish chores. This remedy is useful when feeling as if one's "nerves are at end."

Silica is useful when your child is fearful of having a shot or blood drawn, and has particular anxiety about pointed objects or pins. Using *Silica* prior to the event can help ease the tension. *Silica* is also useful for test phobia when there is over concern about small details.

Gemmotherapy

Lime Tree, a gemmotherapy remedy, is known for its calming influences and is equally beneficial for children and adults.

Bach Flower Essences

Rescue Remedy is excellent for stressful and anxious times. Place 2 drops in a glass of water and sip.

APPENDICITIS

See *Stomachache.*

ASTHMA

Asthma and other problems with difficulty breathing can be life threatening and require a practitioner's care. All of my patients with asthma and lung conditions have inhalers and other standard forms of treatment available to them. In addition, the use of homeopathy, gemmotherapy, and other forms of natural medicine can greatly improve a child's breathing. As a result, patients are less likely to be dependent on prescription medicine. See your practitioner for the treatment of conditions such as asthma and wheezing. But for children whose asthma comes with a cough, some simple remedies may help. See *Cough.*

BEE STINGS

See *Insect Bites and Stings* and *Hives and Allergic Reactions.*

BLADDER INFECTIONS

Bladder infections, also known as cystitis or urinary tract infections (UTI), can involve any part of the urinary system, including the urethra, bladder, ureters, and kidneys. They are more common in girls than boys (5 percent and 1 percent respectively), and many doctors believe these percentages an underestimation, given the number of UTIs that go undetected.

A bladder infection occurs when the bacteria begins to grow in the urinary system, eventually infecting the urine. Repeated UTIs in children may be due to a congenital abnormality in the urinary tract, or to constipation, in which case the stool pushes up against the bladder, making it more difficult to empty the urine. Certain children are more prone to bladder infections, just as others are to ear infections, and parents can take the measures listed below to effectively cut down on the frequency and severity of childhood UTIs.

Symptoms of UTIs can include lower abdominal pain, pain or burning with urination, frequent urination, strong smelling or foul smelling urine, and a sense of urgency with urination. A UTI in an infant or toddler can easily go undetected because it may be accompanied by nausea, vomiting, fussiness, and lack of appetite (in other words, the common symptoms of many infections). Fevers do not usually accompany a bladder infection unless it is severe, and at that point it has probably progressed to the kidneys. Other indicators of a kidney infection are pain in the back, under the rib cage, or in the side. If you suspect your child may have a UTI, it is best to visit your practitioner.

Care and Treatment

Conventional Treatment

In standard medicine, UTIs are treated with antibiotics. If your child has had several UTIs, your doctor may order additional tests to look for any abnormalities in the urinary tract. It is not uncommon for children to be placed on a daily-low dose antibiotic regime for six to twelve months for recurrent UTIs. At the onset of uncomplicated mild symptoms, many parents prefer to begin with a natural approach towards treatment, and many times, families are able to treat the infection without having to resort to antibiotics.

Prevention and Home Treatment

To prevent and to treat bladder infections naturally:

- Make sure your child drinks plenty of liquids, especially cranberry juice (without added sugar). Cranberry is known for its antibacterial properties, which helps fight off bladder infections by adhering to the lining of the bladder. The important ingredient in cranberry juice is a carbohydrate called mannose.
- Try D-Mannose, a nutritional supplement. Mannose is also found in peaches and apples, and is considered safe for young children. Take ½ teaspoon once or twice a day, or as per instructions on the bottle.
- Give your child foods rich in Vitamin C. If taking a supplement, give 150 mg/day.
- Place a hot water bottle on the lower abdomen and back
- Use onion poultice socks overnight (see *Cold*).
- Use clean underwear and avoid synthetic fabrics and tight pants.
- Teach girls to wipe from front to back when using the toilet.
- Avoid irritating products, especially the commercial soaps, shampoos, and bubble baths.
- Bathe in warm baths.
- As always, if symptoms persist or worsen see your doctor immediately.

Homeopathic Medicines

Apis mellifica is indicated for burning, stinging, and soreness in the urethra and while urinating. The child feels better in a cool bath. There can be a desire to urinate frequently, but the urine comes out in scanty amounts, drop by drop. The urine smells foul and can be bloody or milky in appearance. The child is not thirsty.

Cantharis is one of most common remedies to use for acute bladder infections as well as kidney infections. The indications for *Cantharis* is severe burning during urination, however the child may also experience burning before and after. Each drop of urine passes as if it were scalding water, and the child has a constant desire to urinate. There can be large amounts of blood in the urine, and the child's mood is anxious and agitated.

Sarsaparilla is recommended for the frequent urge to urinate, with burning pain at the end of urination often causing the child to scream out. The child may need to stand in order to urinate, though there can be dribbling while sitting.

Staphysagria helps in bladder infections accompanied by the frequent urge to urinate and a sensation of urine dripping in the urethra. Burning sensations in the urethra may persist when the child has not urinated as well. *Staphysagria* is indicated for children who experience bladder infections following sexual abuse or who have a tendency towards suppressing their emotions, especially anger.

Gemmotherapy Remedies

Wineberry and **Black Honeysuckle** are gemmotherapy remedies indicated for the urinary tract and bladder infections.

BOILS

A boil, known as a skin abscess, is a localized, pus-filled inflammation located deep in the skin. It often begins in a hair follicle. Commonly caused by the bacteria Staphylococcus aureus, boils occur on the buttocks, thighs, groin, face, neck, and armpits. A cluster of boils joined together with one or more openings is known as a carbuncle (or furuncle). This may be accompanied by fever or chills.

In general, symptoms usually begin with redness, tenderness, and a lump. The area is warm to touch. The lump hardens followed by a softening in the middle as the boil fills with pus and blood—which contains white blood cells, part of the body's immune response to the infection. With time, it comes to a head.

Children can become susceptible to boils from scratching the skin or a prick injury, which exposes the body to bacteria. Normally, the bacteria live on the skin without a problem. Boils can heal on their own or may enlarge, becoming filled with pus and uncomfortable for the child. When they become too full, they burst, drain, and then heal. **If a boil is getting bigger and the pus is not draining on its own, visit your practitioner; it may need to be lanced (cut open and drained). See your practitioner for boils that persist more than two weeks, recur, and are**

accompanied with fever. Due to vulnerable locations, boils in the middle of the face or near the spine also require medical attention.

Care and Treatment

Conventional Treatment

Boils that do not heal on their own may need to be lanced by a medical practitioner. According to the *Pediatric Infectious Disease Journal*, antibiotics are not necessary in children who have a boil that is adequately drained and dressed by a physician.

Home Treatment

Apply warm compresses, as they encourage the boil to come to a head. Place the warm, moist cloth on the boil several times a day. Keep the area clean, and avoid squeezing the area to prevent infection. In addition:

Add ***Calendula* mother tincture** to warm water or chamomile tea to use for the warm, moist compress. Use 1 part Calendula to 4 parts liquid.

Onion poultices and **raw potato slices** help draw a boil to a head, and speed healing. Place raw potato slices directly on affected area and wrap area with cheese cloth.

Take **Vitamin C** to help treat infection. Give your child foods rich in Vitamin C. If taking a supplement give 150 mg/day.

Homeopathic Medicines

Hepar sulphuris is indicated for skin conditions with a tendency to become infected, such as a boil or abscess. The area is red, swollen, and exquisitely tender to touch. *Hepar sulphuris* can be used in the early stages as well as after pus has begun to form. The discharges and pus smell offensive. Typically, the areas are slow to heal. The child is chilly and sensitive to cold and drafts, and is better with warmth.

Mercurius is for boils that tend to spread and become ulcers. The child perspires easily, and salivates excessively with bad breath. She is worse at night and sensitive to both extreme heat and cold. She craves bread and butter and has an aversion to sweets.

Silica, known as the "homeopathic surgeon," has the power to push out foreign substances from the body. *Silica* is known to help drain pus from abscesses, expel splinters, and help break down scar tissue. It is indicated for boils and abscesses in which the pus smells foul. The child may be timid and sensitive, yet willful and obstinate, and a fear pointed objects like pins. *Silica* should not be taken by people who have a history of tuberculosis. The child is better with warmth and worse in the cold.

Sulphur is indicated for children whose skin easily becomes infected after every little scratch. The skin is slow to heal and is sore after the boil has burst. There can be a yellow, bad-smelling discharge and the skin is oily. *Sulphur* is also indicated for recurrent boils. Other indications for *Sulphur* include dry skin and itching made worse from bathing, warmth, and while in bed. There is a characteristic general aggravation of symptoms in the child at 11 A.M. known as a homeopathic centrifuge, *Sulphur* drives toxins from the interior of the body to the surface, usually the skin. For this reason, if you are using *Sulphur*, use in a low potency, 6C or 6X, and employ conservatively and slowly.

Gemmotherapy

Briar Rose helps strengthen your child's immune system during times of infection.

European Walnut is useful for boils and all types of deep-seated infections.

BROKEN BONES

See *Injuries.*

BRONCHITIS

See *Cough.*

BRUISES

See *Injuries*.

BURNS

Burns are one of the most common household injuries in children, leading to nearly 100,000 visits to the emergency room in the United States each year. Most burns are preventable, and most occur in children less than age four. Burns can result from sun exposure, fire, household appliances (irons), chemicals, electricity, and child abuse, though the most common burn in younger children is scalding, or wet burn, caused by contact with hot liquids. Commonly a toddler reaches up and knocks over a cup of hot coffee or a pot of boiling water.

Burns are categorized by the severity of the injury. First-degree burns are the most superficial and mild. A common first-degree burn is the mild sunburn where the burn is limited to the outer layer of the skin. The skin looks red and can be painful. Second-degree burns, or partial thickness burns, are more serious and include blisters on the skin. They are more painful than first-degrees, and the skin can be weepy or moist, taking up to six days to heal. Second-degree burns often require medical treatment, and usually heal within three weeks. Even more severe is a third-degree burn, a full thickness burn. Here all the layers of the skin have been destroyed, including the nerve endings, which may numb the affected area. The skin is white, charred, and leathery. Depending upon the extent of the burn, your child may go into shock. Third-degree burns may require surgery and skin grafting. A fourth-degree burn is so severe that it has damaged the underlying bone or muscle.

Call your health practitioner for moderate to severe first- and second-degree burns that are painful or weepy. Third- and fourth-degree burns require immediate hospitalization.

Care and Treatment

Prevention

To prevent burns, keep hot food, liquid, candles, and matches out of the reach of your child. Keep cooking handles inwards to avoid being grabbed. Run a bath with the cold water first. For tips on preventing sunburns, see the section on "Sun Safety" in Chapter 10.

First Aid Treatment

First aid treatment is intended to provide pain relief, clean the area, avoid infection, and encourage healing. Your first attention should focus on cooling the burn. For mild first- and second-degree burns, soak the affected area in cool running water or lightly cover with a cool, moist cloth for 10 to 15 minutes. For more severe burns, keep re-soaking or spraying the area with water until you reach the hospital. Do not break blisters. Do not place butter or ice to the burn. Although you can gently remove clothing around the burn, do not remove any clothing that is stuck to the skin.

For mild burns that do not require medical attention, clean with soap and water, soak, and keep open to the air when possible. Cover mild burns if there is difficulty keeping the area clean or free from rubbing. When using bandages, apply ointment or salve and use a sterile non-adhesive bandage that will easily come off. For more questions about dressing changes, contact your practitioner.

Conventional Treatment

In the practitioner's office, the standard treatments for burns are Silvadene or Bacitracin, both antimicrobial ointments. More severe burns may require cleaning and debridement (removing the tissue around the burn) and frequent trips to the practitioner for dressing changes. Pain medication may also be prescribed, along with tetanus shots for children with severe burns.

Homeopathic Medicines

Natural and homeopathic remedies may be used in conjunction with standard treatments for all mild and severe burns.

Apis mellifica can be used for first-degree burns that are red, puffy, painful, and better with cold applications.

Cantharis is useful for burns with rawness, smarting, and severe burning pain. There is restlessness with the pain and relief with cold applications. It is useful for burns from scalds and electrical exposure.

Causticum is also indicated for old burns that are not healing. The person benefiting from *Causticum* may say before taking the remedy, "I've never been well since the burn."

Phosphorus can be useful for electrical burns (including lightening) and burns from x-rays. For electrical burns, seek medical attention.

Urtica urens is indicated for first- and second-degree burns and scalds (including the tincture applied topically in 1:4 dilution). The child may complain of severe burning and itching.

Herbal Remedies

Aloe vera, the succulent plant, is soothing and therapeutic as a topical remedy for sunburns, first-degree burns, and minor second-degree burns with unbroken skin. The gel can be used directly from the plant (preferable) or from commercial preparations. If you are unable to use the plant, aloe is available as a gel, spray, lotion, liquid, cream, or juice. Be sure to look for a commercial topical preparation containing at least 20% aloe vera. If your child is able to bathe, consider preparing a bath of lukewarm water and 1 to 2 cups of aloe vera juice.

Calendula officinalis is an excellent topical for sunburns and second degree burns where the skin has opened. It works as an antiseptic and astringent and helps soothes the pain. As a topical, *Calendula* is available as a cream, gel, tincture, spray, and ointment. After washing the area, dilute *Calendula* tincture in 1:4 dilution with water and soak affected area.

St. John's wort (Hypericum perforatum), well known for healing nerve injuries, can be soothing as a topical treatment for minor burns that are painful and can be prepared in the same manner as *Calendula.*

CANKER SORES

See *Mouth Sores.*

CHICKENPOX (VARICELLA)

The chickenpox virus is part of the herpes family, similar to shingles (herpes zoster). It is considered a mild disease in childhood, but becomes more severe in adults. Chickenpox is highly contagious. Half of the cases of chickenpox occur in children from ages five to nine. Symptoms of chickenpox include fever and runny nose, followed by an intensely itchy rash that crusts over within two to three days. The rash appears in crops on the body and sometimes in the mouth. It is usually extremely itchy and uncomfortable. The disease lasts two to three weeks.

The most common complication is a secondary bacterial skin infection. More severe but very rare problems include encephalitis, septicemia, and osteomyelitis. **Contact your practitioner if your child's condition worsens.**

Care and Treatment

Prevention

The conventional approach is to vaccinate which is up to 85% effective in preventing the disease, albeit only for several years following the shot.

Some parents are eager for their children to get chickenpox, which renders the child immune for life. Chickenpox parties are gatherings which parents deliberately expose their children to chickenpox have been commonplace over the years. For more information about the vaccine, see Chapter 14.

Conventional Treatment

Mainstream medicine uses calamine, caladryl lotion, and acyclovir, an antiviral medicine.

Home Treatment

An oatmeal bath can be very soothing. See *Hives and Allergic Reactions* for more information. *Calendula officinalis* is useful for infected pox. Dilute *Calendula* tincture in 1:4 dilution with water and apply to affected area.

Homeopathic Medicines

Antimonium crudum is for stinging, thick hard honey-colored scabs that itch. The rash feels worse with warmth, and at night in bed. The child is in an irritable mood and does not want to be touched.

Antimonium tartaricum is useful when the eruption gradually is appearing. The crusty rash leaves a bluish red mark. Known as a strong bronchitis remedy, *Antimonium tartaricum.* is also indicated when there is rattling of mucus in the chest and a cough, not uncommon with chickenpox.

Pulsatilla is also used for chickenpox when the rash is crusty, burning, and itching. There can also be cold symptoms with yellow-green mucus. Typically, the child feels worse in a warm stuffy room and better in open air. The mood is weepy and emotional.

Ranunculus bulbosa is more commonly used for shingles (also of the Herpes family). I include this remedy here, because while I was writing this book, both my children had chickenpox, my 6th grader worse than his younger brother. *Ranunculus bulbosus* was the remedy that greatly helped his discomfort. This remedy is called for when the rash itches and burns with shooting pains.

Rhus toxicodendron is the most common remedy used for chickenpox. This rash is intensely itchy, and the child feels better in a hot bath. They can be fidgety from the itching, and often worse at night.

Sulphur is for a chickenpox rash that is moist, itchy and annoying. The pox takes a long time to heal. Worse with bathing, at night, and with the warmth of the bed.

Gemmotherapy

Briar Rose is indicated for strengthening the immune system

Hedge Maple and **English Elm** are specific for the treatment of herpes.

CIRCUMCISION

See *Surgery.*

COLD SORES

Common among both adults and children, cold sores, or fever blisters, are caused by the herpes simplex type 1 virus. Often confused with canker sores, which occur inside the mouth, cold sore blisters appear mostly on the border of the lip, and less often on the nose, chin, and other parts of the skin. Often outbreaks are heralded by tingling, itching, or burning, then the blisters form, burst open, crust, and eventually heal. Children can experience swollen glands, malaise, and low-grade fever with the outbreak. Cold sores are contagious during the first four days, and can last up to ten days.

Unlike canker sores, cold sores are caused by a virus and can be passed from person to person. Other herpes viruses include herpes zoster (chickenpox and shingles) and herpes simplex virus type 2 (genital herpes). Outbreaks only occur from a flare-up of a previous herpes infection, which means that children will not show blisters the first time they are infected with the herpes virus. Approximately twenty percent of five-years-olds are affected, and eighty percent of adults. Once infected, the virus can remain dormant for long periods of time. Outbreaks can be triggered from the sun, colds, illness, fever, stress, weakened immune system, fatigue, extreme temperature exposures, allergies, and around the menstrual cycle. **See your practitioner if the lesion is extremely painful or appears infected.**

Care and Treatment

Conventional Treatment

Standard treatments focus on relieving pain through the use of topical anesthetics and oral or topical antiviral medications. Do not use corticosteroid creams on cold sores. The American Academy of Pediatrics' Committee on Infectious Diseases recommends that children with cold sores cover the affected area with a bandage when going to school. Many parents prefer to avoid antivirals in children as they only suppress the condition and have side effects including nausea, vomiting, diarrhea, or headache.

Home Treatment

During an outbreak eat healthfully and eliminate nuts, seeds, chocolate, carob, raisins, grains, and dairy, all of which are high in L-arginine, an amino acid known to trigger the viral replication. Instead, choose foods high in the amino acid lysine, which possesses antiviral properties and interferes with arginine metabolism in the body. Foods high in lysine include fish, cheese, chicken, lima beans, potatoes, milk, soy, and brewer's yeast. Topically, use Vitamin E as an anti-inflammatory or *Calendula* ointment, an antiseptic, to help to soothe and heal cold sores.

Recurrent cases of cold sores are best treated with professional homeopathic treatments, which can strengthen your child's constitution, reduce the frequency and severity of outbreaks and shorten their course.

Homeopathic Medicines

Mercurius is indicated for yellow-colored blisters accompanied by excessive drooling, sweating, and sensitivity to hot and cold temperatures.

Natrium muriaticum is the most common remedy used for cold sores on the lips. The outbreaks are painful and triggered by emotional stress, illness, and exposure to the sun. There can be a craving for salty foods.

Rhus toxicodendron is indicated for small blisters which contain yellow fluid. They burn and itch. The child is restless and feels better with warm applications.

Sepia works well for cold sores that breakout on the lower lip. There can be cracking of the lip in the middle or at the corners. Outbreaks can occur in relation to a girl's period, and may be accompanied by a craving for vinegar or sour foods.

Gemmotherapy

Briar Rose is indicated for herpes infections and strengthening the immune system

Hedge Maple and **English Elm** are specific for the treatment of herpes infections.

COLIC

Colic is defined by periods of crying, fussiness and discomfort that last longer than three hours a day and are not caused by any discernible medical condition. However long your baby cries, it can feel like hours, and hence colic puts great emotional strain on both parents and baby. Most people use the term *colic* interchangeably with fussiness that stems from discomfort in the belly. Symptoms of colic can include abdominal pain, gas, distention, burping, spitting up, constipation, and diarrhea. It usually presents from approximately three weeks old and dissipates by three to four months old. The cause of colic is unknown.

After endless sleepless nights, the midnight drives around the neighborhood attempting to comfort a distressed baby, and trying "everything under the sun" without success, numerous parents end up in my office willing to try the natural and homeopathic approach. Homeopathy can be effective in alleviating the symptoms of colic, particularly when paired with some of the comforting techniques outlined below. **Contact your practitioner if the condition persists or is accompanied by frequent vomiting or weight loss.**

Care and Treatment

Standard medical treatment for colic includes general soothing and carrying measures, smaller more frequent meals, and use of a pacifier. Medications like Simethicone may be prescribed to relieve gas pains.

Home Treatment

Comfort: Offer comfort to your baby by carrying, wearing, swaddling, and breastfeeding.

Nursing mother's diet: Try avoiding foods that may aggravate the condition, particularly those that other family members are sensitive to. Common culprits include dairy, wheat, eggs, peanuts, citrus, alcohol, coffee, spices, onion, garlic, broccoli, cauliflower, brussels sprouts, green peppers, grapes, and strawberries.

Hot water bottle: If your baby is relieved with warmth, try a wrapped hot water bottle (warm, not hot) on the tummy.

Infant massage: Daily massage may be helpful in preventing or minimizing conditions such as colic. (See the section on "Infant and Child Massage" in Chapter 9.)

Homeopathic Medicines

Aethusa is useful when a baby shows the colicky symptoms of milk intolerance, e.g., when she vomits large curds of milk. She can be weak and sweaty. The child's personality is reserved, she does not look happy, and appears to be in anguish. She may demonstrate a love for animals.

Bryonia is recommended for the infant who is irritable and does not want to be carried. She is worse with movement and touch and tends toward constipation.

Chamomilla is for the "impossible, cranky, irritable" baby who moves about in agony. She cries one minute for something and then pushes it away the next. Both baby and parents are miserable, though baby feels better when carried. Notably, one cheek is often red and the other pale. Stools can be green, slimy, and smell like rotten eggs.

Colocynthis should be considered for severe colic. The baby screams with gas pains and is doubled over. The pain is better with firm pressure on the tummy.

Lycopodium clavatum is indicated for babies who are irritable and constipated. The belly rumbles loudly, is full of gas, and feels relief with massage. Baby's belly gets bloated after feeding, and is uncomfortable with a snug diaper or clothing around the waist. The child is typically worse from 4 P.M. to 8 P.M.

Magnesia phosphorica is used when relief is brought on by gentle abdominal pressure, rubbing, and bending double. The baby also feels better with warmth on the belly.

Nux vomica is good for a fussy baby who is angry, irritable, and sensitive to noise and light. She is worse at 3 to 4 A.M. She does not want to be touched, and when she gets angry she arches her back. Colic symptoms are usually accompanied by constipation and straining.

Pulsatilla is for the affectionate baby who is irritable, weepy, and clingy. Her belly can become bloated and she may have diarrhea. She feels better in the open air and worse in a warm enclosed room.

Herbal Remedies

Gripe water is a European herbal remedy preparation that is helpful for colic. Use as directed by the manufacturer.

COMMON COLD

Colds are the most common reason for doctor visits and account for the majority of sick days taken from school and work. They are caused by a nose virus, which is responsible for those familiar symptoms like congestion, sneezing, tearing of the eyes, sore throat, and in some cases coughing. They usually last one to two weeks. Often a runny nose begins with clear drainage and changes color as the cold matures. Contrary to popular thought, yellow-green mucous is not necessarily an indication for an antibiotic. According to the Minnesota Antibiotic Resistance Collaborative, "Color changes in nasal mucous are a good sign that your body is fighting the virus."

Colds can occur any time of the year, though are more abundant during the flu season from November to March. At times it may be difficult to ascertain if your child has the cold or the flu, since they can present similarly, particularly in the early stages. High fever, muscle aches and pains, weakness, and exhaustion are more characteristic of the flu. Both viruses can cause coughs. Younger children can get as many as seven colds a year, occurring less frequently as their immune system develops with age. **See your practitioner if your child's condition deteriorates, has a fever of 103° for more than three days, or if your child exhibits any problem with breathing such as wheezing.**

Care and Treatment

Conventional Treatment

Because colds are caused by viruses they should not be treated with antibiotics which are for bacterial infections. Practitioners prescribe antibiotics for secondary bacterial infections such as ear infections, sinus infections or pneumonia. Unfortunately, the overuse of antibiotics has led to antibiotic resistance in many infections. Standard medications include antihistamines, decongestants, expectorants, and cough suppressants. Although these medications may provide temporary relief, they are not without side effects. Antihistamines cause drowsiness and dry mouth while decongestants may act like a stimulant. Suppressing the cough interferes with the body's way of clearing the lungs, and these medications should be used sparingly. For preventative measures, see *Flu* entry.

Home Treatment

Hydrogen peroxide, known for germicial properties has been shown to be helpful at the onset of symptoms. Place 4 drops of hydrogen peroxide (3%) into both ears. See *Natural Essentials* in Part V.

Onion. Onion improves circulations and breaks up thick mucus and congestion, making it a great remedy for colds. It helps soften lymph nodes, soothing painful swollen glands in the neck. For colds, an onion pouch in a child's room can help with congestion. Using a cloth or sock, make an onion pouch, securely tied. Place near the child on the nightstand, by the bed, or above the crib, and leave it overnight. You can also use sliced onion: simply place one to two slices on a plate by the bed.

For chest colds, place an onion poultice on the chest and wrap with a scarf. Onion poultices can also be applied to the feet by way of onion socks. To make one, put the prepared onion in a small pouch and place the securely tied poultice in a sock. Fit the sock on your child's foot, so that the pouch stays securely in place on the sole of her foot. Let your child sleep overnight with the onion sock. For swollen glands, place a cloth envelope of chopped onion over the swollen glands and wrap with a scarf. In addition to treating colds, onion poultice socks can be used for earaches, teething, and bladder infections.

Lemon. Like its neat, segmental structure, the lemon's role is to organize and rearrange the conditions necessary to speed healing. Lemon is good for tickle in the throat or chest (tickly cough), watery runny nose or eyes (opposite of onion which is good for thick discharges), sore throat, and high fevers. Lemon can be applied as a throat wrap, throat and chest compresses (line up the lemons in a cloth), foot bath, and room inhalation.

Potatoes. Potatoes draw out toxins and break up congestion, which makes them useful in alleviating sore throats, coughs, headaches, neckache, muscle pain, and chilliness. Potatoes poultices around throat and chest are an excellent source for moist heat and retain temperature longer than a hot water bottle.

Homeopathic Medicines

Aconitum napellus is used in the early stages of an illness, often within hours after exposure to the cold and wind, at the sign of the "first shiver." *Aconite* is helpful for the sudden onset of intense symptoms that range from a profuse runny nose, chills, fever, flu and coughs to earaches and sore throat. The child is thirsty and restless with an anxious look on her face.

Allium cepa is for a watery runny nose that feels like a continuous "faucet of hot water," making it also a strong remedy for hay fever. The nose is red and irritated, and there can be sneezing with a tickle in the throat. The symptoms improve when the child is out of doors.

Arsenicum album is recommended when your child feels chilly and better with warmth. She is tired, fidgety, and anxious, and markedly worse from midnight to two A.M. (when everyone should be sleeping!). Cold symptoms tend to be more severe on the right side, and the runny nose is thin, watery, and irritating to the skin, yet at the same time the nose is stuffed. She may also have a burning sore throat, better with warm drinks.

Belladonna is also helpful during the early stages of colds that are accompanied by a sudden high fever, and sometimes hallucinations. A child who responds to *Belladonna* radiates heat and may have a flushed face and a throbbing feeling. She is hypersensitive to noise and touch, and has no thirst. Often, complaints are worse on the right side.

Chamomilla is well known as a colic and teething remedy, and is also useful for colds. A child who is in a "*Chamomilla* state" is obviously unhappy and uncomfortable—he may be very angry, irritable, impatient, and contrary. The child can be inconsolable, crying, screaming, and arching his or her back. The cold symptoms are watery, hot, runny nose that is also stuffed; the child has difficulty sleeping.

Ferrum phosphoricum is similar to *Belladonna* in that it is indicated when the child's face is flushed and the fever is accompanied by throbbing. But typically, the onset of fever is more gradual and symptoms are mild.

A cold is considered "ripe" when the mucous has become thick and colored. ***Hepar sulphuris*** is good for yellow-green mucous that is thick and creamy. Often there is a sore throat that feels sharp or splinter-like, and the glands are swollen. However, the child is chilly, wants to be covered, and is thirsty for warm drinks. Her mood is irritable, hypersensitive and difficult to get along with.

Mercurius is useful for a child who smells sick with foul breath. She is hurried, restless, and sweaty, and feels hot one minute, cold the next. The sore throat feels raw and burning, the nose will have with thick, runny, and irritating yellow-green mucus. Tonsils and glands can be swollen and tender.

Natrum muriaticum is indicated for colds that begin with sneezing and a copious egg-white discharge from the nose. This is followed by stuffed nose in which it is difficult to breathe, with loss of smell and taste. Sometimes a child may complain of a lump in the throat that makes it easier to swallow liquids than solids. *Natrum muriaticum* is also a good remedy for associated cold sores on the lips.

Pulsatilla is indicated when the mucous is of a creamy consistency ranging from pale yellow to green in color. The child is warm, wants to be undressed, and feels better in the open air. She prefers cold drinks but is not thirsty. The *Pulsatilla* mood is characteristically clingy and emotional, and the child enjoys company.

Herbal Remedies

Echinacea has gained popularity in recent years for its use in boosting the immune system and preventing infection. It has both antiviral and antibacterial properties. Some research studies have concluded that echinacea is not effective in treating children's colds while other studies have found positive outcomes. Despite the conflicting reports, many parents continue to give echinacea to their children and report that it lessens the number of colds.

If you give your child echinacea during the cold and flu season, use it for two weeks on and two weeks off (follow the dosage recommendations on the bottle of commercial brands of echinacea). Avoid using on a daily basis, as the body may become resistant to it. Side effects from echinacea are rare. As with any medicine, if your child experiences any adverse reactions, discontinue usage.

Gemmotherapy

Briar Rose is helpful for alleviating runny nose and congestion in children. It strengthens a child's immune system and works well for conditions involving ear, nose, throat, and sinuses. It is particularly useful for colds. I use this gemmo preventatively two to three times a week as needed during cold and flu season. During an illness, use twice a day.

Black Currant is an excellent remedy for strengthening the constitution during the winter months, especially for adults. It stimulates the adrenals and is good for stress and fatigue.

European Alder alleviates symptoms associated with the early onset of colds, including runny nose and sinus complaints.

Lithy Tree targets the lungs and restores pulmonary function. Lithy Tree is helpful for the coughs and bronchial spasms associated with colds, flus, and bronchitis.

See also *Flu*.

CONJUNCTIVITIS (PINKEYE)

Conjunctivitis (pinkeye) is a common complaint in babies and children and can be caused by a bacterium, virus, allergy, foreign body, blocked tear duct, or trauma. The term implies an inflammation of the conjunctiva (the mucous membrane that lines the inner surface of the eyelids and eyeball); when inflamed, the membrane appears pink. Both bacterial and viral infections are contagious.

See your practitioner for trauma and scratches to the eye, and conditions that do not improve after five days.

Causes or Types of Conjunctivitis

Bacterial or viral infection: Signs of a bacterial infection are redness with yellow and green discharge that can crust over. Lids can become swollen and it may infect one or both eyes. A viral infection usually affects both eyes. With viral infections, however, the eyes can be bloodshot, but there is little to no drainage. There may be a slight crust in the eyes upon awakening. Additional signs and symptoms include tearing, swelling and inflammation of the eyelids, and sensitivity to light. Eye drainage that accompanies cold symptoms may be the sign of a sinus infection.

Plugged tear ducts: Plugged tear ducts occur in six percent of all babies and can be a problem up to one year of age, affecting one or both eyes. By three to four weeks of age, a newborn's eyes begin to tear. Normally, tears drain from the tiny tear ducts located at the inside corners of the eyes into the nose. A thin membrane covers the duct, and usually opens after birth. The blockage occurs when the membrane fails to fully open, and tears become backed up. Persistent tearing is a common symptom of a blocked tear duct, and the condition can lead to infection with redness and discharge. Blockage can recur, though usually by six months of age the duct stays open.

Ophthalmia neonatorum: An infection of the eye in newborns contracted from an infected mother's birth canal. The sexually transmitted diseases gonorrhea and chlamydia are usually the cause. In most cases, an inflammation of the eyelid and cornea which appears within two or three days after birth. Gonorrhea has been known to cause blindness, conjunctivitis, and other infections. For more information, see "Tests and Procedures Following Birth" in Chapter 4.

Care and Treatment

Conventional Treatment

In standard medical practice, mild cases of blocked tear duct are given a wait-and-see approach, as most open on their own. Persistent or severe cases are treated with a minor office procedure using a wire probe, though some may require surgery. Bacterial eye infections are treated with compresses and antibiotic ointments. Allergy eye drops and saline solution are recommended for irritation from viruses and allergies.

Home Treatment

- Wash eye with cool water using washcloth three times a day.
- Place warm teabag compresses on each eye (Chamomile is a favorite).
- Administer euphrasia (Eyebright), commercially prepared eye drops, several times a day. Alternatively, homeopathic eye drops, such as Optique (Boiron) and Similisan, are commonly used.

- Eye massage for blocked tear ducts has been known to open the membrane. Locate the tear duct in the inner corner of each eye. Gently massage in an upward direction toward the nose for one minute. Do this several times per day.
- Don't forget about breastmilk. For generations, mothers have been known to squirt breastmilk in baby's eyes and nose. It works!

Homeopathic Medicines

Apis mellifica is known for conjunctivitis with great puffiness and redness of the eyelids. The eyes sting and burn, and the condition improves with cold compresses.

Argentum nitricum is strongly indicated for conjunctivitis in newborns. There is pus with thick, yellow, profuse discharge. Often, the eyelids are inflamed, with a thick crust. The child acts frightened, hurried, and prefers company, feeling relief in the cool air.

Belladonna is associated with acute, sudden onset of intense symptoms, including pink eye. The eyes are intensely bloodshot. Extreme heat, dilated pupils, and hypersensitivity to noise, light, and touch are characteristic of *Belladonna*. It is also considered a strong remedy for right-sided conditions.

Calcarea carbonica is indicated for pink eye and blocked tear ducts. The eyes are sensitive to light and tear in the open air. Babies and children who respond to *Calcarea carbonica* tend to be large, sweat easily, and are prone to constipation. They are also independent, stubborn, and can play on their own with deep concentration.

Pulsatilla is useful for pink eye with lots of thick, yellow-green discharge. The characteristic *Pulsatilla* mood is weepy, whiney, and clingy. The child may have a desire for open air and rich food (which can also make them feel worse). *Pulsatilla* is also indicated for blocked tear ducts in infants.

Silica is known to be helpful for infection of tear duct or blocked tear ducts in newborns. The *Silica* child may have a history of frequent colds and flu with swollen glands. The inflammation is often accompanied with sensitivity to light. This remedy is also useful for sties.

Gemmotherapy

Briar Rose is for all infections in children.

CONSTIPATION

Although we often equate constipation complaints with adults, it can be a problem for babies and children as well. Constipation occurs when your child has difficulty moving her bowels because the stool has become compacted, hard, and painful to pass. The condition may be accompanied by stomachaches, gas, bloating, a hard belly, cramps, blood in the stool, hard round pellets, foul-smelling stools, straining, sluggishness, and fussiness. The number of stools and frequency of elimination varies and is influenced by how your baby is fed. Your baby may poop daily, every few days, or up to weeks at a time. No fun for baby or family!

Typically, a newborn's first bowel movement, known as meconium, is dark green-black and sticky. A breastfed baby's stool has a soft consistency with a mustard seed appearance, and she will often poop several times a day. A formula-fed baby tends by contrast to have firmer, darker, and fewer stools a day comparatively. Once your baby begins to eat solid foods, her stools will change to become less soft and more formed, and can have an odor. She may also have fewer bowel movements, going from daily to every several days.

Constipation is rare in breastfed babies. However, some babies still have difficulty, straining and getting red in the face with soft stool. This is not necessarily considered "constipation." In general, constipation occurs more often in formula-fed babies: a recent change in brand, overly strong mixture, not enough fluids, the introduction of new foods, or a diet low in fiber can all contribute to hard stools. In breastfed babies, a mother's diet can impact bowel movements, and for all children, lack of activity, medications, emotional factors, and "holding on" following a previous painful bowel movement play a role in constipation. The latter in particular generates a vicious cycle that only complicates matters. **See your practitioner for chronic constipation, painful eliminations, and blood in the stool.**

Care and Treatment

Conventional Treatment

In addition to the home treatment below, practitioners prescribe baby laxatives, Karo syrup, mineral oil, and glycerin suppositories.

Home Treatment

Treatment of constipation usually begins with isolating the cause and avoiding it.

- If you use formula make sure you are preparing it with the correct amount of water. Foods such as rice, bread, bananas, and applesauce are more constipating. For babies eating solids, children, and nursing mothers, increase high-fiber foods such as fruits (plums, peaches, pears, apricots), vegetables (peas), whole grains, and prune juice.
- Encourage fluids to keep stools soft.
- While your baby is lying on her back, simultaneously move her legs in a circular pedaling motion.
- Try infant massage (see Chapter 9, "Infant and Child Massage").
- Encourage activity and exercise.

Homeopathic Medicines

Alumina is recommended for constipation in newborns. Sometimes, the child has no urge to defecate and the stool needs to be mechanically removed. Even a soft stool is passed with difficulty. The child is sluggish and craves dry food, potatoes, and rice. The mouth and anus are dry.

Bryonia is also indicated for constipation with dryness. The stools tend to be large, hard, and dry. The child may experience intense thirst. One of the keynotes for *Bryonia* is an irritable mood and the wish to remain still and not move.

Calcarea carbonica is indicated for constipation with no urge to eliminate. Often, the child is not uncomfortable from being constipated. The stool can be clay colored or sour smelling. The child may crave eggs, sweets, and indigestibles such as dirt. *Calcarea carbonica* is best for children who tend to be large and sweat easily. They are independent, stubborn and can play on their own with deep concentration. This has proven a good remedy for children who try to prevent having a bowel movement following a previous painful episode.

Nux vomica is used when the child strains to pass the stool and only small amounts are passed at a time. The stool is hard and painful, and the child is afraid to move her bowels. She can be chilly, with an irritable and impatient disposition. A desire for rich, spicy foods is common.

Silica is for constipation with no urge. The child has a tendency for a "bashful stool," in which the stool comes out and goes in while straining. The stool is hard and there is the feeling that there is more stool in the rectum. The child is sweaty, especially on the feet, and may crave sweets and eggs.

Gemmotherapy

Wineberry, a gemmotherapy, is good for the intestinal lining and calms the colon.

Rosemary, an important liver and gallbladder remedy, is also useful for constipation.

COUGH

Nearly every parent can recall waking up in the middle of the night to come to the aid of a coughing child. Although most coughs are self-limiting and gone in a few days, some can be disconcertingly severe and persistent. A cough is the body's way of clearing the lungs of mucus, fluid, and other irritants, and can be triggered from infections, lung conditions, irritants, acid reflux from the stomach, allergies, asthma, and nervous habits. Some kids keep on playing despite a cough, while others are prevented from sleeping and are sapped of energy. Remedies, medications, and home treatments can offer relief when the cough is interrupting sleep or interfering with daily activities and breathing. In addition to the variety of coughs that accompany colds and the flu, children can also suffer respiratory difficulty with other infections, including bronchiolitis, bronchitis, pneumonia, respiratory syncytial virus (RSV), croup, and whooping cough.

If your child has a severe cough or serious infection like whooping cough, consult your practitioner. Severe coughs can lead to dehydration, exhaustion, and difficulty breathing, which can be life-threatening. The following guidelines would also be reason to seek medical attention:

- Cough with fever higher than 103°F for more than three days (101°F for five days)

- Chest pain with cough
- Wheezing (whistling) and labored or difficult breathing

Causes or Types of Coughs

Asthma: Asthma can sometimes cause coughing, as well as wheezing and difficulty breathing. In my experience, the use of homeopathy, gemmotherapy, and other forms of natural medicine can greatly improve a child's breathing. See your health-care provider for the treatment of conditions such as asthma and wheezing.

Bronchiolitis and Respiratory Syncytial Virus (RSV): Bronchiolitis is an infection of the smaller air passages in the lungs, called the bronchioles. The infection affects infants (2 to 6 months of age) and is characterized by inflammation in the lower airways, leading to difficulty breathing. Most commonly, bronchiolitis results from the respiratory syncytial virus, known as RSV. RSV is also the most common cause of viral pneumonia in infants. Symptoms of RSV include fever, runny nose, severe cough, fussiness, poor appetite, vomiting, wheezing, and pauses in breathing (apnea). Bronchiolitis is more common in the winter and spring and in infants who are formula fed. Premature infants and multiple-birth babies are more susceptible, as well as those in daycare, those who are exposed to second-hand smoke, and those with older siblings in the home. Boys are more commonly affected than girls. Bronchiolitis is usually treatable at home with supportive therapy, suctioning of mucus, and breathing treatments as needed. RSV is the most common reason for the hospitalization of babies under one year of age. There are no conventional medications used to treat the virus, and antibiotics are ineffective as this is a viral infection.

Bronchitis: Bronchitis is an infection of the main large airways in the upper lungs (bronchi). Acute bronchitis can result from a variety of different infections, including the common cold, sinusitis, and tonsillitis, as well as from irritants such as dust, fumes, and smoke. In children, most cases of bronchitis are viral infections. Pneumonia is a complication of bronchitis. Symptoms of bronchitis include low-grade fever, chills, fatigue, muscle aches, sore throat, and usually a runny nose preceding the cough. The cough often begins dry and becomes more loose-sounding and productive as the illness progresses. The mucus is yellow-green and may be heard rattling in the chest and throat. In severe cases, the cough can cause gagging or vomiting. Bronchitis can last up to several weeks. Conventional treatment for bronchitis is supportive, including rest, liquids, steam, and cough medicine. Antibiotics would be ineffective for viral infections. See your practitioner if your child has difficulty breathing, a fever of 101°F for more than three days, or chest pains.

Croup (Laryngotracheobronchitis): Croup is caused by a virus, allergy, or inhaled foreign body, and most parents initially are unnerved simply by the sound of it. In the typical scenario, your child suddenly wakes up in the middle of the night with a barking seal-like or brassy cough. The barking sound is caused by swelling of the vocal cords in the larynx. Croup may begin suddenly or following a cold. When caused by a virus, it is contagious and more common in the autumn and winter months, and in children less than five years old. Symptoms are usually worse at night, and may include hoarseness and fever. The first two nights are usually the worst, and the illness lasts up to six days. In general, croup is not a medical emergency and is managed at home—often with a phone call to the practitioner for guidance and reassurance. However, if your child is having difficulty breathing as a result of narrowed breathing passages, seek immediate medical attention.

Pneumonia: An inflammation of the lungs in which the small air sacs fill with mucus, pus, and other fluids, pneumonia is classified according to location of the inflammation—either lobar (a lobe or section of the lung) or bronchial (patches throughout the lungs)—and can be due to infection or irritants. While pneumonia can occur any time of the year, it is worse in the winter and spring, affecting boys more than girls. Up to fifteen percent of children with respiratory infections also have pneumonia, which can follow a cough or cold. The usual confirming symptoms of pneumonia are cough, fever, and difficult or rapid breathing. Additional symptoms can include chills, lack of appetite, irritability, headache, chest pain, vomiting, and abdominal pain. Children with pneumonia look and act sick. Seek immediate medical attention if there are any signs of oxygen deprivation such as blue lips or face.

Symptoms of bacterial pneumonia in children include fatigue, productive cough, chest pain, lack of appetite, vomiting, and diarrhea. Antibiotics are the standard treatment for bacterial pneumonia, along with chest percussion and supportive therapies. Viral pneumonia, commonly caused by RSV, is differentiated by a slower involvement in the lungs. Wheezing is usually due to a viral chest cold, and the pneumonia is generally less contagious than the original cold virus that caused it. Walking pneumonia is a milder case in which your child is able to continue her daily activities and does not appear sickly.

Viral infection: Most coughs begin as a viral infection. Often described as a "productive" or dry cough, this cough feels "loose" and makes it easier for your child to bring up the phlegm. In general, younger children will not necessarily spit out the mucus. Most will cough up the phlegm and swallow it. If there is any mucus, it usually begins looking clear in appearance. As the illness matures, the mucus begins to change consistency and color. Over the years, the knee-jerk reaction to the appearance of yellow-green phlegm has been to administer antibiotics, though this tendency is waning due to the overuse of antibiotics and the resultant antibiotic resistance. Keep in mind that viral infections can be as colorful and yellow-green as bacterial infections.

Whooping cough, or pertussis: Whooping cough is caused by the bordetella pertussis bacterium. Within two weeks after the initial common cold symptoms, the cough becomes more severe, with fits of rapid, successive coughs followed by the characteristic long inspiration with a crowing sound or high-pitched whoop. Thick mucus builds up in the lungs, triggering the cough. Depending on the severity of the cough, a child may experience choking, gagging, and vomiting. In between attacks, the child looks normal. For severe prolonged coughs or if you suspect your child has whooping cough, see your practitioner. The pertussis vaccine is given as a part of the DTaP (diphtheria, tetanus, and acellular pertussis) series beginning at two months of age. For more information on whooping cough and the pertussis vaccine, see "Standard Vaccinations" in Chapter 14.

Care and Treatment

Conventional Treatment

Practitioners recommend cough suppressants if your child's cough is preventing sleep during the night, and decongestants if he also has a lot of congestion that interferes with breathing. Expectorants (guaifenesin) help to thin out thick phlegm in the chest, making it easier to bring up.

Whooping cough will usually last approximately six weeks no matter the treatment. Standard treatment includes rest and liquids. Your practitioner will prescribe an antibiotic such as erythromycin, as it is felt that the antibiotic renders your child less contagious. While it remains questionable whether the antibiotic changes the course of the illness, people are generally no longer considered contagious after the fifth day on antibiotics.

For croup, the conventional approach is to treat the fever with ibuprofen or acetaminophen. For severe cases, steroids and breathing treatments are given. Avoid any medication that would dry out the air passages, such as antihistamines or decongestants. Cough medications are usually not used, and antibiotics are of no value in viral infections. Home treatments include parental loving support, which will help calm and relax a frightened child. Mist from the cool night air or steam from a hot shower can often offer relief. When going outside, be sure to keep your child dressed warmly. Other than general home treatment of croup, standard medicine has little to offer for non-emergency cases.

Home Treatment

Poultices and external applications are excellent ways to alleviate the discomfort of a cough.

Onion: Onion helps to break up thick mucus and congestion. As a healing application, it is both versatile and effective: try placing raw slices on a plate near your child's bed, in a chest poultice, or in socks to wear overnight.

Lemon: Lemon is good for watery, thin discharges, tickly coughs, and bronchitis. It can be used as a steam inhalation, warm chest compress, or a throat wrap. Placing lemon slices near a radiator will help disperse oils throughout a room.

Potato: A potato poultice on the chest can help break up congestion in the lungs.

Homeopathic Medicines

Aconitum napellus is useful at the onset of many types of cough. *Aconite* is also helpful for sudden attacks of croup at the beginning stages. Often arising after the child has been playing outside on a cool windy afternoon, the cough is of a hard, dry, barking character, and is usually worse before midnight. The child can be anxious, and can experience difficulty breathing, with a high fever. When *Aconite* is no longer working in cases of a croupy cough, consider *Hepar sulphuris* or *Spongia tosta.*

Antimonium tartaricum is used for rattling in the chest with a strong, loose cough. The chest feels full of mucus, yet the child is too weak to bring up the phlegm (this is not unusual in young children). The child tends to bend backward while coughing and is sleepy after a coughing fit. There can be shortness of breath, a sense of suffocation, and the child feels better sitting up to breathe. The cough can end in vomiting. The child is often irritable, whiney, prefers to be left alone.

Bryonia is an excellent cough remedy for a cough that is dry, racking, painful in the chest and head, and made worse from motion and better from being still. The child often holds her chest while coughing since any movement is painful. Taking a deep breath triggers the cough. This cough is worse from eating and drinking, and often grows worse at 9 P.M. The child's mood is irritable, "like a bear," and she has a strong thirst for cold drinks.

Coccus cacti is a remedy especially noted for winter coughs. The child might have a tickling in the throat, and feels better in the cold open air and drinking cold liquids. The mucus is clear, thick, and ropey, and may hang out of the mouth. The strong fits of coughing can end in choking and vomiting. Coughing spells are common from 6 to 7 A.M. and after 11:30 P.M.

Cuprum metallicum is indicated for violent coughing fits that cause a child to turn blue in the face (cyanosis). In general, *Cuprum* is strongly indicated for spasms and cramps occurring in the calf muscles, hands, abdomen, and throughout the body. Coughs may be so strong that the child can suffer a seizure, and may also be accompanied by a rattling in the chest. The child desires cold drinks and to lie down.

Drosera is another remedy for violent coughing spells ending in choking, gagging, or vomiting. In these instances, the cough is so strong that the child can hardly catch her breath. Often the child is worse when first lying down, and after midnight. She is better in the open air. *Drosera* is indicated for barking coughs, whooping cough and croup. Dryness and tickling in the throat trigger the cough. Bloody nose and a hoarse voice are common.

Hepar sulphuris is for croup that is worse in the morning, as well as the evening (until midnight). Often *Hepar sulphuris* is indicated following *Aconite*, especially with croup with rattling mucus in the chest and worse in the morning. The mood is sensitive, intolerant, and irritable. The child complains of being chilly or worse from a draft. The cough is loose and rattling with mucus that becomes thick and yellow. There is a desire for vinegar, and the child feels better with being warm.

Ipecacuanha is made from ipecac, which is used to induce vomiting. Prepared homeopathically, this remedy is good for whooping cough and other severe suffocative coughs that end in retching, vomiting, or cyanosis with stiffness in the body. The child feels nauseated and has an aversion to food (including the smell of food). There is rattling in the chest with constriction in the throat before the cough. The child may also have bloody nose with the cough. The cough is worse at 7 in the evening and better in the fresh air.

Pulsatilla is useful when there is a cough with yellow-green mucus. The cough is worse at night, interfering with sleep. The cough can be dry in the evening and loose in the morning. The child feels worse in a stuffy room and better with the open air. She typically is not thirsty. The moods are changeable and she can be weepy.

Spongia tosta is indicated for dry coughs that sound like a saw going through wood. Often used for croup, though with a slower onset compared to *Aconite,* it helps in coughs often preceded by cold symptoms. Similar to *Aconite*, *Spongia* is useful for croup before midnight, accompanied by a dry, barking cough that can sound like a seal. *Spongia* follows *Aconite,* when there is no rattling. The child may experience aggravation from a warm room, and indicate a desire to be cool.

Gemmotherapy

Briar Rose strengthens a child's immune system and is useful for conditions involving ear, nose, throat, sinuses and chest. I use this as a preventative 2 to 3 times a week as needed during cold and flu season. During an illness, use twice a day.

European Hornbean is indicated when there is an abundance of mucus. Well known as a sinus remedy, it is excellent for infections of the ear, nose, throat, and chest, as well as for spasmodic coughs and bronchitis.

Lemon Bark is useful for spasmodic coughs.

Lithy Tree targets and restores the lungs. Lithy Tree is helpful for severe coughs, bronchial spasm, and bronchitis.

See also *Common Cold* and *Flu*.

CRADLE CAP

Cradle cap, called seborrheic dermatitis, is usually more annoying to parents than it is to baby. Cradle cap occurs when the skin cells on baby's scalp grow faster than they are shed. This is thought to be due to exposure to mother's hormones in the womb, which stimulate the sebaceous glands on the skin to secrete an oily substance. This leaves baby with patches of flakey skin on the scalp, which looks like dandruff.

Cradle cap is a common occurrence in healthy babies in the first three months. Most often cradle cap is limited to the scalp, but it may spread to the forehead, eyelids, and ears. The symptoms range from simple crusts to large flakes and oozing eruptions. The rash can vary in color from white to yellow. **See your practitioner if the rash becomes irritated, red, or is infected.**

Care and Treatment

Cradle cap does not need to be treated unless it is severe, as it will resolve on its own. Some parents place oil, such as olive oil, on the scalp to attempt to gently remove or brush away the scales. Homeopathic medicines can help speed up the process for stubborn cases that persist longer than three months.

Homeopathic Medicines

Calcarea carbonica is recommended for children who have cradle cap where there is scaling skin on the scalp. There may be foul-smelling, thick crusts. The child's head is large and she perspires easily with a tendency towards constipation.

Graphites is indicated when the skin tends to be dry, rough, thick, and prone to cracks. The rash is moist and oozes a thick, sticky, yellow discharge that looks like honey. The child is prone to eruptions on the scalp, especially back of the head and in the bends in the arms and legs, and may also have skin cracks behind the ears.

Sulphur is a common skin rash remedy indicated for dry skin and itching that become worse with bathing, warmth, and while in bed. The scalp is sweaty. There is a tendency toward diarrhea, especially in the early morning hours, and characteristic aggravation at 11 A.M. Known as a homeopathic centrifuge, *Sulphur* drives toxins from the interior of the body to the surface, usually the skin. For this reason, if you are using *Sulphur*, use in a low potency, 6C or 6X, and use conservatively and slowly.

Viola tricolor is used for many skin conditions in childhood. From large boils to impetigo to cradle cap, the common symptoms that indicate this remedy include intolerable itching with thick scabs and gummy crusts with yellow pus. This causes the hair to become matted. The rash can cover the head and face with burning and itching and symptoms are worse at night. The glands are swollen and urine smells like cat urine. The child is worse in the cold air and in the winter time.

CRAMPS

See *Menstrual Cramps.*

CROUP

See *Cough.*

DENTAL PROCEDURES

See *Surgery and Dental Procedures.*

DIAPER RASH

With the convenience of diapers comes one of the most common frustrations for infants and parents: diaper rash. Whether caused from friction, irritants, allergies, or keeping the diaper on too long, diaper rashes begin because a baby's bottom is warm, wet, and sensitive. The moisture leads to chafing and changes the skin pH, making the skin more permeable. The end result is that the area becomes inflamed—a perfect environment for yeast and bacteria to grow.

Diaper rashes from yeast infections are caused by an overgrowth of *Candida albicans* in the intestine. In addition, yeast infections (fungus) occur following antibiotic use. Typical yeast infection causes red raised patches surrounded by distinct borders, sometimes with white scales over the genitalia. The skin is shiny, smooth, and bright red. Smaller scattered patches may also appear in the groin area. Severe diaper rash can look like a bad sunburn with raw skin, blisters, and peeling.

Rash from friction and contact occurs when a baby's skin is rubbed from diaper edges, elastic, and diapers that are too tight. A common area for friction rash is the inner thighs. Intertrigo is a moist rash that causes redness and irritation in the skin folds and creases. It can appear red, raw, and sunburn-like. Anal redness, which appears as a red ring, can also occur following a bout of diarrhea or from a sensitivity to certain foods. Common culprits include more acid foods such as tomatoes, strawberries, and citrus. If this occurs, eliminate the foods from a baby's or breastfeeding mom's diet. Rash from irritants such as stool, urine, strong soaps, and wipes will cause a local irritation mostly on the buttocks. Your baby can also be sensitive or allergic to ingredients in wipes, soaps, and the diapers. Most diaper rashes remain localized. **For diaper rash that is severely irritated, inflamed, or not improving see your practitioner.**

Care and Treatment

Prevention and Home Treatment

Some babies are more prone than others to diaper rash. Consider the following suggestions, especially if your baby is ultra-sensitive:

- Change your newborn's diaper at least every two hours (and more if needed). With disposable diapers it is not so obvious if your baby has urinated. As your baby gets older and urinates less, changes can be spaced out over longer intervals.

- Wash and dry a baby's bottom thoroughly with each change. When at home, it is best to use warm water with a cloth rag. If using soap, use a mild natural brand. If using commercial wipes, use the unscented natural brands.
- "Air out" your baby's bottom if there is redness. Place baby on her tummy, bottom up. To avoid accidents, place a waterproof cover under her lower side. Do this several times a day for redness.
- Disposable diapers can cause more rashes. Consider trying another brand.
- If using cloth diapers, rinse them in vinegar (add one half cup to the washing machine).
- For yeast infections, eliminate fruit and sweets from a baby's (and breastfeeding mom's) diet, as yeast grows in the presence of sugar.
- Probiotics are useful for diaper rash caused by yeast. Begin with a topical probiotic paste. It can be administered to a breastfeeding mother or infant.
- Grapefruit Seed Extract (GSE) is helpful for diaper rashes and thrush as it is known for its antifungal, bactericidal, antiviral and antiparasitic properties. GSE is highly concentrated and needs to be diluted in water (5 drops of GSE to one ounce of water). Place in a spray bottle, and use as needed in the diaper area after each change.

Calendula is an excellent healing agent for the skin made from marigold. Effective for treating diaper rash, calendula has natural antibacterial properties, making it both soothing and antiseptic. *Calendula* is available in tincture, cream, ointment or gel. Dilute calendula tincture 1:4, and apply to affected area with each diaper change.

Conventional Treatment

Conventional diaper rash creams are widely available; however, if your baby has no redness, there is no need to use a cream routinely. Use as needed for redness. Initial treatment for the first signs of redness includes protective barrier creams (most creams except for antifungals and cortisone). Standard brand creams for mild rashes are petroleum-based ointments. Zinc oxide is used for more moderate breakouts, and, for yeasty rashes, practitioners prescribe anti-fungal creams in addition to the general measures above. Hydrocortisone cream is recommended for severe rashes. In general, many parents prefer to avoid a medication like cortisone as it thins the skin. For more information, see "Diapers" in Chapter 4.

Homeopathic Medicines

Below are some effective homeopathic treatments for diaper rash. Because many rashes are caused by irritants in conventional products, homeopathy proves especially helpful in reducing a baby's exposure to the causes of the rash, while also healing and soothing the area.

Graphites is useful for redness and rawness in the folds of baby's bottom and around the anus. There can be a sticky yellowish discharge that forms a crust, and the skin can be dry with a tendency to crack.

Hepar sulphuris is indicated for moist eruptions in the skin creases, often accompanied by a foul odor of old rotten cheese. Baby is irritable and fussy with the pain, and is sensitive to cold and better with warmth. Cracks in the skin are common.

Mercurius is for diaper rash that is red, raw, and chafed with pimples. The skin is moist, and may also exhibit crusty eruptions with an offensive smell. The child is sweaty and easily drools.

Sulphur, a common skin remedy, is indicated for diaper rash that grows worse with bathing and warmth, and is itchy at night. The child is inclined to rub the area until it is raw. It is also commonly indicated for a bright red anus in children.

DIARRHEA

Anyone who has had diarrhea can attest that it is not a pleasant experience. The term refers to either increased frequency of stool and/or loose, watery stools. Infants and young children can lose a lot of fluid rapidly with diarrhea and need to be monitored to avoid dehydration. Otherwise, most cases of acute diarrhea usually resolve on their own within several days.

Diarrhea is not an illness; it is a symptom resulting from various conditions, such as infections (virus, bacteria or parasite), food poisoning, nervous stomach, and from medications such as antibiotics. In addition, it is not unusual for children to have loose stools while teething. Chronic diarrhea, which lasts more than two weeks, can be an indication of lactose intolerance, food allergies, gluten sensitivity, celiac disease, irritable bowel syndrome, Crohn's disease, ulcerative colitis, and needs to be monitored by a practitioner. Holistic medicine reports many successful treatments for these chronic conditions.

You should seek medical attention if your child has:

- Mild diarrhea (2 to 4 loose stools per day) and otherwise normal appetite, energy and no weight loss that is not resolving after several weeks
- Severe diarrhea especially if there is a rapid weight loss which can be a sign of dehydration. Severe diarrhea is 10 or more loose stools in a 24 hour period. Signs of dehydration: increased thirst, dry mouth, weight loss, dry tears, infrequent urination, listlessness, lethargy, and sunken eyes (sunken fontanelle in babies)
- Diarrhea in babies less than six months old
- Severe abdominal pain
- Bloody stool
- Lack of thirst (loss of appetite for food is not uncommon, though)

Causes or Types of Diarrhea

Rotavirus: Nausea, vomiting, cramps, bloating, and diarrhea with urgency are common symptoms in acute diarrhea. If your child begins with upset stomach, vomiting, and fever followed by watery diarrhea, it probably is caused by the rotavirus. Rotavirus affects children from three months to two years old. A child who has had rotavirus once may have repeat infections, although subsequent bouts tend to be less severe than the original. It is more common in the winter. Also known as acute viral gastroenteritis, there is no specific conventional treatment for it other than supportive therapy such as fluids and rest. The U.S. Food and Drug Administration approved a live virus vaccine (Rotashield) using a genetic human-monkey strain of rotavirus to be given to children beginning in 1998. However, due to severe side effects following the vaccine, including vomiting, diarrhea, and bowel obstruction, the vaccine has been suspended. Currently there are two rotavirus vaccines approved by the FDA for infants.

Shigella, Salmonella, and Other Bacteria: Bacteria can also cause diarrhea, and these include Shigella, E.coli, Salmonella, Campylobacter, Yersinia entercolitica, Vibrio cholera and Clostridium difficile. The latter is found in children who have diarrhea after taking antibiotics. Bacterial infections include symptoms such as bloody diarrhea with mucus, fever, and stomach cramps. Some bacterial infections are treated with antibiotics (Shigella), while Salmonella has become resistant to antibiotics and may actually prolong its contagious period if treated with unnecessary medication.

Parasites: Parasites also account for diarrhea illnesses and include Entamoeba histolytica (amoebic dysentery or traveler's diarrhea), Giardia lamblia (contaminated water), and Cryptosporidium (from pets and day care). Parasitic infections cause illnesses with large amounts of loss of appetite, cramps and watery diarrhea. Conventional treatment for parasites is with antiparasitic medications such as metronidazole.

Food Poisoning: Diarrhea can also occur from food poisoning in which the food becomes contaminated with a virus, bacterium, parasite, or pesticides. Within hours of eating the contaminated food, symptoms of nausea, vomiting, cramps, fever, and diarrhea begin. Within a few days, most symptoms clear.

Care and Treatment

Conventional Treatment

Encourage fluids. Rehydration drinks with electrolytes are recommended, as children can lose electrolytes with diarrhea. Pedialyte is popular; however, it can also be homemade. The Rehydration Project of the Centre for International Child Health Institute gives this recipe: Stir together 1 liter of clean water, 8 teaspoons of sugar (try molasses or natural raw sugar, which have more potassium than refined white sugar), and 1 teaspoon of salt. Make sure the salt and sugar dissolve. For flavor and extra potassium add ½ cup of orange juice and 1 mashed banana. Traditionally, breastmilk, orange juice (½ cup) rice water, carrot soup, or diluted cooked cereal and water (gruel) can prevent a child from becoming dehydrated.

If these are not available, give fresh fruit juice. In older infants and children, slowly introduce solids as diarrhea begins to decrease. The B-R-A-T diet (bananas, rice (including rice cereal and rice crackers), applesauce, and tea or toast) used to be recommended for several days. However, many practitioners have found this limits a child's diet too much and an expanded diet of broth, plain pasta, potato, and steamed vegetables can be introduced as well. For diarrhea illnesses that are not improving, see your practitioner for stool exams. Antidiarrheal drugs are not recommended in children due to unpredictable reactions.

Homeopathic Medicines

A scientific study on acute childhood diarrhea in Nicaragua was published by Jennifer Jacobs, M.D. in the issue of *Pediatrics* in 1994. In the study, Dr. Jacobs confirmed that the group of children who had infectious diarrhea (viral, bacterial, or parasites) who were treated with homeopathic medicines had a significant decrease in the duration of diarrhea compared to the children on placebo. A subsequent study in 2003 combining 3 prior studies confirmed the value of homeopathy for symptomatic care of childhood diarrhea.Below are some of the commonly remedies used for diarrhea, including some of the ones used in the study:

Arsenicum album is one of my favorite remedies to bring while traveling or to use at the first sign of food poisoning. Symptoms include severe cramps and burning pains, vomiting, and diarrhea that is worse at midnight and after eating and drinking. The stools are acrid, watery, and putrid smelling. *Arsenicum* is also indicated for bloody, mucousy stool. The child is typically thirsty for sips, anxious, and prefers company. There can be sweats and chilliness, made better with warmth.

Chamomilla is useful for diarrhea while teething. Consider *Chamomilla* when a baby has green stools that look like spinach and smell like rotten egg. This remedy is strongly indicated for colic, teething, and other conditions where baby is extremely fussy, irritable, and better being carried.

Croton tiglium is for diarrhea that comes in an urgent sudden gush. Gurgling noises can be heard in the belly, and there can be cramps that extend to the rectum. It is worse right after eating or drinking. The child feels better with warm milk.

Podophyllum is recommended for copious, gushing diarrhea which explodes into the entire toilet bowl. There is a sense of urgency and it is worse at four A.M. and in the evening. The stool is watery, and may be yellow, mucousy, and bloody with a bad odor. The diarrhea is also aggravated from eating or drinking. *Podophyllum* can be for diarrhea that is painless or associated with cramps in legs and belly. The child is exhausted and thirsty for cold water. In addition to being used for diarrhea from infection, it can also treat teething-related diarrhea.

Sulphur is useful for painless diarrhea that drives the child up urgently out of bed in the wee hours of the morning. Stool and gas have the odor of rotten eggs. As a strong skin remedy, it is often associated with skin conditions, including redness, itching, and burning around the anus.

Veratrum album, one of the main remedies for cholera, is useful when there is simultaneous vomiting with diarrhea *(Arsenicum album)*. The stool has a consistency of rice water and no odor. The child is debilitated, cold feeling in the belly, and complains of stomach pains.

Gemmotherapy

Wineberry and **European Walnut** are used to restore the intestines following diarrhea caused by a microorganism or after antibiotics.

DRUG ALLERGIES

See *Hives and Allergic Reactions.*

EAR INFECTIONS (OTITIS MEDIA)

According to the Greek philosopher Plato, the ears mark the resonance of divine harmony. In addition to the eyes, they are considered our most perceptive sensory organ. But, as most parents know, a child with an ear infection is anything but harmonious. Ear infections can be painful, and, too often, a chronic aspect of many children's lives, often appearing when they start daycare or preschool. Not uncommonly, a child will be treated with an antibiotic, only to come down with another infection shortly after, requiring a new antibiotic. This cycle can continue for months, with each medication working temporarily until the symptoms flare up again. Unfortunately, the wide use of antibiotics causes bacterial resistance, while lowering a child's immune resistance, setting up a cycle of recurrent ear infections.

Antibiotics, however, remain most pediatricians' medication of choice for treating middle ear infections, medically known as acute otitis media. Swimmer's ear, or otitis externa, is also somewhat common, affecting the ear canal outside the eardrum.

A middle-ear infection can vary from extreme, sharp, stabbing, throbbing pain to a dull ache to no symptoms at all. A cough and runny nose are the most common associated symptoms. Additionally, there may be fever, nausea, or vomiting. Irritability, fitfulness, difficulty sleeping, and tugging at the ear are additional signs, especially in young children who are unable to articulate the location of the pain. Keep in mind, though, that when a baby pulls at her ear she may just enjoy playing with it; teething infants also may tug at the ear.

Ear infections are more common in the winter, in boys, and for children in daycare. Many ear infections begin the week following the common cold and runny nose, The cold and congestion cause blockage in the Eustachian tube which leads to buildup of microorganisms. This leads to an ear infection, most of which are bacterial. Ear infections are not contagious, even though the cold that caused it is infectious. If the pressure in the Eustachian tube builds up, it may cause a perforated eardrum, in which the eardrum ruptures, allowing fluid to drain out of the ear. Although the presence of fluid draining out of the ear (mixed with pus or blood) is disconcerting to parents, it often brings a sigh of relief to the child. Perforated ear drums usually heal well on their own, although most pediatricians prefer to treat with antibiotic cortisone ear drops.

Amongst parents, the main concern regarding ear infection is that the infection will affect the child's hearing. Because of fluid in the middle ear, the child may not be able to hear as well during the infection but the hearing loss is usually not permanent. If the child continues to suffer with repeated ear infections and her hearing problems become chronic (which can also contribute to a speech delay), the doctor may recommend ear tubes (grommets) to be placed in the eardrum to allow the middle ear to drain. The procedure is called a myringotomy, simply known as "tubes."

Complications from middle ear infections are rare; however, they do occur. The following symptoms are cause for concern and should be reported to your practitioner.

- Prolonged and high fever
- Fluid or blood leaking from the ear (symptoms of perforation of the eardrum)

- Swelling pain, redness, or tenderness in the bony region behind the ear (symptoms of mastoiditis)

Care and Treatment

Prevention

A child lying down drinking a bottle (or using a pacifier) is prone to ear infections, because formula flows into the Eustachian tube. Feed your baby with her head propped up slightly while she is in your arms. On other hand, breastfeeding for at least six months or longer in any position is therapeutic and preventive for ear infections. General health and hygiene measures such as hand washing, healthy nutrition, and plenty of rest are beneficial.

Conventional Treatment

The American Academy of Pediatrics has posted guidelines in the treatment of ear infections in an effort to halt the overuse of antibiotics contributing to antibiotic resistance. In an uncomplicated mild ear infection (no fever or severe pain), it is recommended that pediatricians consider a "watchful waiting" option and hold off immediately prescribing antibiotics. Instead, it is suggested that doctors treat the child with pain medication and supportive measures. If the child does not improve after 2 to 3 days, consider antibiotics.

Up until recently, however, practitioners have been prescribing antibiotics (usually a 7- to 10-day course) routinely for all ear infections. In addition, ear infections are often over-diagnosed. Most practitioners diagnose a child with an ear infection if the ear looks red. Just because a child's ear is red, however, doesn't mean she has an ear infection—screaming or a fever can also cause redness of the eardrum without an infection being present. An interesting study found that 33 percent of physicians' equipment lacked the proper lighting to adequately examine the ear.

Antibiotics are also overused in follow-up care. Fluid in the ear and its effect on a child's hearing are big concerns for parents. Following an ear infection, though, fluid in the middle ear can take up to three months to drain. In my experience, the use of antibiotics and other medications weakens the immune system, contributing to chronic congestion, allergies, and enlarged tonsils and adenoids, all of which prevent fluid from draining out of the middle ear through the Eustachian tube, thus muffling the hearing. And before you know it, your child has another ear infection. All too often, antibiotics are given again and again for fluid in the ear—however, antibiotics are for bacteria and usually do not help in draining the fluid.

Some standard practitioners rely more on acetaminophen and ibuprofen for pain, at times also using anesthetic ear drops instead of antibiotics. Unless prescribed by your practitioner, ear drops are not to be used if there is a sign of a perforated eardrum, i.e., liquid or pus coming out of the ear.

Home Treatment

Many patients end up in my office following repeated courses of antibiotics or the threat of having tubes. Homeopathic and natural treatments (herbal, chiropractic, and osteopathy) are successful in treating ear infections and chronic ear conditions, and the following measures can be helpful in strengthening your child's immune system and treating the conditions. For additional tips, see the *Flu* entry.

Breastmilk: Breastfeeding strengthens your baby's immune system, assuring greater resistance to infections, including ear infections. In addition, breastmilk is full of antibodies and can be placed directly in the ear to help treat ear infections. If a baby becomes sick, a mother will receive the organism through the breast from his saliva, and if she has not yet been exposed to it, will make antibodies and transfer them back to baby via the milk.

Diet: Eliminate dairy products. Some parents replace cow's milk with soy or rice milk. Ear infections have been linked to allergies to certain foods, including dairy products. During an acute ear infection, it is best to eliminate common allergenic foods. In addition to dairy products, avoid wheat, eggs, corns, oranges, and peanut butter. Since simple carbohydrates can inhibit the immune system, it is also recommended a child avoid sugar, fruit, and juice.

Mullein-Garlic Ear Drops: Mullein (Verbascum thapsus) is used specifically for ear infections in the form of mullein oil drops. It is also useful for dry, scaly conditions in the outer ear. Mullein oil is often prepared commercially with garlic and other soothing herbs for the ear. Garlic (Allium sativum) has been used since ancient times to treat a wide variety of conditions, including ear infections. The Greek physician Hippocrates described garlic's immune-enhancing properties, and modern science is just now rediscovering its significant broad-spectrum antimicrobial and anti-inflammatory activity. The ear drops can be used at room temperature or warmed under the faucet. Place three drops in the affected ear three times daily.

Hydrogen Peroxide: Hydrogen peroxide is known to be effective in aiding the treatment of colds, flu, and ear infections. Place four drops of hydrogen peroxide (3%) into both ears. The solution will bubble and there may be a little stinging and within a couple minutes the liquid will drain out. This treatment is considered safe for infants. Avoid the eyes. Avoid any ear drops if there is fluid coming out of the ear (rupture of the eardrum). This is best used within the first 12 to 24 hours of illness.

Onion poultice: When my son has an earache, he often asks for the "onion patch" (poultice), which can soothe and alleviate discomfort. I place one small onion envelope in front of the entrance of the ear, and another envelope behind the ear and wrap with a scarf, leaving the wrap on for ten minutes or overnight. Before putting on the applications, I take a little warm onion juice mixed with olive oil, and gently place it in the ear (do not do this if there is any pus, blood, or liquid coming from the ear).

Homeopathic Medicines

Aconitum napellus is for the sudden onset of ear pain, especially after exposure to a draft or chill. The child is anxious, restless, and cries out with pain. *Aconite* is useful the first twenty-four hours of illness.

Belladonna is also for the sudden onset of a painful ear infection. The pain is throbbing, right-sided, and accompanied by a high fever, a red face, and even delirium. The child has a thirst for lemonade.

Chamomilla is useful for painful earaches that can be due to teething. The child is especially angry and irritable and demands to be carried. She may also be inconsolable and difficult to examine. This earache is worse after 9 P.M.

Mercurius is recommended for a painful ear infection often seen with a runny nose with yellow-green mucus. The child smells sick, sweats and drools, and feels worse at night.

Pulsatilla is also for earaches accompanied by yellow-green mucus. The ears feel stopped up, and the child is whiny and desires to be carried. The child feels warm and is better in the open air.

Herbal Remedies

Echinacea is well known for its activation of the immune system and is useful to take during an ear infection and for the common cold. Echinacea has anti-inflammatory properties that help speed the healing process and may also be used as a preventive during the cold and flu season. Children's echinacea (also available in combination with goldenseal) is available at the store; use as directed up to three times a day during illness for 5 to 7 days.

Goldenseal is indicated for severe ear infections and cold symptoms. It is known for its natural broad- spectrum anti-infective and immune stimulating activity. A children's formula with goldenseal (can be in combination with echinacea) can be taken up to three times a day during illness for 5 to 7 days.

Gemmotherapy

Briar Rose, European Hornbean, and **Common Birch** are used for ear infections in children.

EMOTIONAL UPSET

See *Anxiety* and *Grief and Sorrow.*

FEVER

When I was growing up, my mother took the doctor's advice and always gave us medicine at the first sign of a fever. Today, an increasing number of practitioners advocate a different approach to fevers that recognizes the body's own natural healing capabilities. Still, many parents feel panicked when they find their child has a temperature, and will schedule a physician's visit or run to the emergency room when homeopathy and simple home treatments will alleviate a good deal of the child's discomfort.

A fever is a valuable defense mechanism that indicates the body's immune system is stimulated by an infection or other illness. The fever and its accompanying symptoms, while annoying, are vital in helping to strengthen the immune system and ward off future infection. Fever is often accompanied with a faster pulse, more rapid breathing, and flushed skin. Your child may feel hot, sweaty, have chills, and mood changes, ranging from listlessness to irritability, are not uncommon. Febrile seizures occur when the temperature rises quickly or rises over 103°F. Parents report that experiencing a febrile seizure is one of the more frightening events in parenthood. Seizures vary from a simple trance with rolling back of the eyes to a general body convulsion. Fortunately they are usually harmless. Most occur between ages 6 months to five years old, in 2 to 5% of children. Febrile seizures can run in families.

Contact your practitioner if your child has:

- Fever 104°F (40 C) or higher that does not respond to home treatment
- Fever in infants 8 weeks or younger
- Fever 101°F (38.3 C) or higher in infants 8 weeks to 3 months
- Fever that lasts more than three days in all children
- Febrile seizure
- Stiff or painful neck, extreme fussiness, or listlessness

Care and Treatment

Conventional Treatment

The standard approach recommends fever reducers such as acetaminophen or ibuprofen. Acetaminophen (such as Tylenol) reduces fever and relieves aches and pains. Considered a safe drug by the medical community, it can cause serious side effects, including liver damage, if taken in high doses. Ibuprofen (such as Motrin or Advil), is a non-steroidal anti-inflammatory that helps bring down fever and inflammation and reduces pain. Some side effects of ibuprofen are heartburn, stomachache, ulcers, headache, rash, constipation, and diarrhea. Aspirin, also a fever reducer, should not be used in children.

Home Treatment

Although there are many remedies for fevers, I will cover just a few of the more commonly used ones. When your child has a fever, find the remedy that matches his or her symptoms best.

Warmth: Assess your child's condition and temperature. Place your hand on her forehead, belly, arms and legs, and compare warm and cool areas. For cooler areas such as the legs and feet, warm them up with a hot water bottle to help disperse the heat away from the head.

Diet: Simple vegetable and chicken broths, room temperature water, and warm tea can be soothing. Avoid dairy, protein, refined sugars, and heavy foods. During a fever, avoid protein, as your child expends much energy for a healthy immune response, and protein in the diet requires energy for digestion.

Lemon Compress: For high fevers, use a lemon compress wrapped around calf and foot. The lemon will cool and balance temperature throughout the body. If the wrap dries quickly, repeat every 15 to 30 minutes.

Sponge Bath: A good old-fashioned sponge bath with tepid water will soothe and warm your child.

Homeopathic Medicines

Aconitum napellus is useful for the early stages of an intense fever that comes on suddenly. Often the child goes out on a windy day and, a short time later, comes down with a fever. *Aconite* will typically be effective for a fever that's accompanied by anxiety, restlessness, and a thirst for cold drinks.

Belladonna is also useful during the early stages of a sudden fever. However, a child who responds to *Belladonna* radiates heat and may have a flushed face and a throbbing feeling, as well as delirium and a lack of thirst. The head is hot, and the arms and legs cold. If your child's symptoms are not distinct, *Belladonna* is the most common remedy for a simple fever (one without other symptoms).

Chamomilla can be helpful for the fevers that often accompany an infant's teething misery. *Chamomilla* is for the child who is very irritable and difficult to please. Often one of his or her cheeks appears red, the other pale, and the child's fever becomes worse at night.

Gelsemium is good for a child who is trembling with chills and wants to be cuddled. She looks exhausted with drooping eyelids, and may be dizzy with generalized achiness. *Gelsemium* is a common flu remedy.

Phosphorus is useful for the child with chills and sweats during the night, and cold limbs. She characteristically craves ice cold drinks despite being chilly and is often quite hungry.

Gemmotherapy

Briar Rose is an excellent all-around children's remedy. It is useful for strengthening the immune system during a fever.

See also *Flu*.

FIFTH DISEASE

See *Roseola*.

FLU

During November to March, the height of the flu season, numerous children and adults will come down the characteristic muscle aches, fever, and exhaustion. Increasingly, parents are looking to avoid mercury-based flu vaccines, and many turn to homeopathy instead. Because homeopathic remedies are prescribed to the specific set of symptoms rather than a broadly labeled condition, you do not need to worry about whether you are confusing cold or flu: homeopathy will treat your child's specific symptoms. **Contact your practitioner if your child has a fever of 102°F (38.8C) or higher for more than three days, severe cough, or trouble breathing.**

Care and Treatment

Prevention and Home Treatment

Although the flu can't always be avoided, the following measures can aid in preventing and treating symptoms:

- Make sure your child gets plenty of rest. During the holiday season this can be more difficult, but lack of sleep makes us vulnerable to getting sick.
- During illness, avoid radio, television, and videos, as they are over stimulating.
- Wash hands frequently to minimize spread of germs.
- Avoid swimming during autumn and winter.
- Give foods rich in vitamin C to strengthen your child's immune system. If using supplements, give 150 mg daily.
- Garlic is an antibacterial; have your child eat plenty of it.
- Encourage healthy fluids, preferably room temperature to warm. Avoid cold drinks which require the body to spend energy to warm it up inside. Give herb tea, vegetable broths, and unsweetened (diluted) juice. The broths and teas especially help thin the mucous and clear the body. Ginger tea (heat several slices of fresh ginger in three cups of water for ten minutes) or a natural cold and flu tonic (2 to 5 tablespoons apple cider vinegar, 1 cup of hot water, 1 to 2 tablespoons honey, maple syrup or unrefined sweetener, dash of cayenne pepper to taste) can be soothing and therapeutic.
- During illness it is not uncommon for your child to lose her appetite. If your child does not want to eat, don't force it. During acute illnesses, your child's immune system and body is occupied more with fighting the bug and eliminating toxins. For this reason, liquid is more important, so the body does not have to expend energy digesting food, especially protein (meat, fish, legumes, nuts, eggs, and dairy). In addition to avoiding protein, it is best to steer clear of sweets and dairy. Refined sugar compromises the immune system and dairy thickens mucus secretion. When introducing solids, begin with lightly steamed vegetables, grains, healthy crackers, and fruit.

- Dress your child warmly in layers, and cover the feet. Both children and adults should wear thin layers of natural fabrics especially in the cooler months. In colder climates, hats should be worn outside.
- Bring out the hot water bottle for aches, chills, and general comfort. The Wellness Nurses suggest filling a hot water bottle half way with hot water. Carefully press any remaining air out, keep the bottle flat and light and cover it in thick flannel to protect the skin from burns. It should not be too hot to the touch. If hands and feet are cooler than the belly, warm them first. If your child's face is flushed, use the bottle at the feet. For chest congestion, place it by the chest.
- Breastmilk can be used to treat stuffy nose and red eyes. It has antibacterial properties and can be squirted directly in the eye or nose. A few drops of expressed breastmilk can be placed in the affected area with a dropper.
- Hydrogen Peroxide, known for germicidal properties has been shown to be helpful at the onset of flu symptoms. Place 4 drops of hydrogen peroxide (3%) into both ears. See *Natural Essentials* in Part V.
- Lavender, used as an essential oil in aromatherapy, is known for its antiseptic and antibacterial properties. Packaged commercially for children, a lavender aromatherapy bath can help soothe coughs, sore muscles, and calm the nerves.
- Try a lemon compress for fever.
- A potato poultice around the throat and chest is an excellent source for moist heat and retains its temperature longer than a hot water bottle. Potato is useful for headaches, neckache, muscle pain, and chilliness.
- During an acute illness like the flu, your child will often be very precise in what gives him or her relief. Satisfy your child's cravings, within reason. You may hear, "I want a popsicle," "Don't leave me alone," or "I'm not hungry," According to Dr. Samuel Hahnemann, father of homeopathy, "Acutely ill patients rarely crave things that obstruct their cure."

Conventional Treatment

Standard medication can not cure the flu, but it can provide relief. Flu medications include pain relievers, such as acetaminophen or ibuprofen, cough medications and decongestants. Prescription medicine Tamiflu (oseltamivir phosphate) attacks the flu virus and prevents it from spreading if taken at the onset of illness. It can be used in children 1 year and older. Side effects include vomiting, stomachache, nosebleed, and conjunctivitis.

Homeopathic Medicines

Bryonia flu symptoms are characterized by muscles aches that hurt with movement and dryness of the throat and mouth, accompanied with an intense thirst for cold drinks. The child is cranky and likely to say, "Don't touch me."

Eupatorium perfoliatum is excellent for flu symptoms with a deep ache in the bones, as if the "bones are broken." It hurts to move, including moving the eyeballs.

Ferrum phosphoricum is indicated for early flu symptoms with high fever and weakness. The cheeks are flushed and there can be headache, sensitivity to light, and bloody nose with the fever. The child who responds to *Ferrum phosphoricum* can have complaints that are worse on the right side, worse from being touched, and worse from four to six in the morning. They feel better with cold applications. Often there are no other specific local symptoms.

Gelsemium is for the classic flu symptoms of dizziness, weakness, and fatigue. The *Gelsemium* patient is not thirsty and wants to lie down and be left alone. The body feels heavy, any motion is an effort, and even the eyelids droop.

Oscillococcinum, the popular homeopathic flu medicine from France is commonly used in the treatment of flu symptoms such as fever, chills, body aches and pains. For best results take Oscillo at the onset of flu symptoms.

Rhus toxicodendron is good for muscle aches with stiffness, but the child is restless and fidgety.

Herbal Remedies

Echinacea for children helps boost the immune system. Echinacea can be taken for prevention purposes during the winter season two weeks on and two weeks off, or at the first sign of an illness.

Anise and **Mullein,** in tea form, are both natural expectorants.

Gemmotherapy

Briar Rose is useful for many conditions in children, especially infections of the ear, nose and throat. I use it two to three times a week during the flu season as a general strengthener, and twice a day while sick. It can be used in conjunction with homeopathy and all other medicines.

Black Currant is an excellent remedy for strengthening the constitution during the winter months, especially for adults. It stimulates the adrenals and is good for stress and fatigue.

Also for adults, **Common Birch** targets the cleansing of the liver and other organ systems. It is known as the universal drainer and is an excellent general remedy for strengthening the immune system.

See also *Common Cold* and *Fever.*

FOOD ALLERGIES

See *Diarrhea, Hay Fever,* and *Hives and Allergic Reactions.*

FOOD POISONING

See *Diarrhea* and *Vomiting.*

GASTROESOPHAGEAL REFLUX

See *Vomiting.*

GRIEF AND SORROW

Grief and sorrow can be likened to a wound of the heart and soul. Like any injury, it takes time to heal. It is normal to go through a period of pain and suffering following any difficult experience. Children may experience feelings of grief and sorrow after a change in school, a death of a loved one, or divorce. Even an infant will sense the loss of a person who was a consistent presence. Some mothers experience a period of sadness following childbirth.

Children respond differently to a loss than adults. A child's awareness is more concrete and short range, and it is only in adolescence that the abstract concept of the meaning of life and death becomes more developed. Some symptoms of grief and sorrow include sadness, crying, sighing, loss of attention and focus, poor appetite, difficulty sleeping, and withdrawal. **Contact your practitioner if symptoms persist or begin to worsen with unusual behaviors such as hallucinations, anxiety attacks or extreme depression.**

Care and Treatment

Conventional Treatment

For complicated or prolonged periods of unresolved grief, there are books, videos, and counseling that parents can employ to help their children. The conventional treatment can include psychotherapy especially anti-depressants or anti-anxiety medication with older children.

In addition to offering a grieving child love and support, natural medicines can help in dealing with difficult experiences in acute situations—not by suppressing symptoms, but by allowing them expression. A constitutional remedy can alleviate symptoms in chronic cases.

Homeopathic Medicines

Ignatia is the main remedy for loss, sorrow, and grief. It is indicated when sensations include a lump in the throat, sighing, and uncontrollable weeping. I also use this remedy for women with hysterical feelings and sadness in the postpartum period.

Natrum muriaticum is useful for the child who suffers quietly, and keeps her feelings to herself. She tends to be overly responsible and avoids company. She may have difficulty crying and may experience long periods of sadness following a loss through death or breakup of a relationship. She may crave salty foods, lemon, and ice cold drinks.

Phosphoricum acidum, also for grief, is indicated when the child appears more exhausted, weak, and indifferent than sad. Symptoms improve following a short nap, and the child may have a desire for refreshing fruit juices and carbonated drinks. He or she may also experience sadness with homesickness and nostalgia.

Bach Flower Essences

These can be used in conjunction with homeopathic remedies.

Star of Bethlehem helps to relieve sadness associated with loss and grief.

Rescue Remedy is a combination of five flower essences, including Star of Bethlehem. Rescue Remedy can be used for sadness and grief associated with emergency situations and panic, such as a grave accident, earthquakes, or even starting a new school. Place 2 drops in a glass of water and sip.

GROWING PAINS

Growing pains, or benign limb pain of childhood, are known to affect up to forty percent of children. Growing pains usually occur at two peaks—from three to six years old and then from eight to fourteen. Some practitioners don't believe that growing pains are caused by growth but instead attribute them to the general aches and pain from activity during the day.

Whatever the cause, children usually experience growing pains from time to time, and often toward the end of the day and at night in bed. Growing pains occur in the muscle over a generalized area: the pain is felt in the leg, typically the calf or shin, and sometimes in the thigh, foot, or behind the knee. Growing pains, which can be worse in cold or damp weather, are usually relieved with massage, stretching, and sometimes heat. Growing pains are more common in children who are active in sports and other physical activities. Seek medical attention if your child is consistently limping or has swelling, redness, or a tender arm, leg, or particular joint.

Causes and Types of Pains in Growing Children

In addition to general growing pains, Osgood-Schlatter disease and Sever's Disease are other causes of pain in growing children.

Osgood-Schlatter disease: Osgood-Schlatter disease, which causes pain and swelling below the knee cap, caused when the thigh muscle pulls on the patellar tendon, affects children from eight to sixteen years old. It commonly occurs among kids participating in soccer, baseball, basketball, track, and other sports. For painful areas, rest, ice, compression, and elevation (R.I.C.E) is recommended. Strenuous exercise should be avoided, and the child may require leg braces and/or anti-inflammatory medication.

Sever's Disease: A pain at the back of the heel, caused by inflammation where the Achilles tendon attaches to the heel bone,. Sever's also affects children from nine to fourteen. Standard treatment includes heel pads, R.I.C.E., and ibuprofen.

See *Injuries* for more information on R.I.C.E.

Care and Treatment

Home Treatment

Simple home treatments can ease growing pains.

- Rub or massage the affected area.
- Stretch the limb.
- If growing pains consistently bother the child after a particular activity, avoid it for a period of time.
- Provide warmth: during cold damp weather, keep the area covered with long pajamas and socks. Place a hot water bottle or warm potato poultice on the muscle.
- Arnica cream or oil can be massaged into the muscles, especially after exercise.
- For growing pains that are not relieved with general home measures, children are prescribed pain medicine such as acetaminophen or ibuprofen.

Homeopathic Medicines

Calcarea phosphorica is important for soft, growing tissues and bone solidity and well known as a remedy for growing pains. It is also indicated for school headaches and stomachaches in school-aged children. The child is moody, sensitive, and can easily become overwhelmed by school. *Calcarea phosphorica* is my first choice of remedies for growing pains.

Causticum is for growing pains accompanied with stiffness around the joints. The joint feels stiff and tight. Growing pains are more likely to come on when a child is overwhelmed.

Magnesia phosphorica, well known for writer's cramp and menstrual pain, is also useful for erratic, wandering growing pains. The muscle is better from rubbing, heat, and pressure. Right-sided complaints are common.

Phosphoricum acidum is for children and adolescents who experience pains after growing too rapidly. The child also complains of fatigue, depression, and craves fruit juice. *Phosphoricum acidum* is also used for grief and after mononucleosis.

Gemmotherapy

Red Spruce is important for the calcium in bones and growing pains.

Briar Rose is a good general remedy for children.

See also *Injuries.*

HAND-FOOT-MOUTH DISEASE

See *Mouth Sores.*

HAY FEVER

In a medical journal article on spring allergies, an astute doctor writes, "Nasal diseases have sometimes been regarded as disorders that are unimportant . . . to those who do not have them." If you or your children suffer from hay fever (also know as allergic rhinitis), you're one of many who can relate to the good doctor.

Seasonal allergies affect nearly one in ten Americans; some experts estimate that the number is as high as 20 percent. (Strangely, allergic rhinitis appears to be most common among the young and affluent.)

While spring allergies may not pose a life-or-death situation, symptoms can be so severe that they affect a child's quality of life and ability to play and work in school. Allergies can disturb sleep, impair concentration, and lead to emotional problems. Familiar irritating symptoms of hay fever run the gamut and usually center around the nose—watery runny nose, stuffed nose, sneezing, watery eyes, post-nasal drip, itching in the throat, nose, and eyes. In addition, there can be a horizontal crease at the top of the nose from rubbing it, dark circles under the eyes, and coughing or wheezing. There are many different types of allergies which cause symptoms of allergic rhinitis, yet are not hay fever. Seasonal allergies appear at different times of the year, and often in the spring (i.e. due to pollens in the air), while perennial complaints are year-round (dust, mold, animal dander, second-hand tobacco smoke, food allergies including milk and food additives, and pollution). Children who have a family history of allergies are more prone to having allergies. Besides hay fever, eczema and asthma are also common. Allergies can also make a child susceptible to infections in the sinuses or ear. **Contact your practitioner if your child has difficulty breathing or if chronic allergies are affecting the quality of your child's life. Additional reasons to go to your practitioner are, if you unable to determine the cause of your child's allergies or if symptoms persist or worsen.**

Causes and Types of Hay Fever

Allergies occur when a foreign substance, also known as an allergen, typically nontoxic (such as pollen), is misread by the body as harmful. In reaction, the body overreacts with an allergic immune response that can range from mild to severe. It has been suggested that this oversensitivity is caused by a dysfunction in the immune system which may be linked to antibiotics, vaccines, and stress, in addition to family predisposition.

Allergic substances are minute and permeate an environment, making it at times difficult to identify the cause of a reaction. Pollens, yellow grains from the center of a flower, are blown by the wind, while dust mite droppings, which provoke dust-related reactions, spread through the air in similar fashion. Both are more pronounced in warm humid weather. Mold, on the other hand, is found in houses, especially in the cool, dark areas. The spores from mold can trigger allergic reactions.

Care and Treatment

Conventional Treatment

Medications are used as needed for seasonal allergies, while a child with perennial allergies may be prescribed medications year-round. These include antihistamines, decongestants, and steroids, which often have side effects including drowsiness and dry mouth. In addition, the skin prick tests use a small needle test for food and environmental allergens. A positive test will form a bump at the site of the skin prick. The test is uncomfortable for children, and not always reliable. In general, allergy testing is more reliable in children over five years old. Also, a blood test is available. The older RAST test is less accurate than the newer version, ImmunoCAP®; be aware of which lab your doctor uses and which testing the lab does. Allergy shots, meant to make the child less sensitive over time to allergens, are also sometimes recommended by allergists. Allergy shots contain the allergens that cause problems for your child. They may be given on a regular basis over a five year period. This approach is expensive, time consuming, and uncomfortable for the child.

Home Treatment

- Avoid known allergens, when possible.
- If your child is allergic to dust mite droppings, keep a clean environment. Carpets, heavy curtains, stuffed animals attract dust, so avoid these types of fabrics as much as possible. Many of my families with allergies report better results with hardwood floors rather than carpeting. Keep your child's room free of clutter.
- Cover mattress, pillow, and box springs with an allergy-proof plastic cover.
- Use a HEPA (High Efficiency Particulate Accumulator) filter for airborne allergies. It reduces mold, pollen, dust mite droppings, and animal danger.
- Nasal rinses, known as nasal lavage or irrigation, have been shown to be helpful for children with hay fever. The saltwater solution is sprayed into each nostril either by using a bulb syringe or a neti pot. The neti pot, used in India for centuries, has a spout for the nose. The salt-to-

water ratio is 1 level teaspoon sea salt to 2 cups (½ liter) of lukewarm filtered water. Use once or twice a day as needed.

- Bathe (including washing the hair) in the evening to get rid of pollen from the day.
- Lemon is good for watery runny nose or eyes, allergies, and hay fever. Use lemon as a steam inhalation, chest compress, or lemon slices in socks and kept in place on the soles of the feet.

Homeopathic Medicines

Allium cepa is indicated for a runny nose that "drips like a faucet," accompanied by sneezing, which gets worse in the late afternoon and is better outside. Likewise, the nose can also be stuffed. The discharge from the nose burns and irritates the skin, while the tearing from the eyes is mild and bland.

Euphrasia is for allergies which are more centered on the eyes. *Euphrasia* is good for eyes that itch, feel irritated, and burn with lots of tears. In contrast to *Allium cepa*, there can be a mild discharge from the nose. The child blinks frequently and may be sensitive to sunlight and wind. *Euphrasia* is also known as eyebright, and is a common ingredient in homeopathic eye drops useful for redness and irritation.

Natrum muriaticum is for allergies that begin with a watery runny nose and sneezing; the mucus will look like raw egg white. After three days, the nose becomes stopped, making it difficult to breathe. There can be loss of smell and taste. The symptoms are worse at 10 A.M. and in the heat of the sun, but better outdoors. The child tends to be mature, well behaved, and does not like to be consoled.

Nux vomica is recommended for stuffy nose, occurring mostly at night and when outside. However, nose will be runny during the day and in warm rooms. Sneezing and runny nose can also be worse when waking up in the morning. The child is moody, impatient, and easily angered.

Sabadilla is indicated for continuous fits of sneezing with itching and tingling of the nose. Tearing of the eyes is also possible. The child feels better when outside and when she has a warm drink. Discharge from the nose is usually thin and irritating.

Wyethia is for symptoms of extreme itching of the mouth (especially the palate), throat, nose, and ears, along with the desire to "scratch" the roof of your mouth with your tongue. The mouth feels dry, and the throat swollen with frequent clearing of the throat.

Gemmotherapy

Briar Rose is for runny nose and congestion in children.

European Hornbean is for congestion in the sinus, nose, and lungs.

HEADACHES

Sometimes, life can be a headache for us—and for our children, too. Not getting enough sleep at a slumber party, skipping meals, or too much homework all can result in headaches in children. Headaches affect approximately sixty percent of children, and are more common during adolescence. They occur as a sole complaint or as one of the symptoms in an illness, such as the flu or strep throat, or as an adverse effect from a medication. Recurrent headaches, usually tension (stress), migraine, or organic headaches, are less common in children. Nausea is a common symptom with many headaches, as well as irritability, tender teeth, and sensitivity to light, noise, and motion. **See your practitioner for an evaluation if your child suffers from a severe headache, unexplained headache, or recurrent episodes.**

Causes and Types of Headaches

Tension Headaches: Tension headaches originate from tight muscles surrounding the head and back of the neck and are more common in adolescents than younger children. Stresses from school, anxiety, and poor posture are common causes of tension headaches in school-aged children. Often, tension headaches come on during school or after school, and are less common on the weekends. The pain is not throbbing or pounding like a migraine, and may be localized in the front of the head. There is usually no nausea or vomiting.

Migraine Headaches: Migraine headaches affect one in twelve children. In adolescents, migraines are more common in girls, and before puberty, more often affect boys. Migraine sufferers usually have a strong family history of the condition.

Common triggers include lack of sleep, skipping meals, flashing lights from video games or television, and food products such as chocolate, nuts, caffeine, cheese, processed meats like hot dogs, additives in processed meats (nitrates), MSG, and alcohol. Menstruation can also trigger migraines. Migraine symptoms are caused by the dilation or constriction of blood vessels in and around the head, and for this reason are considered vascular headaches. Migraines can be preceded by a visual aura, throbbing or pounding sensations, and may be accompanied by nausea, vomiting, and stomachache. The child can often pinpoint the location of the headache and feels better with sleep.

Organic Headaches: The rarest and most serious headaches are the organic headaches, which originate from illnesses like meningitis, encephalitis, abscess, bleeding after an injury, and brain tumors. In many of these conditions, the headache is caused by increasing pressure in the skull. For this reason, these headaches are worsened by activities that "strain the brain" (increase the pressure), such as coughing and sneezing. The headaches may waken the child during sleep and be accompanied by vomiting. In contrast to a migraine, the pain is more generalized. Sometimes the child may experience loss in vision, change in alertness, tingling feelings, and seizures. If you believe your child may be suffering from this type of headache, see your practitioner.

Care and Treatment

Conventional Treatment

The conventional treatment includes medications such as ibuprofen and acetoaminophen, though practitioners are also more frequently recommending non-medicinal relaxation techniques such as biofeedback. Stronger migraine medications (ergotamine and sumatriptin) are sometimes used in older children. However, parents often hesitate at these measures because of the side effects, which include flushing, dizziness, nausea, and hot flashes. Sumatriptin is not approved for children under age twelve.

Home Treatment

- Encourage your child to lie down.
- Avoid bright light and loud noises—quiet, dark, and calm environments are preferable.

- Avoid known triggers to headaches: fatigue, stress, hunger, heat stroke, motion sickness, lack of exercise, and offending foods.
- Ginger tea and peppermint tea are helpful for headaches, especially those associated with nausea. Use ginger in children two years and older.
- Massage the back of the neck.
- Employ cold compresses.

Homeopathic Medicines

Bryonia headaches are described as bursting or splitting. Because movement worsens them, the person just wants to stay still. The mouth and lips are dry. The child is irritable and thirsty for cold drinks. Pain tends to be concentrated on the left side of the head.

Calcarea phosphorica is often chosen as the remedy for headaches in school-aged children. These children are sensitive and easily overwhelmed by the homework and stress of going to school. They may also complain of stomachaches coming on in the afternoon after school.

Iris versicolor is the remedy for the classic migraine symptoms—visual aura, pain on one side of the head, and nausea and vomiting. The pain is usually on the right side, or alternates sides. A history of being overly tired often precedes the headache.

Natrum muriaticum is used for headaches brought on by loss, grief, or disappointment. Similar to *Calcarea phosphorica, Natrum muriaticum* is helpful for school pressure headaches due to the mental effort of concentrating and working hard in school. The headache feels like little hammers knocking on the brain. The pain may be located over the eyes, tends to worsen around 10 A.M. until the late afternoon, and is especially aggravated by sunlight. A cold cloth on the head, lying down in a dark, quiet room, and fresh air also bring relief.

Sanguinaria migraines differ from *Iris* headaches in that the pain begins at the back of the head and then settles in the right side or behind the right eye. The pain is described as sharp, knifelike, or splitting. This patient feels better after vomiting.

Spigelia is more commonly used for left-sided headaches that feel like a hot needle, poker, or wire in or above the left eye; the pain is piercing and sharp. This headache is accompanied by a stiff neck and shoulders, and is aggravated by the sunlight, motion, and touch. Relief comes with steady pressure.

Gemmotherapy

Lemon Bark is indicated for migraine and tension headaches.

Briar Rose, a common children's remedy, is also helpful for migraines.

HIVES AND ALLERGIC REACTIONS

Hives, also known as welts, urticaria, or nettle-rash, occur when a substance called histamine is released in the body. Histamine works as a defense mechanism when it comes into contact with something foreign, causing the capillaries (small blood vessels) to dilate and form welts on the surface of the skin. Welts are warm, circular, raised, and can be intensely itchy. They look like a mosquito bite, red on the outside and white in the center. The rash often appears in clusters and can come and go lasting from minutes to days. Urticaria is usually the result of an acute allergic reaction from drugs, food, pollen, and occur after exercise and from being in the cold. There are many foods to which your child may be allergic but some of the most common are nuts (especially peanuts), dairy, eggs, and shellfish. Hives can also result from chronic infections, autoimmune diseases, cancer, or other causes. **Severe life-threatening swelling of mouth and throat requires immediate emergency medical care.**

In addition, some children who are susceptible to hives suffer severe anaphylactic reactions to allergenic substances. As a precaution, parents keep an emergency injectable epinephrine kit (EpiPen) to be given to children who have a history of life threatening reactions. Parents should be instructed on how to use it ahead of time.

Care and Treatment

Conventional Treatment

Standard treatment for hives begins with an over-the-counter antihistamine, such as Benadryl. Atarax, also an antihistamine, is available by prescription.

Antihistamines reduce the itching. Side effects for Benadryl include drowsiness, dizziness, stomach upset, irritability, and dry mouth. Atarax can also cause drowsiness and dry mouth. Higher doses of Atarax my cause twitches and convulsion. Severe reactions such as closing of the throat and difficulty breathing are treated with epinephrine.

Home Treatment

Most of the cases of hives I see in the office result from antibiotics given for infections—most of which could have been easily treated with natural remedies, without the side effects! For chronic cases of hives, consider working with a practitioner in the natural healing arts for preventive treatment and constitutional strengthening.

Oatmeal Baths can be soothing for children with hives, as well as relieve dry skin, minor burns, and other sources of itchy rashes. Commercially prepared packets of colloidal oatmeal can be purchased or you can easily make your own. (Colloid means that the oatmeal has been pulverized into a fine powder so that it is completely absorbed in the water.)

To make your own, place 1 cup of unflavored oatmeal (slow or quick) in blender, processor, or grinder. Place at high setting until oatmeal is ground into a fine powder. As a test, stir 1 tablespoon into a glass of warm water and stir. You know you have blended it long enough when the water turns milky and feels silky. With the tub of running water, slowly sprinkle in the blended oatmeal. Use ⅓ cup for infants, and 1 cup for children. With your hand make a figure eight in the tub to insure dispersion. Be careful as the tub will be slippery! Soak up to 15 minutes, using 1 to 3 times a day as needed.

Homeopathic Medicines

Apis mellifica is an excellent remedy for hives where complaints of burning, stinging, and puffiness predominate. The rash may have extreme swelling, with the area red, raised, and warm. One of the keynotes of *Apis* is relief with cold applications. *Apis* is the most common remedy I use following an allergic drug rash, and is also one of the remedies indicated for anaphylactic shock.

Carbolic acid is used for extreme symptoms such as anaphylaxis, collapse, and swelling of face and tongue, especially after an insect sting, or hives with burning and itching sensations and blisters that cover the body, especially the hands.

Rhus toxicodendron is indicated for hives with small blisters that are intensely itchy with prickly, burning pain. The child may also experience a feeling of bodily stiffness, which is alleviated by moving around and frequently changing position. *Rhus* rashes feel better with scalding hot water, and worse in the cold.

Urtica urens comes from the stinging-nettle plant. It is often used for reactions to shellfish, but also for hives following insect bites, stings, and from becoming overheated. The skin stings, prickles, burns, and itches violently. *Urtica urens* is also used for first- and second-degree burns. The hives feel worse with cold.

Gemmotherapy

Black Currant, a gemmotherapy remedy, has strong anti-inflammatory properties and is indicated for allergies and urticaria.

European Alder, used with *Black Currant*, is also helpful for hives. Use together three times a day.

Bach Flower Essence

Rescue Remedy can be used for agitation. Place 2 drops in a glass of water and sip as needed. As a cream, apply to affected area.

INDIGESTION

See *Stomachache*.

INJURIES

Bumps, bruises, and skinned knees are rites of passage in childhood and any active child will experience their share of minor scrapes and contusions, less often serious injuries such as broken bones and sprains. Injuries can result from direct impact, such as with a fall, or from movements that twist or strain joints, tendons, and ligaments, leading to sprains and pulled muscles. Repetitive stress injuries resulting from overuse are rare in children; isolated incidents like bumps, sprains, and muscle strains are more common. Following an injury, the area may be painful, swollen, bruised, red, weak, and warm. Your child may not want the area touched or may have problems moving in a normal fashion, limping or otherwise favoring the injury.

If you suspect a fracture or a severe injury call your practitioner. All severe injuries, including head injuries, require immediate medical attention. After a moderate to severe accident or injury, many patients visit the practitioner for a full evaluation including an X-ray.

Causes and Types of Injuries

As your baby begins to roll over, crawl, fall, walk, and fall again, she will be prone to all types of bumps and bruises. Older children tend to injure themselves from climbing, running, playing, and sports. A bruise, caused by a bump or direct blow, is also known as a contusion. Some of your child's everyday injuries will be accompanied with bruising of the area. The marks are caused when the blood from the damaged underlying capillary leaks into the tissue, leaving the skin looking "black and blue."

Joints are particularly vulnerable to injury due to their complexity and frequent use. At the joint, the bones are connected to each other by ligaments, which are made of long collagen fibers that can stretch slightly. Ligaments function to provide stability and protect the joint from doing certain movements that could lead to injury, while tendons connect bones to muscles, and are made of a fibrous connective tissue—the Achilles tendon, for instance, is the largest in the body.

A strain is caused by twisting, tearing, or overstretching a muscle or tendon and can result from lifting a heavy object or from trauma to an area. Common areas of strain include lower back and hamstring. A sprain, on the other hand, results from a strong pulling or twisting action on the ligaments, forcing the joint out of its alignment. The knee and wrists are common areas for sprains, while the most frequently injured joint is the ankle. With both sprains and strains, your child can experience pain, swelling, and sometimes limited movement of the joint. Older children are more prone to strains and sprains than younger children, whose growth plates are weaker comparable to their muscles and tendons and hence more flexible. This makes younger children more prone to broken bones, however.

An often overlooked cause of trauma is the minor "fender bender." At a recent homeopathic medical conference, osteopathic physician Maud Nerman, D.O. presented research showing that injuries from motor vehicle accidents occur in collisions as slow as 7 to 8 miles per hour! In fact, these seemingly simple traumas can progress to chronic problems, especially the older we get.

Care and Treatment

Prevention

Accidents happen, but parents can cut down on the frequency and seriousness of injuries by taking preventative measures. Make sure that your child wears a helmet (and protective pads when needed) when bicycling, skateboarding, snowboarding, and skiing. Protective gear functions most importantly to minimize the chance of head trauma, but it also helps to stabilize joints (such as at the knees and elbows), lowering the risk of strains and sprains.

First Aid Treatment

R.I.C.E. (rest, ice, compression, and elevation) is basic first aid for sprains, strains, and bruises.

- **Rest:** Have your child rest after an injury. Avoid all activity that causes pain.
- **Ice:** Apply an ice pack (or a pack of frozen peas) to the injured area. Ice for 15 to 20 minutes at a time repeating every 2 to 3 hours as needed. For children who find it difficult to sit still for the ice to be kept in place, try for 5 minutes at one time. Use a towel to prevent ice burn and avoid heat for the first 36 to 48 hours after injury.
- **Compression:** Use compression for visible swelling. Elastic bandages work well, and should preferably be applied by someone who knows how to wrap. Avoid bandages that are too tight!
- **Elevation:** Elevate the area above heart level and place on a pillow or chair.

Conventional Treatment

The standard treatment for basic injuries includes home therapy, such as rest and ice, as well as medication—typically non-steroidal anti-inflammatories like ibuprofen. Not everyone can tolerate these medicines, and some of their side effects include ulcers, bleeding of the stomach, heartburn, rash, and hepatitis.

Additionally, the FDA (Food and Drug Administration) has recently issued health advisories on several non-steroidal anti-inflammatory medications that are known to increase the risk of heart attacks and strokes and many parents prefer to avoid them altogether. Depending on the injury, your child may also be given crutches, a splint, and a cast.

In general, young children are amazingly resilient and often impervious to minor injuries. However, as your child moves into adolescence, she may experience and complain about more various symptoms following an accident or injury, such as stiffness, sore muscles, and pain. Chronic or persistent injuries are a danger in adolescence, so be sure that your busy teenager properly rests and recuperates following a trauma.

Homeopathic Medicines

Homeopathic medicines can be used following an accident to minimize injury and speed the healing process, and are effective both before an accident (as preventative medicine) and following, working months and even years after the initial injury. Chiropractic, osteopathy, physical therapy, massage and other hands-on treatments also offer a significant amount of relief, especially for adolescents and adults who may not bounce back as quickly as a child.

Aconitum napellus is useful for the feeling of anxiety and panic resulting from an accident or from frightening or shocking events. This child is nervous, agitated, and can't sit still. *Aconite* can be used during an S.O.S. (emergency), which is why I keep *Aconite* 30C in my purse along with *Arnica.*

Arnica montana is the first medicine to think of for all trauma and injuries. *Arnica* is indicated for bruises, swelling, muscle soreness, sprains and strains, falls and blows, overexertion from lifting, or everyday activities such as biking, sports or skateboarding. In addition, *Arnica* helps reduce after-surgery swelling, and may be administered following dental procedures and surgery. I keep *Arnica* 30C in my purse, because you never know when someone will need it. And it is not always the kids! In addition to the pellets taken by mouth, *Arnica* can be used simultaneously as a rub over the injury. *Arnica* is available as a cream, gel, ointment, and oil. Do not use topical *Arnica* on open wounds.

Bellis perennis is used for trauma similarly to *Arnica*. Both alleviate soreness, swelling, and bruising in cases where the injury feels better with movement and rubbing. *Bellis* is also particularly indicated for deep tissue injuries following surgery, or bruising after having blood taken. If *Arnica* is not providing relief for bruising, give *Bellis*.

Bryonia is useful for sprains, dislocations, injuries to tendons, and fractured ribs. The pain feels worse from the slightest movement, including being jarred or bumped, and also grows worse with cold. The injured child feels better keeping still and when pressure is applied to the area. *Bryonia* keynotes also include irritability, desire to be alone, and dry mouth.

Calendula officinalis is a remarkable healing agent recommended for open wounds, scrapes, minor burns, and sunburns. *Calendula* can be used as a cream, gel, tincture, spray, and ointment.

Hypericum perforatum is excellent for injury to nerves, especially in the neck, back, fingers, toes, nails, and brain. The characteristic pains are shooting and sharp, and the injury is very sensitive to the touch. *Hypericum* is also indicated for puncture wounds (including at the site of an injection). For severe back injuries, I often begin with *Hypericum*, alternating with *Arnica*.

Ledum palustre is the primary remedy for puncture wounds (e.g., stepping on a rusty nail), as well as for insect bites and stings. The person feels better from ice cold applications. Often, the wound appears purplish and swollen, which also makes this a good remedy for a black eye. I like to use *Ledum* before any procedure that requires an injection—for example, amniocentesis, epidural, vaccination, or needle biopsy (i.e. liver, breast).

Rhus toxicodendron works well for injuries associated with stiffness that feel better with movement. Often the child is fidgety, and improves with heat therapy, such as taking a hot bath. *Rhus toxicodendron* is a good remedy for sprains, tendonitis, whiplash, and ligament injuries.

Ruta graveolens is used for injuries and bruises to flexor tendons and the periosteum (the covering of the bone), and is also indicated in the overuse of tendons (including tennis elbow), sprained ankle, bursitis, and nodular growths in the wrists. There may also be weakness and stiffness. *Ruta* works well after *Arnica.*

Symphytum officinale, known as knitbone, is used to speed the healing of broken bones and bone bruises. For fractures, use after the bone has been set or is in a cast. *Symphytum* is also good for injuries to the eye, along with *Arnica.*

Herbal Remedies

Tea tree oil (Melaleuca alternifolia), grown in Australia, is known for its antiseptic, antibacterial, and antifungal properties. It is useful for treatment of insect bites, bee stings, cuts, scrapes, minor skin infections, and wounds. Chronic skin conditions, including toenail fungus, are best treated using a constitutional homeopathic remedy.

To use, clean the skin with soap and water. Use a preblended commercial brand. If familiar with essential oils mix 1 drop of tea tree oil with 1 teaspoon of carrier oil (i.e. olive oil, wheat germ, sweet almond, etc.) and apply with to affected area twice a day. Discontinue use if skin becomes irritated. Tea tree oil is not to be taken internally.

Bach Flower Essence

Rescue Remedy contains five flower essences useful for emergencies and crises following an accident. Place 2 drops in a glass of water and sip as needed.

INSECT BITES AND STINGS

From raising a simple welt to prompting a possibly life-threatening swelling, a mosquito bite or bee sting has the potential of ruining a perfectly fun time outdoors. Bites and stings are not the same. Common bites come from mosquitoes, fleas, chiggers, ticks, and spiders. Some insect bites carry disease. Stings considered venomous include bees, fire ants, yellow jackets, wasps, and hornets. Compared to stings, bites tend to be milder. Bites usually itch and may have some redness. Pain and allergic reactions are uncommon. Stings are often less itchy but are more painful, with stinging and burning sensations and more intense swelling and redness. Severe reactions, although rare, are almost always caused by venomous insect stings though bites from black widow or brown recluse spiders are more serious and require medical attention. **If there is swelling in the throat and the child has difficulty breathing, the reaction can become life-threatening and requires emergency medical attention.**

As a precaution, if your child has a history of life-threatening reactions to stings, you can carry an emergency epinephrine kit (EpiPen) the urgent treatment of choice for children who have a history of life-threatening reactions to bee stings. Make sure you know how to use it ahead of time.

Although the bites are usually only a mild nuisance, they sometimes spread disease like malaria, yellow fever, typhus, West Nile virus, and Lyme disease. Lyme disease, the most common, is caused from the bite of the Ixodes tick (deer tick) infected with the *Borrelia burgdorferi* bacteria. Symptoms usually begin within a week following infection. The early stage of infection begins with a painless, red-ringed bull's-eye rash and flu-like symptoms. Chronic symptoms appear from 2 to 4 months after infection and may include arthritis, Bell's palsy, nerve symptoms, heart block, and meningitis. The last stage, which can occur up to years following a tick bite, can cause arthritis (knee), mood swings, and disturbances in thinking, mostly in adults. Lyme disease is usually treated with antibiotics but adjunctive therapy with homeopathy Chinese medicine, naturopathy, or osteopathy are extremely helpful. **Consult your practitioner if your child has any symptoms of Lyme disease.**

Care and Treatment

Prevention

Insect repellants work against biting insects, but are not helpful against stingers. Standard chemical repellants and coils may contain DDT (dichloro-diphenyl-trichloroethane), DEET (N, N-diethylmeta-toluamide) permethrin, and other chemicals. DEET is considered quite effective against mosquitoes, fleas, and ticks, and is found in most commercial brands. However, DEET has dangerous side effects that range from localized rash to more severe conditions such as twitching, seizures, shortness of breath, and confusion. Permethrin is toxic to the nerves and brain, and more dangerous to children than adults. It is meant to be used on clothing and camping equipment, not to be used directly on the skin.

It is difficult to justify the use of these harmful chemicals on children and adults. If you use these products consider the following recommendations:

- Use the product sparingly and avoid applying to your child's face or hands.
- Wash off with soap and water after done for the day.
- Do not use DEET in children less than two years old.
- Do not use DEET on open cuts or wounds.
- Do not apply more than once a day.
- Avoid concentrations of more than 10% on children.

As an alternative, consider natural DEET-free repellents. Some of these include the citronella, cedarwood, eucalyptus, lemongrass, castor, rosemary, clove, neem, geranium, and peppermint. They may need to be reapplied more often than the commercial chemical brands, but they are well worth it. Burn citronella candles or incense during picnic outings. For increased protection, apply the natural repellant to clothing, shoes, tents, and nets.

In addition, here are tips for avoiding insects:

- Think location, location, location! Avoid areas where insects are more prevalent. As mosquitoes breed in wet areas, don't stay by swamps or standing water. Ticks are more common in dense woods.

Ways to avoid stinging insects:

- Don't dress your child in bright colors
- Don't use creams with scent
- Keep a clean picnic area, free of garbage and odors:

Ways to avoid mosquitoes, ticks, and other critters:

- Cover up: Dress your child in a hat, and a long-sleeve shirt tucked into pants with shoes and socks. This is more important especially in the evening when most insect bites occur.
- After playing outdoors in a wooded area, inspect your child for ticks. The tick can be removed with tweezers; grab the tick at the head. Early removal of a tick may help prevent infection.
- Use insect repellant, preferably the natural ones.

Conventional Treatment

The standard approach to treating insect bites and stings is with topical creams for itching, pain, and swelling. These may contain antihistamines, anti-inflammatories, analgesics, and steroid cream. Topical anti-bacterials are prescribed to prevent infection from moderate stings.

Home Treatment

As an alternative, try the following:

- If your child has been stung, examine the area. Brush off the stinger (using the straight edge of a credit card or your nail). Avoid pulling out the stinger with your finger, as it may release more venom into the skin.
- Clean the area with soap and water. Use *Calendula officinalis* mother tincture, an antiseptic.
- Apply *Calendula* cream to the bite, after cleaning.
- Apply baking soda paste (baking soda with water) over affected areas.
- Soak in an oatmeal bath.
- Place ice packs on the area to reduce pain and swelling.
- Throw some rosemary or sage on the barbeque to help repel mosquitoes.
- Garlic (capsule or raw) may reduce the risk of insect and tick bites. Garlic juice (diluted 1:5 in water) sprayed on legs and arms is known to be effective. As an alternative, consider saturating cloth strips and strategically placing them around your outdoor areas.
- Vitamin B1 (thiamine) has been reported to repel insects, though this is not approved by the Food and Drug Administration (FDA). It is thought to work by providing an unpleasant odor and taste in perspiration. Although some people use this during mosquito season, it is suggested to take at least one day before exposure (100 mg in adults) Food sources of vitamin B1 are found in whole-grains, green leafy vegetables, legumes, sweet corn, brown rice, berries, yeast, sunflower seeds, oats, avocado, pasta, tofu, artichoke, tuna, and salmon.

Homeopathic Medicines

Apis mellifica is an excellent remedy for stings, especially bee stings. The bee sting is painful, burning, stinging and feels better with cold applications. The area is red, raised, warm, and swollen. *Apis* is a also a good remedy for hives with the similar presentation. See *Hives and Allergic Reactions*.

Carbolic acid is used for extreme symptoms such anaphylaxis and collapse associated with swelling of the face and tongue, especially after an insect sting. Hives with the sensations of burning and itching and blisters cover the body, especially the hands.

Ledum palustre is a common remedy for mosquito bites and stings, often accompanied with significant swelling. Sometimes the inflammation appears puffy and purple. Typically the bites are relieved with cold applications. According to the late British physician Noel Puddephatt, "*Ledum* is unsurpassed for dealing with the effects (recent and past) of all animal bites and stings and all punctured wounds. Into this category come dog bites, and bites from other animals, insect bites (mosquito especially) and tick bites with the resulting tick bite fever, scorpion bites and all insect stings and bites." If your child comes home with a tick bite, or you suspect one, give *Ledum* 30C twice a day for 3 days.

Urtica urens comes from the stinging-nettle plant. It is often used for reactions to shell-fish, but also for hives following insect bites, stings, and from becoming overheated. The skin stings, prickles, burns, and itches violently. *Urtica urens* is also used for first- and second-degree burns. The hives are worse with cold.

INSOMNIA

When my son is having a problem going to sleep out of excitement or fear, he sometimes requests his "dream drops" to ensure a good night's sleep. Insomnia, difficulty in falling asleep or staying asleep, can affect children from time to time. A fitful night of sleep can impact your child's mood, energy level, and school performance the next day (not to mention yours!). Common interruptions to sleep include illness, teething, or the need for a diaper change. The most common is a transient insomnia, which can last up to four weeks, and when it occurs is more common in school aged children. It may be due to anticipation, fears, emotional upsets, or stress prior to or accompanying an event such as the beginning of school, a performance, or sports competition. For more information, see Chapter 11 "Poor Sleep".

Care and Treatment

Sleeping pills for children have not been approved by the Food and Drug Administration. However, children are being prescribed medications, such as clonidine, for sleep. Many of these children are also on medications for attention deficit hyperactivity disorder (ADHD) which can cause sleep difficulties at night. Common side effects include dizziness, constipation, drowsiness, dry mouth, and decreased heart rate.

Home Treatment

Hot Water Bottle: Some children find a hot water bottle soothing during the cooler months of the year.

Warm Milk: Warm milk, which is high in tryptophan, is known for its calming properties. Use sparingly, as some children are sensitive to milk and prone to mucus production.

Chamomile Tea: Known to calm and to encourage sleep. Drink before bedtime. It can also be used for calming the nerves as a bath. Avoid chamomile if there is an allergy to ragweed.

Lavender: Used for calming nervous tension and stress and for inducing sleep. Use lavender as an essential oil in an aromatherapy preparation for the bath.

Homeopathic Medicines

Aconitum napellus is indicated for sleeplessness and restlessness from sudden onset of anxiety or fear, or from a frightening event. The child tosses about in bed with feelings that she will soon die.

Arsenicum album is for fitful sleep with anxious feelings and dreams. The child wakes at approximately midnight to 2 A.M. She is chilly, worries about her health, and feels better with company.

Chamomilla is useful for insomnia in children with the characteristic keynotes of fussiness and irritability, and improvement with carrying. The child may also start and twitch during sleep. The head is sweaty, with one cheek red and the other pale. The difficulty sleeping can be due to colic, teething, or illness.

Coffea cruda is for sleeplessness and difficulty falling asleep. The child is over stimulated, restless, and wants to play. She is sensitive to noise, stimuli, and touch. She is an extremely light sleeper and wakes at 3 A.M.

Ignatia is known for being an excellent remedy for insomnia following a loss. *Ignatia* is also used for sleepiness following a grief. The child is a light sleeper, and the arms and legs jerk on falling asleep. The child is prone to sobbing, is easily offended, and frequently sighs.

Kali phosphoricum is useful when a child has difficulty sleeping from an over-active mind, including thinking about school activities. The child is anxious, nervous, and overly sensitive. She can suffer from frightening dreams. The child is sensitive to hearing about bad news and unpleasant world events.

Nux vomica is recommended for a child waking at 3 or 4 A.M., and for sleepiness during the day. In addition, there may be difficult with sleep due to stressing about school and overworking. The child may talk or weep during sleep. Known as the Type A remedy in adults, *Nux vomica* is for children who are impatient, competitive, and sensitive to noise and light. There can also be chilliness and constipation.

Gemmotherapy

Lime Tree is a good general remedy for insomnia, known in our house as "dream drops." Lime Tree is also used for its calming effects.

JAUNDICE

Jaundice is not uncommon in newborns and is caused by an accumulation of bilirubin, a substance excreted by the liver. It is normal for newborns to be slightly yellow, but excessive levels of bilirubin can cause medical alarm. **If your baby is sleepy, lacks interest in nursing, or is dehydrated, see your practitioner.** Excessively high levels of bilirubin can lead to deafness, cerebral palsy, or brain damage.

Care and Treatment

Prevention

Babies who experience a difficult birth are at higher risk for jaundice, and in these cases, the homeopathic medicine, *Arnica montana* is the first choice for both baby and mom. Since *Arnica* speeds up recovery for bruises and swelling caused by trauma, it is also a terrific preventive for jaundice.

Parents can also take other measures to minimize or avoid jaundice in their babies. If levels are slightly elevated, babies usually do not require any treatment. Your pediatrician may suggest an increase in the frequency of breastfeeding, which will aid in eliminating the bilirubin.

Conventional Treatment

Light therapy (also referred to as bili lights, or phototherapy) helps break down bilirubin in baby's skin. Phototherapy has been traditionally done in the hospital over the course of one to two days, where the baby is placed naked under lights specifically designed to counteract bilirubin. The treatment, however, can also be done at home using a fiber-optic blanket or band that wraps around the baby. The latter takes longer than the conventional hospital treatment and is more commonly recommended for babies with less severe cases of jaundice. Adverse effects of phototherapy include burns (similar to sunburn), skin rash, loose stools, temperature problems, damage to the retina if the eyes are not properly protected, and dehydration.

Home Treatment

Check your baby for any changes in coloring: It is best to observe in natural daylight. Gently press your finger on the tip of your baby's nose or her forehead.

If the skin looks pale when pressing, there is no jaundice (this can be done on babies of all skin colors), while a yellow hue indicates jaundice. If this is the case, don't panic! Call your practitioner to discuss a course of action to take, if any.

Frequent nursing is helpful in flushing out the bilirubin: For slight levels, increasing your breastfeeding can often be effective in eliminating bilirubin.
Sunbathe your baby: Both of my sons were slightly yellow during their first week, so as a precaution, I let them "bask" in the natural daylight. If the weather is cloudy or cold, a blue incandescent light or "grow light" may be used.

- Place baby in diaper only on a blanket next to a closed window in direct light.
- "Sunbathe" for approximately fifteen minutes, three times a day.
- Avoid allowing baby to become chilled (through exposure to drafts), overheated, or sunburned.
- Cover baby's eyes.

Homeopathic Medicines

Aconitum napellus is used for jaundice that appears acutely and suddenly. It is also useful in soothing fright, either a mother's or a baby's.

Arnica montana is indicated for jaundice that is caused from a difficult or traumatic birth. If a baby is bruised or swollen, use this remedy as a preventive.

Chelidonium maius is a prominent liver and jaundice remedy recommended for babies who are tired with sluggish bowels.

Lycopodium clavatum babies are irritable and constipated. The belly rumbles loudly and is full of gas, and symptoms are worse from 4 P.M. to 8 P.M.

For more information, see "Jaundice" in Chapter 4.

LEAD POISONING

Lead poisoning is a major health hazard in children, especially up to the age of six years old when brains are still growing and developing. Children's bodies are not able to purge toxins like adults' bodies, and nearly 60% of the lead they consume is retained and accumulates. With significant exposure, lead may permanently injure the brain, resulting in learning disabilities, reduced IQ, attention deficit hyperactivity disorder (ADHD), short stature, hearing impairment, loss of appetite, stomachaches, constipation, fatigue, headaches, seizures, irritability, muscle weakness, and death. See your practitioner if you suspect your child may have been exposed to lead. Your practitioner can order a blood test which is done with a simple finger-prick.

Lead is a toxic metal prevalent in many household environments. It was added to paint, appears in residential soil, and now is used in lunchboxes. In previous decades, paint was a common source of lead poisoning, as children could easily consume chips and even small amounts of lead dust particles. Lead paint was banned in 1978, though some older homes still contain it. In addition, the Center for Environmental Health (CEH) has found lead in the lining of some vinyl lunchboxes, where it is added to the PVC vinyl for color or as a stabilizing agent. Although most of the lunchboxes investigated did not contain lead, you cannot know without testing them. Kits to check for lead are available and easy to use. In the meantime, the CEH has advised parents to avoid use vinyl lunchboxes. It is uncertain whether lead is also present in hard plastic or metal boxes. Best bet—use a cloth bag!

Care and Treatment

Conventional Treatment

Treatment of lead toxicity begins with avoiding further exposures. If your child has been exposed to high levels of lead, increase calcium and iron in the diet, as deficiencies allow the body to absorb lead. Decontamination for removal of lead from the body includes oral medication and chelation therapy, which removes lead or other toxic metals from the body. Chelating agents are given by injection, intravenous infusion or taken by mouth.

Homeopathic Medicines

Consider also seeing a homeopath or holistic doctor as there are many remedies and additional treatments to be used in conjunction with standard protocols. Homeopathic medicines such as *Causticum*, *Alumina* and *Plumbum* have been used to treat the effects of lead poisoning.

LICE (PEDICULUS CAPITIS)

One day while I was helping out in my son's kindergarten class, I was summoned along with the other grownups to do a head lice check in another classroom. Apparently, a child was just sent home with them. Head lice, popularly known as cooties, are dreaded by both teacher and parent, as they are very contagious and bothersome. However, they do not spread disease and are not dangerous. The common head lice complaints are a crawling sensation, tickling and itching of the scalp, and loss of sleep. Persistent scratching can cause the skin to become raw and irritated. The nearby lymph glands can also be swollen.

Head lice are small wingless insects that live on the human scalp, attaching themselves to the shafts of hair. Head lice are often over diagnosed in schools so make sure your child does indeed have lice before beginning any treatments. Examine your child's scalp and part the hair section by section. Lice eggs, known as nits, which appear as little white to yellow dots on the scalp, are more common than actual lice. Once hatched, they look like sesame seeds. Lice are more common in girls than boys, from ages 3 to 12 years old. Some children are more susceptible to head lice than others, regardless of hygiene and socioeconomic status. **If you suspect that your child has lice, see your practitioner.**

Care and Treatment

Conventional Treatment

Pediculicides, lice medicines, are available as shampoos, creams, and lotions. If the skin becomes infected from scratching, your doctor will prescribe an antibiotic (topical or oral). Lice medication should not be used in children less than 2 years old. There are a variety of over-the-counter and prescription medications that include Pyrethrin, Permethrin, Lindane, and Malathion. All have side effects. Lindane can cause rash, hair loss, itching, headache, seizures, and even death. Malathion (Ovide) is poisonous to the brain, immune system, and may cause cancer.

Home Treatment

Many parents prefer to try the more natural, gentle, and non-toxic approach before resorting to toxic pesticides. In addition, many of the standard brands are considered ineffective due to some recent strains of lice becoming resistant to their effects.

- Use a fine-tooth comb (preferably a nit comb) to remove the nits, along with a magnifying glass and proper lighting. Grooming is considered an effective way to eliminate lice. It is easier to comb out lice when the hair is wet. While this is also time-consuming, there are no side effects! Combing towards the scalp, against the hair grain, makes it easier to dislodge them. Clean comb after each use. Do this daily for several nights, and then every three nights as needed.
- Check other family members for lice, and treat immediately.
- Encourage your child to avoid sharing hats, hairbrushes, and other personal items.
- Traditionally, some parents shave a child infested with lice. Although it may make it more difficult for lice to find a warm, comfortable spot, and easier for parents to search for lice, this may draw unwanted attention to the child.
- Vacuum carpets and upholstery in the house and car. Clean combs, brushes, and barrettes. Wash them in hot water for 20 minutes, soak in rubbing alcohol for one hour, or discard.
- Machine-wash linens, bedding, and clothing in hot water. Place in a hot dryer cycle for 30 minutes. Dry-clean stuffed animals or put away in an airtight plastic bag for three weeks.
- Oil may be helpful in eliminating lice by covering and suffocating them. Coat the entire scalp and hair with olive oil or mayonnaise after combing out the nits. Cover the head with a shower cap or towel and leave on for at least two hours. (I would recommend leaving it on for six to eight hours.) Shampoo the hair, which may take several washings. Examine the scalp and remove any existing nits. Repeat every four days, as needed, for three weeks.
- In a study from the Israel Medical Association Journal, a natural head lice remedy with essential oils proved very effective in controlling head lice without serious side effects. The remedy, which contained coconut oil, anise oil, and ylang ylang oil, was applied every five days on three occasions.

There are commercially prepared essential oil treatments containing lavender, lemon, rosemary, tea tree, and other oils that may also be effective.

Homeopathic Medicines

Consider also seeing a homeopath or holistic practitioner as there are many medicines and additional treatments which can be used in the treatment of lice.

LYME DISEASE

See *Insect Bites and Stings.*

MASTITIS

Mastitis is an infection or inflammation of the breast. Mastitis can be extremely painful and is usually associated with hard, swollen, engorged breasts. There can also be a discharge from the nipple. **If you experience severe pain with breast-feeding, fever (higher than 100.6° degrees F (38.1 C), flu-like symptoms (chills, body ache), or red streaks in the breast, consult your practitioner immediately.**

Care and Treatment

Prevention and Home Treatment

To prevent engorgement, usually a common cause of mastitis:

- Nurse frequently at least every 1½ to 2 hours during the day, and up to 3 hour stretches at night. Begin by nursing at least 15 minutes or longer on each side.
- Use breast pumps if your newborn is not feeding as often as two hours.
- Cold compresses between feedings may reduce swelling, congestion, and improve milk flow. Wrap in cloth, and place on the breast and underarms, avoiding the nipple or areola. Use for 15 to 20 minutes every 1 to 2 hours if needed for swelling.
- Warm compresses can be used just prior to breastfeeding or pumping to help your milk let-down if you are engorged. Moist heat, such as a warm, wet cloth, is preferable. Avoid using warm compresses for more than five minutes as they can increase swelling.
- Gently massage breasts while taking a warm shower or bath, immersing breasts in a basin of warm water, or using a hot water bottle wrapped in a wet cloth.

- Place a few drops of olive oil on the breasts (avoid the nipple) while doing gentle breast massage prior to breast feeding.
- Use cabbage leaves for mastitis. Personally I used raw green cabbage leaves to help relieve fullness and sore nipples in between feedings. Trust me, it feels soothing! Clean the inner leaves of a green cabbage and place on breasts inside bra. They can be room temperature or chilled. Change every two hours or when wilted.
- Get plenty of rest and stay around the house, including taking naps with baby.
- Nursing or sports bras without under wires may be helpful for support. Avoid binding the breasts, which can lead to plugged ducts.
- Increase fluids, and drink lots of water. Eat healthy, including a diet low in saturated fats.

Conventional Treatment

The standard prescribed care for pain and swelling is an anti-inflammatory drug, like ibuprofen or stronger pain medication. In the case of a moderate to severe infection, antibiotics are prescribed. Nystatin may be given if your doctor suspects a yeast infection (thrush) on the nipple.

Homeopathic Medicines

Belladonna is indicated when breasts are red, hot, swollen, and very tender. Symptoms can come on suddenly, and may be accompanied by high fever. Often pain occurs on the right side, with a throbbing sensation. The breast is extremely sensitive to touch or being jarred, with streaks radiating from the nipple.

Bryonia is helpful in relieving breasts that are hot, painful, hard, and engorged. Symptoms may include stitching pains that are greatly aggravated by any motion, as well as a dry feeling and irritable mood.

***Calendula* Ointment** or **Cream.** Use prior to childbirth for several weeks, and in the first weeks of nursing. *Calendula* is an excellent natural topical and will help condition nipples and minimize cracking. Wash off before nursing.

Castor equi is recommended for nipples with painful cracks or ulcers, and extremely tender, swollen breasts that are sensitive to clothing and which feel worse going down stairs. Breasts may also itch with redness of the areola.

Hepar sulphurs is a useful remedy for boils and abscesses in general, as well as for sore and cracked nipples especially for pus forming organisms. The woman's mood is irritable, and she tends to be chilly.

Phytolacca is indicated for inflamed or swollen breasts that are also full of lumps. Nipples may be cracked and excoriated, and the mother will often experience intense suffering on putting child to breast, with pain radiating from the nipple all over the body. She may also have a sore throat with swollen glands.

Pulsatilla is a versatile remedy used to prevent breast engorgement, *Pulsatilla* also helps to dry up mother's milk when weaning. Recommended for women whose mood is changeable and weepy.

Silica. I use this remedy routinely after birth for several days to prevent or minimize sore nipples. It is recommended to relieve soreness and cracks on the nipples, accompanied by sharp, splinter-type pain (extending from breast to shoulder), and/or inflamed breast with constant burning.

Gemmotherapy

Black Currant is ideal as a general strengthener, and **European Walnut** is good for deep seated infections.

MEASLES

Measles, also known as rubeola, is a contagious viral illness. Measles begins with cold-like symptoms, high fever, red sensitive eyes, and a hacking cough. On the fourth to fifth day, a rash appears. Characteristically, Koplik spots, small white spots in the insides of the cheek, appear before the rash. The rash begins faintly behind the ears and within twenty-four hours becomes darker as it spreads to the face, neck and arms. In two to three days the rash reaches the legs, while the rash on the face correspondingly fades. With the onset of the rash, the child begins to feel better. Occasional complications of measles are due to secondary infections manifesting as severely high fevers, deafness, blindness, ear infections, pneumonia, and encephalitis. **If you suspect your child has measles, contact your practitioner.**

Care and Treatment

Prevention

Measles is given as part of the trivalent vaccine, MMR (Measles, Mumps, and Rubella) and is usually given at 12 to 15 months with a second dose given between 4 to 6 years old. For more information about the measles vaccine, see "Standard Vaccinations" in Chapter 14.

Conventional Treatment

Standard medicine has no specific treatment for measles. The symptoms of high fever and cold do not respond to antibiotics, aspirin, or cough medicine, though supportive treatment, such as rest and fluids are helpful. Homeopathy, naturopathy, traditional Chinese medicine have all been useful in the treatment of measles and in strengthening the body's natural ability to heal. For general home treatments, see *Flu.*

Homeopathic Medicines

Aconitum napellus is an excellent remedy to use at the onset of measles to relieve the sudden onset of high fever, red eyes, light sensitivity, runny nose, sneezing, and dry barking cough. It is also helpful for skin that itches and burns. The child is typically restless and fearful.

Apis mellifica can be taken when the skin eruptions are burning, red, and puffy. There is a feeling of heat on the skin, and the child feels better with cold compresses. The throat can be painful, stinging, and red.

Belladonna during measles is helpful for sore throat (often right-sided), dry barking cough, restlessness, vomiting, and fevers with delirium.

Euphrasia is considered the remedy par excellence for measles when eye symptoms are the most bothersome. *Euphrasia* is indicated when the eyes tear and eyes and lids itch, burn, and are swollen. It will also treat an accompanying sneezing and runny nose.

Gelsemium is useful for many conditions including measles. Three common symptoms that would indicate the use of *gelsemium* are dullness, dizziness, and drowsiness. *Gelsemium* is often useful at the onset of measles with a fever when there are frequently muscle aches, croupy cough, headache, and an absence of thirst.

Pulsatilla is also indicated to treat measles after the fever has begun to decrease and the rash begins to fade. *Pulsatilla* can be used for the frequently changeable symptoms in measles that include the rash, respiratory symptoms, eye discharge (yellow-green), diarrhea, cough, and earaches. Typically, the child may be moody, weepy, and want company.

Sulphur is commonly used for measles. Common indications for *sulphur* include a rash appearing dusky or purplish in color, an itchy rash, and rough, coarse skin.

Gemmotherapy

Briar Rose is a good general strengthener for a child's immune system.

See *Fever* and *Flu*.

MENSTRUAL CRAMPS AND PMS

One of the big milestones in an adolescent girl's life is the onset of her period. With early puberty on the rise, her period may begin as early as nine years old or as late as sixteen, with an average age of twelve. In my experience, a girl's first period is rarely met with indifference but rather with a myriad of strong feelings ranging from excitement to despair.

Some, but not all, girls experience painful cramps, caused by hormones called prostaglandins, which in turn are stimulated from the hormone progesterone, released by the ovaries after ovulation. As girls get older, the cramps usually diminish. Many of the women in my practice report that their period was more painful during the teen years, although this is not always the case.

Also commonly associated with the period is the well-known *premenstrual syndrome* or PMS. PMS is an all-encompassing term used to define many symptoms associated with the week or days just before the period. In addition to cramps, the symptoms of both PMS and menstruation may include irritability, tearfulness, depression, anxiety, food cravings, headaches, back pain, nausea, bloating, skin breakouts, sleep disturbance, breast tenderness, and more. At least 30 percent of females suffer from PMS and probably every woman at some time in her menstrual history has experienced it in varying degrees. Painful periods and difficulty with PMS can greatly affect an adolescent girl's life and interfere with daily activities such as school, sports, and social life.

Care and Treatment

In standard medicine, painful cramps are treated with non-steroidal anti-inflammatory (NSAID) medications such as ibuprofen or naproxen. Following the NSAID, it is commonplace for practitioners to prescribe the birth control pill. In addition, the pill has been prescribed for young women with irregular periods. Used since the 1960s, most pills contain the synthetic hormones estrogen and progesterone.

From my professional viewpoint, I consider the Pill (and alternatives like hormonal shots and patches) an unhealthy medication made of synthetic hormones. Like many other conventional medications, the Pill only treats the symptoms and not the deeper underlying problem. The Pill works by blocking the natural process of ovulation, thus tricking the body into thinking it is pregnant. Among the Pill's side effects are bloating, weight gain, breast tenderness, increased risk to breast cancer, fatal blood clots, stroke, migraine headaches, gall bladder disease, liver tumors, and mood swings. The Pill is known to deplete the body of B vitamins (especially B6 and folic acid), vitamin C, magnesium, and zinc, which can contribute to heart disease. There are safer methods of handling menstrual cramps, as well as avoiding unwanted pregnancies.

Home Treatments

Hot Water Bottle: A hot water bottle can be comforting for complaints that are relieved with warmth.

Diet: As the saying goes, "We can be our own worst enemy." Not uncommonly we crave foods such as caffeine, chocolate, salt, and sugar around the time of period which may aggravate symptoms. Try to avoid these foods prior to and during menstruation.

Exercise: Get out and walk, run, or swim! Exercise has been shown to relieve symptoms of PMS and menstrual cramps.

Homeopathic Medicines

Belladonna is useful for intense cramps that come on suddenly. These throbbing pains are relieved when a woman straightens her body. *Belladonna* is indicated if the pains worsen when she bends over or applies pressure to her abdomen.

Chamomilla is indicated with painful spasmodic menstrual cramps that have been compared to contractions during labor. Think of *Chamomilla* when there is hypersensitivity to pain, and anguish and anger with the cramps. The intense pain can extend to the back and down the thighs.

Colocynthis, in contrast to *Belladonna*, works better for young women whose cramps are relieved by applying pressure or warmth or by doubling over. The cramps are bearing-down in nature. Usually an adolescent with these symptoms also suffers from PMS anger, irritability and indignation.

Magnesia phosphorica also is useful when the cramps improve with warmth and gentle pressure and when the woman feels irritability or anger. *Magnesia phosphorica* is the first remedy to think of for general menstrual cramps.

Pulsatilla is indicated when the onset of the period is delayed in puberty, the flow starts, stops and starts again, or is easily suppressed from nerves. There is a scanty amount of blood. The period is preceded by severe gripping menstrual cramps. *Pulsatilla* improves a wide variety of PMS symptoms, and is often chosen for the adolescent who feels weepy and depressed and wants to be comforted. Other keynote symptoms include complaints of feeling warm, faint, diarrhea, better in the open air, and lack of thirst.

Lachesis mutus is one of the remedies that I prescribe for complaints of strong PMS symptoms, which are relieved once the period begins, or are better with the flow. Other *Lachesis* symptoms are pain on the left ovary, palpitations, feelings of jealousy, and sensitivity to tight clothing around the belly and neck.

Gemmotherapy

Raspberry in gemmotherapy form is an excellent for painful spasmodic menstrual cramps and PMS. Take three times daily at the onset of the period. Raspberry can also be used once daily throughout the month.

MILK SUPPLY

Reasons for low milk supply include stress, fatigue, poor nutrition, inadequate water intake, infrequent nursing, nipple confusion from bottle or pacifier, supplementation with formula, or anatomical conditions in mother or baby. Many mothers jump to conclusions about their milk supply, however if your baby is gaining weight while exclusively on breastmilk, then your milk supply is probably adequate.

Care and Treatment

Conventional Treatment

Prescription medications like Reglan can be used to increase milk supply. Most of my patients prefer to use the plethora of remedies and basic measures available rather than beginning with prescription medication.

Homeopathic Medicines

Lac defloratum helps restore flow of milk when there is deficient production. Often the low milk supply is due to small atrophic breasts. The patient who responds well to *Lac defloratum* tends to strongly fatigued and worn out, is often allergic to milk, and has a history of migraines.

Pulsatilla can increase milk when it is deficient, and restore milk supply after a breast infection.

Ricinus communis is used to increase the quantity of milk in nursing women. It is indicated in women with large breasts. There may also be diarrhea.

Herbal Remedies

In addition to homeopathic medicines, herbs can increase milk supply. Used for centuries in a variety of cultures, these prepared herbal remedies are known as galactagogues. Unlike homeopathics, herbal remedies may carry side effects. For this reason, I recommend you start with herbal tea. See your practitioner or lactation consultant if you are not getting the desired results.

Mother's Milk Tea, which contains fenugreek and other herbs, helps boost milk supply. As a tea, it is a milder galactagogue, but can still work effectively. Drink several cups a day as needed either warm or cooled. Fenugreek is commonly used to increase milk supply and has been known to work very quickly. Employed for centuries in Ayurvedic and Chinese medicine, fenugreek's many indications include improving metabolism, managing diabetes, and reducing cholesterol. If you have a tendency to hypoglycemia or history of diabetes, monitor blood sugar levels closely when taking fenugreek, since it can affect blood sugar levels.

Bach Flower Essence

Rescue Remedy can be helpful in triggering the let-down reflex and is known as well for its calming influence during stressful times. If feeling overwhelmed, Rescue Remedy can help with relaxation, which will increase milk flow. Place 4 drops in a drink prior to pumping or nursing.

MOTION SICKNESS

Motion sickness, whether from a car, plane, boat, or amusement park ride, can be a particularly unpleasant experience, both for a child and an adult. Motion sickness can also be aggravated from riding on winding mountain roads, turbulence in the air, or rough ocean waters. Motion sickness is caused when the brain receives conflicting messages about the environment from the inner ear (the center for balance) and the eye. As a result, some children can begin to feel queasy.

Common in childhood, motion sickness mostly affects children between the ages of four and ten years old. Symptoms of motion sickness include dizziness, headache, dry mouth, queasiness, nausea, vomiting, increased saliva, yawning, and cold sweat.

Care and Treatment

Prevention

- Avoid reading while en route.
- Avoid large meals prior to travel; small snacks are preferable.

- Avoid the smell of gasoline, tobacco, or strong-smelling foods.
- Face forward in a car (for children over 20 lbs) with a view of the horizon.
- In a plane, sit over the wing, where the ride is less bumpy.
- Distract your child with music, song, or chat.
- Direct your child's gaze outside of the car.
- Be prepared: Keep an empty bag handy, just in case.
- Acupressure wrist bands are known to be helpful in preventing motion sickness. There are no side effects and they can be worn by both children and adults.

Conventional Treatment

The conventional treatment of motion sickness includes over-the-counter medications, such as the antihistamine, meclizine (Antivert, Bonine). It can help with the nausea; however, the side effects of drowsiness, dry mouth, and blurry vision can be as unpleasant. See your practitioner prior to using any medications.

Home Treatment

Here are simple measures to deal with motion sickness:

- Stop the activity. Get out of the car or off the boat or plane as soon as possible.
- Get your child into fresh air.
- Place a cold washcloth on the face.
- Unbuckle the pants and loosen tight clothes.
- Have your child lie down.

Give your child tea and crackers to soothe the stomach. Ginger tea can be especially effective. To make ginger tea, mix ⅛ teaspoon powdered ginger in a cup of hot water, or place two slices of raw ginger in one cup of water, and boil for 10 minutes. For children over age two, dilute ¼ cup of ginger tea in 8 ounces of water. (Ginger should not be given to children less than two years old.) Sweeten with natural sweetener and cool slightly before serving.

Homeopathic Medicines

I am particularly prone to seasickness and will take several measures to avoid feeling ill. I have had excellent success using a combination of the acupressure wrist bands, ginger (capsules for adults), and homeopathic remedies. The following are some of the commonly used homeopathic remedies for motion sickness:

Cocculus indicus is indicated for motion sickness provoked from a car, boat, train, or plane. The nausea can even be aggravated by looking at a boat or car in motion. There is an aversion to food, with an aggravation at the thought or smell of food. The child is worse in the fresh air and better lying down. *Cocculus* is also useful for people who are tired from having been up in the night caring for family (nightwatching), and also have the above symptoms.

Petroleum is also for nausea from a car or boat. There can also be dizziness, headache at the back of the head, and an excess of water or saliva in the mouth. A sensation of emptiness in the stomach with pain is relieved by constant eating. The child feels worse in the cold.

Sepia is recommended for nausea intensified by the thought or smell of food. The child is worse in the morning, and desires vinegar, sours, and pickles. She feels better with strong exercise and is chilly, even when in a warm room. There is an empty feeling in the stomach.

Tabacum is for motion sickness with tremendous nausea. There can be violent vomiting. The child is pale, cold, and clammy with much spitting of saliva. She feels better being in fresh air, uncovering the belly, and closing the eyes. She is made worse from motion.

MOUTH SORES

Mouth sores can make it difficult for your child to eat, drink, and brush her teeth. Some, like canker sores, are not contagious, but do run in families and are often confused with cold sores, which are fever blisters caused by the herpes simplex type 1 virus. Others, like herpangina, may be accompanied by other symptoms like sore throat and fever. In most cases, mouth sores will heal on their own within a week or two. **See your practitioner if a sore persists for more than two weeks.**

Causes and Types of Mouth Sores

Canker Sores: Also known as aphthous ulcers or aphthous stomatitis, canker sores are small sores inside the mouth along the inner lining of the cheeks, lips, tongue, gums, throat, or palate. Researchers do not know the cause of canker sores, though evidence indicates they are triggered by eating certain foods, such as salty or sweet foods, chocolate, and nuts, by nutritional deficiencies, especially in folic acid, vitamin B12, and iron, and by abnormalities in the immune system, stress, menstrual cycle, and local irritation caused from injuries and habitual biting on the inside of the cheeks and lips. Canker sores are more common in females than males, and in teenagers and young adults in the early twenties. Canker sores typically manifest as painful small red spots, resembling little craters, and occur one or a few at a time. They begin as swollen red spots which burst, and once ruptured, are surrounded by a red halo and covered with a white or yellow film. The size ranges from one eighth of an inch and, in more severe cases, as large as one inch in diameter (2.5 cm). Most of the time, discomfort is the main symptom, which lasts the first 3 to 4 days, and fever is rare. It can take up to two weeks for a canker sore to disappear.

Herpangina and **Hand-Foot-Mouth Disease:** Herpangina, caused by the coxsackie virus, is a painful condition consisting of blisters in the mouth accompanied by sore throat and fever. The illness usually begins with loss of appetite and a high fever. Additional symptoms may include runny nose, drooling, vomiting, diarrhea, headache, and rash. If blisters appear on the palms and soles, it is called *hand-foot-mouth disease.* The rash consists of tender red spots, which blister (not on the buttocks), and do not itch. The virus can be confused with strep throat, ear infection, and chicken pox. Up to fifty percent of children may have no symptoms, and some children may only have a few characteristic symptoms. It lasts from three to seven days and, like chickenpox, your child will only get it once (though there can be other strains of coxsackie virus). It is a contagious infection that spreads from unwashed hands (i.e. daycare) and is more common in children under age five. It peaks in the summer and early fall.

Care and Treatment

Conventional Treatment

For canker sores, most treatment is aimed at providing relief. Medications such as Zilactin, a topical anesthetic, Mylanta to coat the sores, and anti-inflammatories for pain are often prescribed . Severe cases are treated with cauterization of the canker sore, steroids, or immunosuppressive drugs.

Conventional treatment for herpangina and hand-food-mouth disease is to provide pain relief if needed and general home therapy measures such as rest and fluids. Antibiotics are of no value, as this is a viral infection. Frequent hand-washing can be helpful in reducing it.

Home Treatment

While your child has a mouth sore, avoid irritating foods such as salty items, nuts, tomatoes, pineapple, grapes, plums, and all citrus. Use a mild toothpaste and soft bristled tooth brush. Throw away old toothbrushes. Give your child bland soft food, and use a straw if necessary with liquids.

Many parents prefer to begin with treatments that are natural and have no side effects. The following treatments and remedies can be helpful in alleviating the discomfort and speed the healing process. In general, they should be used four times a day for the duration of symptoms.

Lukewarm Water: Rinse the mouth four times a day.

Hydrogen Peroxide: 2 ounces hydrogen peroxide diluted with 2 ounces water (1:1). Use as a rinse for older children or dab the affected area with a cotton swab for infants.

Baking Soda Rinse: Mix 4 ounces of water with 1 teaspoon salt and 1 teaspoon of baking soda.

Black Tea: Place a wet black tea bag over the canker sore. Tannin, an astringent found in tea, can help reduce pain.

Cold Popsicle: Cold liquids can provide temporary relief.
***Calendula* mother tincture:** 1 tablespoon tincture diluted in ½ cup warm water. For older children, use as a mouthwash; for younger children, spot dab with a cotton swab.

Homeopathic Medicines

Borax is one of the first remedies I use to treat mouth sores, and is particularly recommended for sores on the mouth and tongue that bleed easily. The ulcers are painful, and the mouth feels hot and tender. A child who is easily startled and frightened or has a fear of downward motion (i.e. being laid down in the crib) will generally respond to this remedy. It is also a common remedy for thrush.

Calcarea carbonica is indicated for recurrent mouth sores in infants. Often, the infant is chubby and sweaty with a big head.

Mercurius is helpful for mouth sores associated with excessive drooling. The child has bad breath, sweats easily, and is sensitive to both hot and cold. The tongue is yellow and indented.

Natrum muriaticum is useful for sores on the mouth and tongue. They smart and burn when in contact with food and drink. The lips can be dry, and there is a craving for salty food. The mood is sensitive, with a desire to be left alone. This is also a common remedy for cold sores.

Gemmotherapy

Briar Rose is useful for general conditions and for strengthening children.

Prim Wort is for mouth ulcers and **Hedge Maple** is specific for treatment of viruses, and can be used for herpangina and hand-foot-mouth disease.

MUMPS

Mumps is a mild viral infection that is contagious. Mumps begins with the common symptoms of fever, headache, and fatigue. Within 24 hours, it leads to the characteristic swelling of the cheek (one or both sides) caused by inflammation of the salivary gland. The illness lasts a week. Complications from mumps are rare and may include inflammation of the ovaries, testicles (more common in adults), deafness, encephalitis, and meningitis. If you suspect your child has mumps, contact your practitioner.

Care and Treatment

Prevention

The MMR (Measles, Mumps, Rubella) vaccine is given at 12 to 15 months and from 4 to 6 years old. For more information, see "Standard Vaccinations" in Chapter 14.

Conventional Treatment

Treatment for mumps infection includes bed rest, and a bland diet with fluids. Other health care therapies such as homeopathy, naturopathy, traditional Chinese medicine, and chiropractic care are effective in aiding the healing process.

Homeopathic Medicines

Abrotanum is a useful remedy, especially when the swelling in the parotid gland (cheek) starts to lessen, and testicles begin to swell. The child feels chilly.

Belladonna is helpful for mumps when there is high sudden fever, especially in the afternoon, and when the face and eyes appear red. There can be difficulty with swallowing. Belladonna is especially indicated if the swelling of the cheek goes down followed by a lethargy, deliriousness, and headache.

Carbo vegetabilis is indicated if the swelling in the cheek is hard and the fever is low, accompanied by hoarseness. It is also useful when the swelling changes location from the parotid gland in the cheek to the testes in boys or breasts in girls. The child may have a desire to be fanned or have open air.

Mercurius is the first remedy to consider for most cases of mumps. Typical *Mercurius* symptoms are night sweats, chills, fever, and drooling. The parotid gland is swollen, inflamed, and painful.

Phytolacca is excellent for swollen glands including mumps infection. The swelling is hard and painful, and worse at night. Typically the child who responds to *Phytolacca* feels better with cold drinks. The neck can be stiff and worse with motion.
Pulsatilla is used when the swelling has wandered to another gland, including enormously swollen testes in boys and swollen breasts in girls. Typically the child is not thirsty, worse in a warm stuffy room, and enjoys company.

Gemmotherapy

Briar Rose is a good general strengthener for a child's immune system

See also *Fever* and *Flu*.

NAUSEA

See *Motion Sickness*.

NOSEBLEEDS

Nosebleeds happen, and often when you least expect them. Although the sight of a child bleeding from the nose is disconcerting, the amount of blood lost during a nosebleed is usually mild. Nearly every child has experienced a nosebleed, and some up to several times a month. The mucous membrane in the nose is thin and delicate and susceptible to bleeding from picking the nose, sneezing, swelling caused by allergies, and dryness in the winter months. Nosebleeds are painless and usually begin without warning in one or both nostrils. **See immediate medical attention if the bleeding is heavy or doesn't stop after two trials of applying pressure on the nose for 10 minutes at a time.**

Care and Treatment

Prevention

- Winter nosebleeds can be caused by dryness. Minimize central heating that would aggravate the condition.
- Place ice pack or cube of ice on the nose or upper lip.
- Avoid picking the nose. Picking the nose can be irritating, and may trigger nosebleeds, especially during allergy season. Keep your child's nails cut short.

Conventional Treatment

No medical treatment is necessary for mild nosebleeds. For severe nosebleeds, standard doctors use prescription nose drops and dressings. Sometimes, they will cauterize the vessels.

Home Treatment

During a nosebleed, have the child sit down, leaning forward to avoid swallowing blood, which can trigger vomiting.

Pinch nostrils together at the tip of the nose with the thumb and forefinger for up to ten minutes with continuous pressure. For severe bleeding, apply pressure below the nostril just above the upper lip. Place a small piece of wet cotton under the upper lip and apply pressure for ten minutes.

Homeopathic Medicines

Homeopathic medicines can be helpful during a nosebleed. If your child is prone to recurrent nosebleeds, consider seeing a homeopath who can prescribe a constitutional medicine, which can remedy the situation.

Arnica montana is for bleeding following an injury. It can also be used for nosebleeds after exertion, trauma, fits of coughing, and during a growth spurt. The child wants to be left alone and says there is nothing the matter with her. She is better lying down and worse with motion, being touch, and in the damp cold.

Belladonna is known for sudden onset, intensity, and throbbing sensations associated with bleeding. There is tingling in the tip of the nose, and the face is red. Your child is extremely sensitive to being touched, jarred, and to noise, and is better reclining propped up. *Bellladonna* more often affects the right side and is strongly indicated in sudden high fevers. There is a great thirst for cold water. *Belladonna* is strongly indicated for nosebleeds in bed at night, or on waking in the morning.

China officinalis (Cinchona officinalis) is best for great weakness and anemia following the bleeding. The child easily bleeds from the nose, especially upon rising from 6 to 7 A.M. She is better with hard pressure, open air, and warmth, and worse from drafts. Bleeding can occur like clockwork every several days. The child can be in a sensitive, touchy mood.

Crotalus horridus is strongly indicated for bleeding from the nose, and widespread bleeding from any orifice in the body. Bleeding is characterized by slow oozing of dark, unclotted blood. There is an intolerance for collars and turtlenecks and a craving for pork, stimulants, and sugar. The child can appear quite ill, with trembling and weakness, and is worse on the right side.

Ferrum phosphoricum is indicated for bleeding of bright red blood. The child feels better with cold applications and is worse at night, from 4 to 6 A.M., and with motion. The face looks flushed, the pulse is quick, and the child may be restless. *Ferrum phosphoricum* is also a strong remedy for weakness and anemia. The child is usually thirsty for cold drinks. Along with *Arnica* and *Hamamelis, Ferrum phos* is good for bleeding after operations.

Hamamelis is excellent for healing veins, including those associated with nosebleeds, hemorrhoids, and bleeding following surgery. Bleeding from the nose is profuse, with a slow, steady flow of dark, unclotted blood. There is a feeling of tightness in the bridge of the nose and can be a bad odor from the nose.

Lachesis mutus is for the bleeding of thin, dark blood. Symptoms are worse on the left side. In *Lachesis*, all symptoms, including bleeding, can be aggravated before the period in adolescent girls. The child feels better after bleeding (including a nosebleed), and with hard pressure and open air. She is worse from sleep, warmth, and in the spring and fall seasons. The child is emotional, jealous, and talkative.

Phosphorus is for the child who suffers readily from nosebleeds, and bruising and bleeding gums while brushing the teeth or after visiting the dentist. The blood is bright red, thin blood and is apt to come in the morning or upon blowing the nose. In adolescent girls, a bloody nose may occur instead of her period. They are friendly children who are anxious with many fears. They crave icy cold carbonated drinks, and are better in the open air and after washing with cold water. The child is worse after exertion, a change of weather, and lying on the left side.

OSGOOD-SCHLATTER DISEASE

See *Growing Pains.*

PINKEYE

See *Conjunctivitis.*

PINWORM

Pinworm, while annoying, is usually considered harmless. Caused the enterobius vermicularis parasite, pinworm is one of the most common parasitic intestinal infections, and affects up to 50 percent of children. The worm looks like a piece of thread less than a half inch (2 cm.) in length. For this reason, it is also called threadworm. Pinworms make their home in the large intestine and live off of feces. Most children who have pinworm have no symptoms at all. When a child is affected, the common complaint is intense itching around the anus at night. In girls, the infection can extend to the vagina, causing itching with discharge. Pinworm has also been linked to grinding of the teeth, hyperactivity, poor appetite, and bed wetting, which is caused by an irritation in the urethra from pinworm.

A pregnant female pinworm will travel from the colon out of the anus, laying her eggs around the child's buttocks. This causes the child to be intensely itchy around the bottom at night. A vicious cycle is set up when the child scratches her bottom, and unknowingly transfers the eggs on fingers and under nails. Pinworm is contagious, as the eggs can land on a variety of surfaces and easily end up in the mouth, which allows the eggs to hatch in the child's intestine.

To determine if your child has pinworm, examine the buttocks with a flashlight during the night. To further confirm the diagnosis, place transparent tape (scotch tape test) by the skin near the anus in the morning. The tape can be analyzed for eggs under the microscope. See your practitioner if you suspect your child has pinworm.

Care and Treatment

Conventional Treatment

The standard treatment for pinworm is anti-pinworm medication, mebendazole (Vermox)—administering one dose with a second dose two weeks later. Side effects to Vermox include allergic reactions, hives, diarrhea, and fever. Some doctors also recommend treating the rest of the family members, washing the bedding and pajamas following treatment, frequent hand-washing, and keeping short fingernails.

Home Treatment

- Wash hand when coming indoors, after using the toilet, and before eating.
- Keep your child's nails clipped.
- Change underwear and bedding daily during treatment.
- Bathe daily.
- Spread olive oil or vaseline on the anus and buttocks, including the skin folds, which can be helpful in stopping the eggs from getting hold on the skin.
- Add raw garlic, pumpkin seeds, carrots, beets, and pomegranates to the diet, as they have anti-worm properties.
- Eat healthy. Avoid dairy, refined foods, and sugars. Add acidophilus to the diet.

Homeopathic Medicines

Cina is one of the common remedies used for pinworms. In addition to itching of the anus, the child can show a tendency to pick her nose and grinding her teeth during sleep, and is generally restless. The child is touchy and angry, which can lead to tantrums.She can also have night terrors and yawns frequently.

Nux vomica is also indicated for itching and tickling around the anus from pinworm. The child who responds to *Nux vomica* is angry, impatient, and competitive in school and sports. The digestive system is often affected, causing colic, irritable bowel, and constipation. They are chilly and can easily awaken at 3 or 4 A.M.

Sabadilla is associated with pinworms and a crawling sensation with itching at the anus. It is known as a strong remedy for hayfever, and the child may also suffer with sneezing fits and runny nose.

Spigelia is indicated for pinworms when there is a feeling of itching and crawling in the rectum and anus. Yet the child's worst complaint is pain around the navel. The child is restless, anxious, easily offended. There is a tendency to have bad breath, constipation, and itching of the nose. The child is also worse from touch and walking in open air, and may be afraid of sharp, pointed objects, such as a shot. *Spigelia* is also a common headache remedy.

Teucrium is indicated for terrible anal irritation and itching caused by pinworm. Nose symptoms are also marked with irritation, stuffiness, and desire to pick the nose. There can be difficulty sleeping,

PMS

See *Menstrual Cramps.*

PNEUMONIA

See *Cough, Fever,* and *Flu.*

POISON IVY, POISON OAK, AND POISON SUMAC

Growing up in the canyons in Los Angeles, many of the kids in my neighborhood suffered from poison ivy after hiking in the brush. Although I was spared, I know it is not fun! Poison ivy is found throughout the United States and grows as a shrub or vine. Poison oak, a shrub, is more common in the western United States, and poison sumac is the least common nationwide. All three plants can cause the same reactions, which occur when oil from the leaves touches the skin. Symptoms include extreme itching, redness, and blisters that appear in patches, starting on areas of the skin that were exposed to the plants. The rash itself is not contagious, though any residual oil that remains on clothes can affect those who come into contact with it. Symptoms can appear within a few hours of contact or after several days, and last approximately two weeks. **Contact your practitioner if your child has a severe case of poison ivy.**

Care and Treatment

Conventional Treatment

The standard treatment includes calamine, cortisone cream, and antihistamines. Oral steroids are reserved for severe cases.

Home Treatment

Itching and irritation can lead to secondary infections. To avoid this, apply Calendula topically over the rash (as a cream, lotion, ointment, or dilute as a tincture in a ratio of 1:4).

In addition, applying cool cucumber slices or rubbing the inside of the banana peel on affected area can offer relief from itching. Oatmeal baths are also helpful. See *Hives and Allergic Reactions* for more information.

If you suspect exposure, wash the skin with soap and water. Clean hands, including under the fingernails, and remove and wash affected clothing. To prevent further contact, teach your children to avoid the plants; show pictures so they know which ones to avoid.

Homeopathic Medicines

Anacardium is indicated when there is horrendous itching relieved with scalding hot water. The itching is worse after scratching and the blisters are filled with yellow fluid. Children who respond to *Anacardium* are known for their "angel and devil" personalities, and can be prone to cursing and getting into fights.

Croton tiglium is recommended for intense itching, where the skin feels tight. The skin burns, and scratching is painful. The blisters ooze and form crusts. There can also be gurgling in the intestines with sudden diarrhea.

Graphites helps when the rash is moist and oozes a thick, sticky, yellow discharge that looks like honey. The child is prone to eruptions on the scalp, especially on back of the head and in the bends in the arms and legs. The child is worse with the cold, at night, and in warmth of bed. She is better in open air.

Rhus diversiloba, made from California poison oak, is for sensitive skin characterized by intense itching, burning, and swelling. The swelling can be on both the skin and genitals and the rash looks like chicken pox. There is relief with cold, and symptoms are worse from the warmth. The child is often exhausted and wants to sleep. Similar to *Rhus toxicodendron* below, there is joint stiffness made better with motion.

Rhus toxicodendron is indicated for a rash with small fluid-filled blisters that burn and are intensely itchy. The rash feels better under hot water, and is worse in the cold. The child can also be stiff and feels better with motion, and, in general, is fidgety and restless. A craving for cold drinks and milk is common. Like *Rhus diversiloba*, *Rhus toxicodendron* is made from poison ivy. Both *Rhus* remedies can be used for any type of rash, regardless of the origin, as long as the symptoms match.

Sulphur is a common skin rash remedy. Indications for *Sulphur* include dry skin and itching that are worse from bathing, warmth, and while in bed. There is a characteristic aggravation at 11 A.M. Known as a homeopathic centrifuge, *Sulphur* drives toxins out of the body to the surface, usually to the skin. For this reason, if you are administering *Sulphur*, use in a low potency, 6C or 6X, conservatively and slowly.

See also *Chickenpox* and *Hives and Allergic Reactions.*

RASH

See *Diaper Rash* and *Poison Ivy, Poison Oak, and Poison Sumac.*

ROSEOLA AND FIFTH DISEASE

Prior to the use of vaccines, viral childhood infections causing skin rashes (usually accompanied with fever, fatigue, and aches) were more commonplace than today. These skin rashes, known as exanthems, used to be lumped together as measles, but are now distinguished as different conditions. The most common viral childhood exanthems include measles (rubeola), rubella (German measles), chickenpox, erythema infectiosum (fifth disease), and roseola (sixth disease).

Causes and Types

Roseola infantum is a mild viral infection. It is known as *sixth disease* due to the fact that the childhood rashes were sequenced according to numbers.

Following exposure to roseola is an incubation period that lasts up to 10 days. Also referred to as baby measles, roseola is contagious and caused by the human herpes virus. Roseola occurs in children from six months to two years of age and by age two, most children have had it. Antibodies from the mother protect babies younger than six months old. The symptoms of roseola often begin with mild respiratory symptoms, followed by a high fever that lasts several days. When the fever ends, a rash begins on the trunk and spreads up to the neck, face, and to the arms and legs. The rash can last from several hours to a few days and can be flat or raised and rose-pink in color. Some areas have a light halo. Upon touching the rash, the spot will turn white (blanch). The disease can last from 3 to 7 days, and resolves on its own. It is more common in the spring and fall. Roseola does not require any particular treatment other than supportive care for fever.

Fifth disease, known as erythema infectiosum or "slap cheek syndrome," is also a mild viral exanthema. Fifth disease starts with a low grade fever, headache, and malaise. Similar to roseola, these symptoms pass as a bright, rosy-red rash appears on the cheeks, which spreads to the trunk, arms, and legs. The rash lasts up to 5 to 7 days. There is no specific conventional treatment for fifth disease, and most cases resolve without complications. Fifth disease is considered a mild illness and many children have either mild symptoms or no symptoms at all. It is more common in school-aged children from ages 5 to 12 years old, and outbreaks occur in the winter and spring, occurring every three to four years.

See also *Fever, Flu,* and *Measles.*

RESPIRATORY SYNCYTIAL VIRUS (RSV)

See *Cough.*

RUBELLA (GERMAN MEASLES)

German measles is a mild viral childhood illness, also known as the *three-day measles*. Rubella is a mild rash and fever that lasts for two to three days. Common symptoms include a low-grade fever, swollen glands, rash, and fatigue for a few days. A rash appears on the face and then spreads downward, fading by day three to five.

Care and Treatment

Prevention

Nowadays, rubella is rare in the United States due to the vaccine (MMR). The purpose of the rubella shot is to prevent Congenital Rubella Syndrome, which can affect a fetus whose mother contracts rubella early in her pregnancy. If she is not immune to rubella (either through having the illness or through vaccine), her fetus is at risk for birth defects, including deafness and mental retardation. In addition, she may suffer a miscarriage. For more information, see "Standard Vaccinations" in Chapter 14.

See *Fever, Flu* and *Measles.*

SEVER'S DISEASE

See *Growing Pains.*

SINUS INFECTION

Just like adults, children can suffer from sinus infections, although symptoms in children are not as painfully obvious. Sinuses are air-filled cavities in the bones of the face, located behind the cheeks (maxillary sinus), between the eyes (ethmoid sinus), and behind the forehead (frontal sinus). The sinuses connect with passages to the nose and are not fully developed until twenty years old. The small size of a young child's sinuses coupled with her immature immune system can make a child susceptible to sinus infections. Sinus infections are precipitated by a variety of triggers, such as the common cold, allergy, or exposure to smoke. When infected, the sinuses fill with mucus or pus and can become blocked.

Symptoms of sinus infection in children involve a long-lasting cold (up to two weeks), low-grade fever, fatigue, fussiness, nasal congestion, cough, mouth breathing due to stuffed nose, drainage of yellow-green mucus, and post-nasal drip. Additional symptoms can include nausea, vomiting, sore throat, swelling or drainage of the eyes, malaise, and bad breath. A cough that worsens while lying down for a nap or at night is probably due to mucus drainage from the sinus and nose irritating the throat. Older children and adolescents will also tend to experience the more familiar adult-like sinus symptoms of pain in the face and headache. See your practitioner if your child has a persistent nasal discharge or cough for more than ten days.

Care and Treatment

Conventional Treatment

The common cold, which is caused by a virus, also causes inflammation of the sinuses. When the symptoms of congestion and cough (worse at nap and at bedtime) last up to two weeks, the diagnosis usually is a bacterial sinus infection and the practitioner often prescribes antibiotics. In addition, she may give your child decongestants, including nasal sprays and saline nasal rinses.

Chronic sinusitis includes prolonged symptoms that last for more than three months or recurrent bouts of acute sinusitis (four to six a year). Sometimes the ear, nose, and throat specialist may recommend surgery to correct chronic sinus blockage, which can include removing the adenoids in the back of the nose.

Home Treatments

Nasal rinses, known as nasal lavage or irrigation, have been shown to be helpful in clearing and thinning secretions for children with sinus infections, as well as any condition with congestion, such as the common cold and hay fever. The saltwater solution is sprayed into each nostril either by using a bulb syringe or a neti pot. The neti pot, used in India for centuries, has a spout for the nose. The salt to water ratio is 1 level teaspoon sea salt to 2 cups (½ liter) of lukewarm filtered water. Use once or twice a day as needed. Steam inhalation with chamomile is also useful for treating sinus infections.

Homeopathic Medicines

Hepar sulphuris is useful for sinus conditions with extreme tenderness of the nostrils and thick nasal discharge that smells like old cheese. The child is worse in the cold, and the nose stops up when in the cold. She feels better with warmth, moist heat, and in damp weather. There can also be a post-nasal drip. The mood is irritable and sensitive.

Kali bichromicum is the most commonly used remedy for sinus infections. The child experiences pain and pressure at the root of the nose, which is alternately stuffed and runny. The mucus is thick and stringy, like glue, and sneezing is common in the morning. *Kali bichromicum* can also be used for a stuffed nose in infants (see *Stuffed Nose*). The child is worse in the cold, the damp, and in open air, but feels better with motion, heat, and pressure.

Mercurius treats the sinus infections where the child's nose looks red, raw, and dirty. She may be sneezing frequently with a yellow-green, thick, pus-like discharge. The child has bad breath with excessive drooling and can also be sweaty. She feels worse in the extreme heat and cold temperatures.

Nux vomica treats symptoms of sinusitis where sneezing and runny nose are frequent by day. During the night, the nose is stopped up, and it is not uncommon for a child to wake up with complaints around 3 to 4 A.M. The keynotes of *Nux vomica* also include an angry and impatient child.

Pulsatilla is recommended for sinus infections with a bland, yellow-green discharge. The nose is stuffed and aggravated by lying down, and the child feels better in the open air. She is worse in a warm, stuffy room and after eating rich foods. The mood is weepy and clingy.

Gemmotherapy

Briar Rose and **European Hornbean** are helpful in treating sinusitis.

See also *Common Cold, Flu,* and *Stuffed Nose.*

SORE THROAT (PHARYNGITIS)

Nearly every child will experience a raw, scratchy, or painful throat at least once year, and many on a more frequent basis. Known also as pharyngitis, sore throats are typically caused by infections and can be contagious. Viral infections are responsible for nearly 90% of sore throats, especially in association with common cold or flu viruses. Bacterial infections account for the remainder, approximately 10%, with the majority of these caused by group A *Streptococcus* (commonly known as strep throat). As most sore throats are caused by viruses and heal on their own, there is no need for antibiotics. Sore throats can be aggravated by coughing, post-nasal drip, and breathing through the mouth. For children with seasonal allergies or a stuffed nose, breathing through the mouth during the night can contribute to sore throats in the morning upon awakening. Usually the condition improves throughout the day.

Causes of Sore Throat

The sore throat from the common cold or flu is usually accompanied by other symptoms such as a runny nose, congestion, cough, hoarseness, body aches, and fever. Other viruses that can cause sore throat include chicken pox, measles, whooping cough, Coxsackie viruses, and mononucleosis.

Mononucleosis (Mono): Also known as glandular fever, mono is usually caused by the Epstein-Barr virus. It is also known as the "kissing disease" because it is contractible through saliva, and more common in adolescents and young adults. Common symptoms of mono include painful sore throat, fatigue, sore muscles, fever, cough, swollen lymph glands (in the neck, armpit and groin) and an enlarged spleen. Mono is diagnosed with a blood test called the mono spot test. Standard medical treatment for mono includes rest, and most people heal on their own.

Mono can take some time for recovery (from several weeks to months).

Coxsackie Virus: This virus spreads from unwashed hands and occurs more frequently in the summer and early autumn in children up to age ten. While nearly half of children have no symptoms, Coxsackie can present in different parts of the body and general symptoms include fever, aches, mild sore throat, and stomachache. The types of Coxsackie that can cause sore throat are *Hand, Foot, and Mouth disease,* and *Herpangina.*

Strep Throat: Diagnosis of strep throat is based on history, a physical exam, and, if needed, a throat culture or rapid strep test. Many sore throats are considered *probable* strep and treated with antibiotics. If your doctor believes your child has strep, ask for a Rapid Test in the office to confirm and avoid taking antibiotics unnecessarily. The throat culture, which takes up to 48 hours to process by the lab, is up to 99% precise. Parents who are concerned about waiting several days for a result can be reassured that antibiotics for strep throat can begin up to nine days after onset. In fact, beginning treatment too early can increase the chances of re-infection later. Strep throat is accompanied by a fever that tends to be over 101°F (38.3°C) and lasts more than three days). Children with strep throat usually have painful swollen glands, pain on swallowing, and redness and inflammation with white patches and pus in the throat (pharynx). Additional complaints include nausea, vomiting, chills, body ache, headache, and lack of appetite. If your child has a cough, runny nose, hoarseness or conjunctivitis, she most likely has a viral infection and not strep throat. Strep is most common in school aged children from 5 to 15 years old, especially in the cold winter months, and is rare in children under three years old. On rare occasions, strep throat can result in damage to the heart valves (rheumatic fever), joints, kidneys (glomerulonephritis), and other organs several weeks following the infection. Antibiotics are up to 80% effective in eliminating a strep infection, and you can still use homeopathic medicines in conjunction with a regularly prescribed course.

Scarlet Fever: Strep throat accompanied by a bright red sandpaper-like rash, most prominent in the skin folds, is known as Scarlet Fever. The rash is caused by production of a toxin from the bacteria and often lasts from the second to the sixth day. Scarlet fever is rare and is treated in the same way as strep throat.

Care and Treatment

Conventional Treatment

In standard medicine, treating your child's sore throat begins by determining whether it is a viral or bacterial (i.e. strep throat) infection. If your practitioner suspects strep, she will begin your child on antibiotics, typically penicillin. Sore throats can result in chronically enlarged tonsils and adenoids, which can impede breathing and lead to difficulty sleeping. Treatment usually begins with medications such as antibiotics and decongestants to help bring down the inflammation. If the condition persists, surgery is recommended to remove the tonsils and adenoids.

When possible, avoid surgery, as the tonsils and adenoids are considered an important part of the immune system. Many patients come to my office wanting to try homeopathy before considering surgery. Constitutional homeopathy for chronic conditions can be successful in alleviating the condition.

Home Treatments

- Older children can be encouraged several times a day to gargle with warm salt water (¼ teaspoon in 8 ounces of warm water) and *Calendula* tincture (10 drops) mixed together. Both have antiseptic properties.
- Change the toothbrush monthly at least during the cold and flu season, as the toothbrush is a refuge for bugs.
- Keep the throat covered with a scarf.
- Try potato poultice or lemon compress around the neck three times a day.

Homeopathic Medicines

Aconitum napellus is useful for painful sore throats that come on suddenly and intensely (for similar indications, see *Belladonna* below). The throat is red and can sting, burn, or feel prickly. Symptoms may come on after exposure on a windy day or following a frightening event or accident. The child is restless, anxious, and fearful, and is usually thirsty for cold drinks. She may feel better in open air and is typically worse at evening and at nighttime.

Apis mellifica also works for intense sore throats. The keynote to using *Apis* is a sore throat that feels swollen or that stings and burn. Often, the soreness diminishes with cold drinks. In general, children who respond to *Apis* feel worse in heat. The throat looks fiery red with swollen tonsils and the pain tends to be predominantly right-sided.

Belladonna is useful when the sore throat comes on suddenly and intensely. The sore throat tends to be right-sided, and the throat and tonsils are bright red in color with swollen tonsils, often accompanied by high fever. The throat feels dry, hot, and constricted with pain upon swallowing. The child is sensitive to light, noise, and being jarred. Although there is not much thirst, the child craves lemonade. She is typically worse at 3 P.M., 11 P.M. and after midnight. *Belladonna* is indicated for strep throat and scarlet fever. It can be used in conjunction with antibiotics.

Hepar sulphuris is recommended for sore throats and swollen tonsils that feel like a fish bone or splinter is lodged in the throat; the sensation can typically be felt in the ears. The glands are swollen, filled with pus, and sensitive to touch and cold, including drafts. Appropriately enough, children who respond to *Hepar sulphuris* also tend to be overly sensitive and irritable. There is a craving for vinegar and other acids.

Lachesis mutus is indicated for left-sided sore throats, which may move to the right side. The throat feels dry, very swollen and painful, and is purplish in color. There is pain on swallowing, with food easier to swallow than drinks. The child may experience a choking feeling, with sore throat pain extending to the ears when swallowing. The child does not like anything tight around the neck. He can experience waves of heat, and is better with cold drinks.

Lycopodium clavatum relieves sore throats that begin on the right side and move to the left. The child usually feels better with warm drinks, and craves sweets. The tonsils can be chronically swollen. The throat feels contracted and restricted, leading to frequent swallowing.

Mercurius is recommended for an inflamed sore throat that can be present with ulcers and pus on the tonsils and back of throat. The child complains of the throat feeling raw, burning, and smarting. The glands in the neck are swollen and painful. The child has bad breath, is drooling and sweaty, and has a constant desire to swallow. Left-sided pains can be treated with *Mercurius iodatus ruber*, and right-sided with *Mercurius iodatus flavus*.

Phytolacca is for sore throats that are dark red or bluish in color. The throat and tonsils feel hot, burning (like a hot ball), and swollen, with shooting pains that extend into the ears on swallowing. The throat feels better with cold drinks and is aggravated by hot. The neck glands are hard, painful, and swollen.

Gemmotherapy

Briar Rose strengthens a child's immune system and is useful for conditions involving ear, nose, throat, and sinuses.

Red Spruce targets the tonsils, throat, and nose.

See also *Flu*.

SPRAIN

See *Injuries*.

STOMACHACHE

Aches and pains in the digestive system are commonplace in children, and result from a whole variety of causes that include gas pains, indigestion, stomach flu, food poisoning, emotional upset, lactose intolerance, food allergies, overeating, and constipation. In infants, pain is often dismissed as a colicky phase. **For any persistent stomachache for more than two days or if your child is having severe complaints, contact your practitioner.**

Causes and Types of Stomachaches

Gas: The most common cause of abdominal pain in a child who does not have fever, vomiting, or diarrhea is trapped gas. Gas may be due to eating certain foods, swallowing air, or digestive conditions. There is usually relief from burping or passing gas.

Heartburn: Some children may complain of stomachaches that originate in the upper abdomen beneath the breastbone. Often referred to as indigestion or heartburn, this condition is characterized by a burning or warm feeling of discomfort that may extend up to the throat. Heartburn can be accompanied with burping, nausea, bloating.

Appendicitis: A more serious yet rarer cause of abdominal pain is appendicitis. The appendix is a small accessory piece of intestine located in the lower right side of the belly. Its purpose is unknown, but when infected can cause intense pain and potentially serious consequences. Symptoms of early appendicitis usually centered around the belly button and may resemble a number of other common illnesses, so avoid jumping to conclusions. If your child has appendicitis, the pain becomes more severe and localized in the lower right part of the belly. The child will have a nausea, vomiting, diarrhea or constipation, fever, and loss of appetite, and the pain is constant and continues to worsen. She must lie down curled in a fetal position. There may be vomiting, but diarrhea and frequent vomiting are rare. A commonly used test in medicine is the jumping test. If your child is able to jump, she probably does not have appendicitis. Appendicitis is more common from ages ten to thirty. An appendectomy, or surgical removal of the appendix, is the usual treatment once it is diagnosed.

Care and Treatment

Conventional Treatment

When general home treatments fail to offer relief and a serious condition is ruled out, most practitioners prescribe an array of medications for gas pains and stomach acid. Common medication that lessen intestinal gas are Mylicon and Gaviscon. For heartburn, your child may be prescribed an antacid such as Mylanta or Maalox.

Home Treatment

- Hot water bottle placed on the belly.
- Abdominal massage (see "Infant and Child Massage" in Chapter 9).
- Peppermint tea and chamomile tea are good for soothing an upset stomach. Sip as needed. Ginger tea can be used for children over two years old (see *Motion Sickness*).
- Young infants should be fed in a semi-upright, 45-degree angle while held in your arms. Some swallowing of air is inevitable but bottle feeding may contribute because of the design of the bottle or nipple. Switch one or both.
- Burping baby in a vertical position will help the air bubbles come out, instead of going down into the intestines causing discomfort.

Gently pat your baby's back, while she is lifted up resting comfortably against your chest with her head peering over your shoulder. In an upright position, the air in the stomach stays above the milk level and makes it easier to burp. Avoid placing baby on your lap to attempt to burp baby. The horizontal position can lead to more air bubbles going down into the intestines rather than up and out.

- Encourage your child to chew slowly and avoid gulping. Prevent your child from playing, roaming, or watching television while eating—better to sit at the dinner table with the family.
- Avoid gas-producing foods. Big offenders are carbohydrates, while fat and protein cause less gas. Foods to watch out for include cauliflower, Brussels sprouts, broccoli, cabbage, beans, and sugars. Rice is the only starch that does not cause gas. Dried beans will be less gassy if they are soaked for several hours before cooking. Be sure to change the water several times while soaking. Children who are lactose intolerant should avoid dairy products because they contain the sugar lactose.
- Breastfeeding mothers and children can avoid foods that may cause indigestion, such as rich, greasy, fast foods (and soda pop, too).
- Avoid overeating or eating too quickly.
- Juice has a lot of fructose, a sugar that produces gas. Juice can lead to gas and diarrhea. If your give your child juice, dilute it at least 50 percent, and allow no more than one glass per day.
- Minimize chewing gum as it contributes to increased gas. It also accounts for increased swallowing of air. The artificial sweetener sorbitol, a sugar, is difficult to digest and ferments in the intestines, leading to increased gas.

Homeopathic Medicines

Arsenicum album is indicated for stomachaches with burning pain that extends into the throat. The pains are relieved with drinking milk and warm beverages. *Arsenicum* is well known for alleviating nighttime aggravation from midnight to two A.M., that causes a child to wake up with complaints. *Arsenicum* also treats food poisoning, gastritis, and ulcers, as well as vomiting and diarrhea. The child feels nervous in the stomach and likes to have company. She may experience the sensation that food gets lodged in the esophagus and crave sour foods.

Calcarea phosphorica is for stomachaches in school-aged children. These children are sensitive to the demands of school and may also complain of headaches. They are worse at the end of a school day. There may be diarrhea, aggravated during dentition, as well as a craving for smoked meats such as hot dogs and bacon. The child is irritable, fussy, and demanding of attention.

Carbo vegetabilis can be used for indigestion from rich, fatty foods. It is helpful or children with tremendous bloating, belching, gas, and gas pains. The child feels better propped and worse lying flat. Clothing must be loosened around the waist. The child improves with open air or a fan, despite being chilly, and feels tired and weak. A desire for carbonated drinks is common.

Lycopodium clavatum is also indicated for bloating with relief from belching and gas. The child is worse eating small amounts of food, and she gets full quickly. The belly is noisy and rumbles and feels better with rubbing. The child craves sweets and is hungry, waking at night to eat. Pains tend to be right-sided (or go from right to left), and worse from 4 to 8 P.M.

Nux vomica is for stomachaches caused by overeating favorite foods, especially spicy, fatty food. In our house, *Nux vomica* is the remedy to use when one has eaten "too much." The child is chilly, constipated, and can waken at 4 A.M. with stomach cramps. Stomach pains are worse from tight clothes and in general better with warmth and hot water bottles. The mood is angry, irritable, and impatient. The child feels relief after using the toilet.

Pulsatilla is for the child who gets indigestion and gas from eating greasy, rich foods. There is no thirst and the stomach is bloated and feels heavy. There is a tendency toward loose stools. The mouth is dry, yet the child is not thirsty. She feels warm and gets relief with gently walking in the open air. The child is easily brought to tears, and is shy and clingy.

Sulphur is for a child who has a big appetite, and suffers from indigestion and heartburn. The belly is sore and sensitive to pressure, better bending forward. The child is suddenly hungry at 11 A.M. with an aversion to eggs and fish. She is awoken early in the morning with a sense of urgency caused by smelly diarrhea or loose stools. The child may also have a tendency towards itchy skin rashes.

Herbal Remedies

Gripe Water is a European herbal remedy preparation that has been used for generations for colic, stomach aches, gas pains and cramps for babies and children. Although there are different brands with varied formulas, most of them contain some of the following ingredients all of which are helpful for the digestive system: anise, angelica, cardamom, chamomile, dill, fennel, ginger, and sodium bicarbonate. Use as directed by the manufacturer.

Gemmotherapy

Fig Tree is soothing for conditions of the stomach while normalizing stomach acids.

Wineberry helps ease the intestine from bloating, diarrhea, or constipation.

See also *Colic, Diarrhea, Motion Sickness,* and *Vomiting.*

STREP THROAT

See *Sore Throat.*

STUFFED NOSE

A stuffed or blocked nose is extremely uncomfortable and can result in seemingly endless hours of lost sleep for you and your child. Typically a stopped up nose forces your child to breathe by mouth. This can get tricky especially while nursing because a baby frequently has to stop feeding in order to take a breath through the mouth. Stuffed nose can be the result of a cold, runny nose, or sinus infection, or can occur chronically due to allergies or enlarged tonsils and adenoids.

Care and Treatment

Conventional Treatment

For stuffed nose caused by the common cold, your practitioner may prescribe decongestants. If it is caused by a sinus infection, she will also prescribe antibiotics.

Homeopathic Medicines

The following homeopathic medicines are for acute conditions of stuffed nose. For chronic nasal stuffiness and enlargement of the tonsils and adenoids, see your practitioner for natural ways to clear the air passages and reduce swelling.

Dulcamara is for a completely stuffed nose that is worse in the cold, damp weather, or during the changes of temperature common in the autumn months. Nose and eyes can also have thick yellow mucus crusts. There is a desire to keep the nose warm, as cold air stops the nose.

Lycopodium clavatum is indicated for stopped up nose that is predominantly right sided (or right going to left). There is an aggravation of symptoms especially from 4 to 8 P.M. and symptoms are worse at night in bed. *Lycopodium* is also indicated for tummy upsets and colic.

Nux vomica is well known as a remedy for moodiness with irritability, anger, and impatience. Effective in treating colic and constipation with hard painful stool, *Nux vomica* is also useful for colds with stuffy noses and snuffles. A child can be sneezing with a runny nose in the morning and stuffed up at night, and is especially worse around 3 to 4 A.M.

Sambucas nigra is one of my favorite remedies for snuffles. *Sambucas* is indicated for a completely stopped up nose that makes it extremely difficult for baby to nurse or breath. There can be sweatiness, anxiety, and hoarseness. The child feels better sitting up in bed, with motion, and being wrapped up. *Sambucas* is also used for croup, whooping cough, and bronchitis.

Gemmotherapy

In addition to **Briar Rose, European Hornbean** is effective for stuffiness of the nose caused from infections and allergies.

See also *Common Cold, Flu* and *Sinus Infections.*

SUNBURN

See *Burns.*

SURGERY

Over 7 million procedures and surgeries are performed in the United States each year. Surgeries both minor and major place great strain on the body, and homeopathic remedies can be helpful for both postoperative and post-anesthetic healing. They can be used in conjunction with pain medication, and most patients find they heal quicker and require less pain medication when using homeopathic remedies.

Care and Treatment

Conventional Treatment

Depending upon the procedure, most patients are prescribed pain medication and sometimes antibiotics to prevent infection.

Homeopathic Medicines

The following list represents some of the commonly used homeopathic medicines for postoperative healing. It is best to have the chosen remedies on hand before so that they can be used immediately following the procedure. Unlike some herbs and medications, there are no contraindications for using homeopathic medicines right after surgery. A correctly chosen remedy can help with pain relief , speed healing, and may help avoid infection.

Except for *Arnica*, all of these medicines can be taken at a 30C strength. With improvement decrease to 1 to 2 times a day, then discontinue. Major surgery may require the remedy be used for several days. With improvement, the remedy should be used less often. Homeopathic medicines can be used in conjunction with other medications.

Arnica montana is the first medicine to use following dental procedures and surgery. In addition, *Arnica* is useful for bruises, swelling, muscle soreness, sprains and strains, falls and blows, overexertion from lifting, sports and childbirth. Use *Arnica* 30C (or a higher dose 200C for major injuries and operations); have your child take 3 tablets 4 times a day after surgery for several days.

Bellis perennis is indicated for post operative pain and bruising, especially of deeper tissues such as the abdomen and pelvis. If *Arnica* is not providing relief following surgery, give *Bellis*.

Hypericum perforatum is excellent for injury to nerves, especially in the fingers, toes, nails, teeth, brain, and spinal cord. The characteristic pains are shooting and sharp, and very sensitive to the touch. *Hypericum* is also indicated for puncture wounds, including epidural spinal anesthesia.

Ledum palustre is also recommended for puncture wounds with much swelling and inflammation, particularly when the inflamed the area looks purple, puffy, and is cold to the touch. I use both *Ledum* and *Hypericum* following epidural anesthesia.

Staphysagria is useful for surgical wounds and lacerated tissues requiring stitches, as well as for wounds that remain painful and sensitive after a procedure since it helps to quickly reduce the pain and inflammation and allow the wound to heal. The child's mood may be sensitive. *Staphysagria* can also be used to speed up recovery following episiotomies in childbirth and caesarean sections.

Phosphorus can be used to treat the ill effects from anesthesia and is indicated for nausea and vomiting. The child may be fearful and prefer to have company around. There is a craving for cold drinks or ice chips.

TEETHING

Just when you think you've made it through the newborn period with its fussiness and colic-like symptoms, you discover that teething waits right around the corner. By around six months many infants have begun to teeth and some may have their first teeth. For others, it can take months. Symptoms of teething include painful swollen gums, drooling, diarrhea, fever, irritability, increased nursing, fussiness, and difficulty sleeping. Often baby has her fist in her mouth (or anything else she can chew on!). Symptoms of runny nose and fevers higher than 101°F (38.3C) are traditionally not associated with teething according to most practitioners. However, I believe that teething with all its symptoms can render an infant susceptible to becoming sick.

Care and Treatment

Conventional Treatment

Standard treatment for teething includes topical pain medicines that temporarily numb the gums. Sometime the topical may touch the throat interfering with the gag reflex, which is one reason why many parents prefer to avoid this medicine altogether. Most practitioners recommend acetaminophen or ibuprofen for basic teething discomfort.

Home Treatment

Many babies find relief with cold objects and gentle pressure placed on the gums. This can be done by massaging the gums with your clean finger or by providing a rubber-tipped spoon, chilled moistened washcloth, chilled teething ring, or teething biscuits to bite on. Avoid small objects and other choking hazards.

Many European families place an amber necklace on their babies (both boys and girls) during the teething phase. Amber, the fossilized resin of ancient trees, is known in European folklore for its healing properties. Traditionally, wearing amber is thought to have natural calming, relaxing, and analgesic properties for teething pains. Keep in mind that any child wearing a beaded necklace should be supervised. Remove while sleeping.

Homeopathic Medicines

Homeopathy can work wonders on little ones with teething discomfort. In fact, many parents are initially introduced to homeopathic medicines during the teething stages. Camilia (made by Boiron) and Hyland's Teething Tablets (made by Hyland's and Standard Homeopathic Company) are two popular homeopathic teething products that contain a combination of several teething medicines. This is appealing if you are not familiar with homeopathy or if you have difficulty finding the right remedy.

Belladonna is recommended for teething accompanied by sudden fever. The pain is intense and the face is red, throbbing, and radiates heat. The gums are swollen and the mouth is hot and dry. The baby feels better biting on objects, and may twitch and jerk during sleep.

Calcarea carbonica is indicated for teething babies who are chubby and sweaty, especially while nursing or during sleep. Teething is painful and delayed. They have a tendency towards constipation.

Calcarea phosphorica is also for delayed teething, though this child constantly wants to be carried, and is whiny and more irritable than in *Calcarea carbonica.* The teeth are sensitive to chewing and tend to be soft with easy decay.

Chamomilla is one of the most common remedies for teething babies. Typical indications are swollen inflamed and tender gums. One side of the face may be flushed. In addition, the child is angry, irritable, impatient, and contrary, and can also seem inconsolable, frequently crying, screaming, and arching his or her back. The child desires something then refuses it, and is relieved by being carried and rocking. Her stools can be green and look like spinach.

Gemmotherapy

Use **Briar Rose** for additional support during the teething phase.

TETANUS

Tetanus (*Clostridium tetani*) bacteria exist in soil as spores. Tetanus is not a contagious disease, but enters the body through a break in the skin, such as a puncture wound, burn, or major injury, where it then affects the nervous system. Early symptoms include difficulty swallowing, painful spasms, and tightening in the jaw (also called lockjaw) as well as in the neck and abdomen. These symptoms can progress to severe muscle spasms and contractions in the neck, chest, belly, and back. Complications associated with tetanus include pneumonia, fractures (from severe muscle spasms), and brain damage. Tetanus is a serious illness. See your practitioner for preventive treatment of tetanus in the first 48 hours following an injury such as stepping on a rusty nail, animal bites, or any other significant injury like gangrene, crush injuries, or frostbite.

Care and Treatment

Prevention

In children tetanus is part of the DTaP vaccine (diphtheria, tetanus and pertussis). If a child has received a series of three tetanus shots, or is older and has had a booster within the past ten years, she may not need a tetanus shot following an injury. However, if your child is not vaccinated against tetanus, she can receive the tetanus immune globulin (TIG) shot which will neutralize the toxin from the bacteria. The TIG will give your child passive immunity and protect her at the time of injury. This will not provide protection in the event of future injuries. For more information on the tetanus vaccine, see "Standard Vaccinations" in Chapter 14.

Conventional Treatment

Tetanus is treated in the hospital with an antitoxin, antibiotics, and sedation. The wound may require surgical cleaning. Supportive measures include bed rest in a quiet dark environment.

Home Treatment

Clean the wound with soap, hot water, and *Calendula officinalis.* According to an article from the *Journal of the American Medical Association*, "Good wound care is probably the single most important factor in the prevention of tetanus in fresh wounds."

Homeopathic Medicines

Ledum palustre is commonly indicated for puncture wounds. The area around the wound may be cold to touch and feels better with cold applications.

Hypericum perforatum is also used for puncture wounds and injuries to nerves. There may be extreme sharp shooting pain.

See also *Injuries.*

THRUSH

I have received distress calls from new parents who call to report their beautiful baby has white spots in the mouth. What is it? Most likely, it is thrush: yeast (candidiasis) overgrowth in the mouth. During childbirth, babies can be exposed to yeast in the birth canal. Approximately 5 percent will come down with thrush by a week to 10 days of age. Thrush is a result of an imbalance in the body that leads to an overgrowth of yeast which is a fungus. These imbalances can be caused by antibiotics (given to babies or their breastfeeding moms), which kill the normal bacteria in the digestive tract, contributing to potential yeast overgrowth. Pacifier use, extensive use of the bottle, stress, difficulty with nursing, and a weak immune system can also lead to imbalances.

Thrush can be passed back and forth between baby's mouth and mom's nipples (or an artificial nipple on a bottle). The symptoms of thrush are varied. Thrush is easy to spot in a baby, as there are white to gray plaques visible on the inside of the mouth—on the inner cheeks, tongue, gums, palate, or lips. After feedings, baby's tongue can have a thin, whitish coat; this is not thrush. Usually thrush spots come in groups in several different places and can stay for weeks. For some babies, there are no symptoms other than the plaque, and for others the areas can be tender, painful, and cause baby to be irritable and avoid feeding. An overgrowth of yeast can also cause diaper rash, vaginal yeast infection, and rash between the skin folds.

For breastfeeding mothers, thrush can be an equally painful experience. Breast symptoms include itching, soreness, burning, and redness of the nipple, with stabbing pain that extends throughout the breast while nursing, Nipples can become flaky, cracked, and can bleed. Thrush is not considered dangerous, and will heal on its own if left untreated. See your practitioner for stubborn cases of chronic thrush.

Care and Treatment

Conventional Treatment

Although most cases of thrush will usually disappear without treatment after a month, most conventional practitioners prescribe treatment for pain or discomfort. Conventional treatments for thrush include topical antifungal medicines. In addition, the mother may be prescribed an oral anti-fungal (Diflucan). One of the topical antifungals, *gentian violet*, is the purple solution that stains everything; or an oral nystatin antifungal solution. Both can be used in baby's mouth and on mother's nipples. See your practitioner for more information. If there is no improvement after three days, discontinue use.

Home Treatment

Before resorting to the conventional treatments, many parents prefer to begin with the more natural approaches. These remedies can be used for both mother and baby:

- Keep clean and dry. Wash hands, breast, and nipples after each feeding. In addition, consider rinsing the nipples with one of the following:
- Raw apple cider vinegar. Dilute 1 tablespoon of apple cider vinegar to one cup of water. Rinse and dry. Calendula mother tincture can also be used instead at the same dilution.
- Lactobacillus acidophilus and lactobacillus bifidus. These bacteria belong to a group of microbes known as probiotics; they fight harmful germs and produce nutrients and vitamins. Acidophilus or plain yoghurt can be taken orally and also applied to nipples and dabbed on patches in baby's mouth. Dissolve bifidus (⅛ teaspoon) in baby's bottle. Lactobacillus acidophilus is also useful after a course of antibiotics and to treat vaginal yeast infections, diarrhea, and other conditions of the intestine such as ulcers, irritable bowel syndrome, or Crohn's disease.
- Avoid unnecessary antibiotics.
- Breastfeed, minimizing use of bottles and pacifiers. After using bottles or pacifiers, boil for 20 minutes to sterilize.
- Eat healthy. Avoid sweets, fruit, yeasty foods, and dairy (except for live-cultured yoghurt).
- Yeast thrives on moisture and sugar, so avoid both. Gently rinse and air dry breast and nipples after each feeding.
- Treat mother and baby simultaneously to avoid passing it back and forth.
- Sunbathe for 10 minutes several times a day (preferably with bare breasts). This can even be achieved indoors by a window. The light kills the yeast which loves moisture and the dark.
- Do not store breast milk while infected.
- Visit with a lactation consultant to ensure proper breastfeeding positioning, latching, and to avoid further irritation.
- Natural ointments include Lansinoh (pure) and Calendula ointment.
- For stubborn cases of thrush, clean bras, undergarments, towels, and breast pads after each use. For laundry, use hot water and add ½ cup of vinegar to rinse cycle. As sunlight kills yeast, dry items in the sunlight when possible.

- Increase vitamin C for mothers to several grams a day. Vitamin C is known to stop yeast growth.
- Grapefruit Seed Extract (GSE) known for its antifungal properties is helpful for thrush and diaper rash. GSE is highly concentrated and needs to be diluted in water (5 drops of GSE to one ounce of water). Swab on mothers nipples and inside baby's mouth several times a day.

Homeopathic Medicines

Borax is the most common remedy used for sore mouth from thrush. The mouth feels hot and tender and the affected areas are painful and can bleed. While feeding, the baby lets go of the nipples, and cries while nursing. *Borax* is also useful for canker sores. Another key to *Borax* is that the child does not like downward motion, such as being laid down. This makes it also a good remedy for motion sickness. Likewise, *Borax* can be given to breastfeeding mothers who experience sore or ulcerated nipples. There is a stitching pain in the chest and a sensitivity to noise.

Mercurius is used for similar sore mouth symptoms as *Borax*; however, there is increased saliva with a foul odor. Consider *Mercurius* if the patches spread, making the whole mouth looking like it is covered with flour. The baby may have additional symptoms of night sweats, and colic with greenish diarrhea.

Sulphur is indicated for thrush symptoms that are painful while eating. The inside of the mouth looks red, dark, and swollen. The tongue is coated with a thick white or brownish coating. There is excess saliva which can be bloody and also a tendency to morning slimy diarrhea. This can irritate the diaper area leading to diaper rash. The child wakes often and is unable to nap.

Gemmotherapy

Prim Wort is an excellent remedy for mouth sores and infections in the mouth.

Wineberry treats candidiasis and yeast infections. Both can be used orally for mother (25 drops twice a day), and baby (5 to 8 drops diluted in 2 to 4 ounces of breast milk or water).

VACCINE SAFETY

Care and Treatment

Conventional Treatment

Typically, your doctor will recommend acetaminophen before and after the shot for prevention and relief of fever and fussiness. Because medications like acetaminophen suppress symptoms, however, they make it difficult to choose a proper remedy if there is any type of reaction.

Home Treatment

In an attempt to use a more natural preventive approach, I prefer a different course of action. Before any vaccination, I recommend administering the following seven days before and after the shot for general strengthening of the body. They may help reduce side effects following the vaccine if there would be any. Remember, your child should not receive a vaccination if she is cranky or ill. Contact your practitioner if any unusual symptoms occur following the shot. You can use this protocol in conjunction with the acetaminophen or any personal remedies that you give your child. On a daily basis for 7 days before and after the shot give your child the following:

- Black Currant alternating days with Briar Rose.
- Constitutional remedy: A constitutional medication is a homeopathic remedy or treatment plan that has been specifically chosen for your child according to her total symptoms and disposition. Use as prescribed by your homeopath or holistic practitioner.
- Vitamin C (less than 2 years of age: 100 mg daily—over 2 years old, 150 mg a day).

Homeopathic Medicines

On the day of the shot,

***Ledum palustre* 30C:** 1 hour before shot, and 2 doses after shot (every 12 hours)

***Thuja occidentalis* 30C:** 3 pellets twice a day for 3 days following shot

***Chamomilla* 30C:** as needed for fussiness following shot

See "The Safe Shot Strategy" in Chapter 14.

VOMITING

It is as unpleasant for parents to watch their child retch as it is for the child to experience it. Vomiting is an all-encompassing reflex in the body, prompted by triggers in the gut, infection, pain, motion sickness, odors, and emotions. Nausea and vomiting are symptoms, the result or part of a condition; they are not a disease.

A common concern among parents is to prevent dehydration, which happens more easily in infants and young children than adults. It is not unusual for most children who are vomiting to lose fluid, causing an electrolyte imbalance in the body and mild dehydration. A child who has normal energy, watery tears when crying, moist mouth, and is urinating every four hours is not dehydrated. Signs of mild dehydration include dry mouth, chapped lips, dry tears, increased thirst, less frequent urination, and a dry diaper. As it progresses, signs of severe dehydration include weight loss, sunken eyes, fast heart rate, parched mouth, cold extremities, listlessness, and lack of alertness. This requires immediate medical attention.

If there is frequent severe vomiting that does not taper and lasts longer than 8 hours in a baby or 12 hours in children older than one year old, you should also seek medical attention. Repeated bouts of vomiting can cause small tears in the throat, which can result in a slight amount of blood-tinged vomit. This will heal on its own. **If there are signs of moderate to severe dehydration or a large amount of bloody vomit, seek medical attention.**

Causes and Types of Vomiting

Vomiting is the body's attempt to rid itself of stomach upset caused by conditions such as the stomach flu (rotavirus), food poisoning, motion sickness, bladder infection, intestinal obstruction, and, in infants, gastric reflux. Other times, vomiting is not related to the stomach at all, such as after a strong cough, or emotional upset.

Stomach Flu: With the stomach flu, the child also has a high fever and cramps. In general, vomiting usually tapers by 12 to 24 hours (e.g., the 12-hour stomach flu), though occasionally will go on for several days.

Food Poisoning: Food poisoning comes on a few hours after eating spoiled food. Common culprits are chicken, mayonnaise, fish, or beef. Vomiting is usually not accompanied by a fever and can last up to 12 hours. This may be followed by diarrhea.

Reflux: Up to fifty percent of babies spit up following a feeding for the first three months. Although this may be a hassle for both baby and parent, requiring frequent clothing changes, most of the time, spitting up resolves on its own, and baby is happy, thriving, and continues to gain weight. If your baby spits up continuously, though, she may have gastroesophageal reflux. Reflux occurs when baby's milk and food are regurgitated back into the esophagus and throat, caused by a laxed closure of the sphincter (entry-door valve) leading into the stomach. Symptoms of reflux include frequent spitting up, fussiness (aggravated by lying down and while and after feeding), bad breath, and poor weight gain. In fact, reflux may be originally confused with colic-like symptoms. In addition, it may irritate the breathing passages and cause cough, wheezing, or asthma. More than fifty percent of infants at three months old regurgitate at least once daily. Reflux usually resolves on its own as your baby gets older, due to improved neuromuscular control and the ability to sit up. If symptoms are particularly severe, your practitioner will usually begin an evaluation. The standard approach is to prescribe medication for stomach acid. If the condition persists, surgery may be recommended.

Pyloric Stenosis: Pyloric stenosis is a common cause of intestinal obstruction in infants due to a narrowing in the digestive tract where the contents of the stomach empty into the small intestine. Often there is persistent projectile vomiting in which a baby can spit up clear across the room. The belly is hard and distended after feeding, which comes down after vomiting. This can lead to weight loss and dehydration. It occurs in around three out of 1000 infants in the U.S., with symptoms beginning around three weeks of age. The standard treatment for pyloric stenosis is surgery.

Care and Treatment

Conventional Treatment

In addition to fluid replacements to prevent dehydration, anti-nausea and vomiting medications are available. However, these medications have side effects which can complicate healing; and within a short period of time and appropriate liquids, the condition usually resolves itself.

Home Treatment

Typically in an illness, your child will usually vomit more frequently for a period of time before it eventually tapers. At this stage, minimize drinking (don't offer any food), as it will probably come right back up. If your child is thirsty, offer 1 to 3 teaspoons of liquid at 5 to 10 minute intervals or more. As the vomiting begins to lessen (from of several times an hour to every 1 to 2 hours), your child can begin to take a sips at 5 to 10 minutes intervals, albeit slowly.

Rehydration drinks with electrolytes are recommended, since the right combination of salt and sugar can help children replace electrolytes lost from vomiting and diarrhea. Breastmilk, Pedialyte, white grape juice, or healthy popsicles are popular choices. In addition, you can make a rehydration drink at home. See *Diarrhea* entry for a recipe.

After vomiting has stopped for 8 to 12 hours and your child is tolerating fluids, slowly resume an age-appropriate normal diet. If your child is taking solids, begin with small amounts of nutritious bland foods, simply prepared and preferably consisting of complex carbohydrates. These include potatoes, rice, whole grain bread, and healthy cereals. Include steamed vegetables, nondairy soups, and live active-cultured yogurt. Avoid fried foods, too much juice, and junk food, including soda pop. Once popular, the strictly BRAT diet (bananas, rice, applesauce, and toast) is okay to eat, but also considered overly restrictive.

For babies who spit up frequently, make sure your baby is in the upright position while feeding, and offer smaller more frequent feedings. Breastfeed your baby, as mother's milk is easier to digest. Research has shown that reflux is more common in formula-fed babies. Carry, comfort, and calm your baby, as agitation and crying can increase spitting up and reflux.

Other tips:

- For treatment of nausea, try an acupressure wristband. (See *Motion Sickness.*)
- A hot water bottle may offer relief for a child with chills.
- Peppermint tea and chamomile tea are good for soothing an upset stomach. Sip as needed. Ginger tea can be used for children over two years old. (See *Motion Sickness.*)

Homeopathic Medicines

Aethusa is useful for babies who are milk intolerant. They vomit large curds of milk soon after drinking. It is also recommended for severe, explosive projectile vomiting with diarrhea in newborns who also show extreme prostration. The baby is weak, nervous, and cries easily. The child is worse in the heat, during teething, and after vomiting, and feels better in the open air, while resting, and while covered.

Antimonium crudum is also useful for a baby who throws up curds of milk. She refuses to nurse, is easily angered, and does not want to be touched. There is frequent belching and the tongue is coated white, giving it a furry or snowy appearance. She feels better in open air and worse in the evening.

Arsenicum album is strongly indicated for extreme nausea with vomiting. The child is chilly, weak, and exhausted, and aggravated by food and water. There is burning in the esophagus and stomach, and although the child is thirsty, liquids are soon vomited. Aggravation is common between midnight to two A.M. *Arsenicum* is a also a strong diarrhea remedy.

Calcarea carbonica, similar to *Aethusa*, is indicated particularly for vomiting milk, which looks like white, yellow, or green curds. It is also indicated for sour, loud belching, heartburn, and vomiting. Cramps in the stomach are common and worse after eating. The child craves indigestibles such as chalk and pencils. Exhausted after vomiting, the child immediately falls asleep.

Ipecacuanha comes from ipecac, which is used to induce vomiting for certain oral poisonings. Homeopathically prepared, *Ipecacuanhua* soothes a child who has constant nausea and vomiting. The tongue is clean with much saliva, and there can also be hiccoughs. The child is worse with motion, does not feel better after vomiting, and has an aversion to food, including the smell. There may be cramps and a rattling cough. The child feels better in the open air.

Nux vomica is also recommended for vomiting occurring with stomach pains. The child is angry, impatient, and arches her back. *Nux vomica* is often indicated for vomiting after eating too much, so that the child feels better after vomiting. She is oversensitive to light, music, and odors, and feel worse in tight clothes, in the cold, and at four A.M. She feels better with warmth and when covered.

See also *Diarrhea, Motion Sickness,* and *Stomachaches.*

WARTS

Every culture has its cure for warts, the most common skin condition in children. Warts occur in nearly 50% of all children and are caused by the human papillomavirus. Common places for warts in children are on the fingers, elbows, knees and feet—areas susceptible to small cuts and breaks in the skin. Regardless of injuries, some children are more vulnerable to warts than others. Children tend to get warts more than adults, probably because of their physical play and because their immune system is still developing.

Causes and Types of Warts

The **common wart (verruca vulgaris)** appears like a thick bump on the skin and is common on hands (especially around the nails, periungual), knees, and elbows.

Flat warts (verruca plana) are smoother and flat-topped; they commonly are found on the face, and plantar warts are found on the soles of the feet.

Genital warts, considered a sexually transmitted disease, are contagious once sexual activity begins.

Plantar warts are easily confused with calluses as they grow into the skin rather than outward as a bump like other warts. A plantar wart is identifiable by a central black dot, caused by a small blood clot. Most warts are painless, except for plantar warts which may be uncomfortable with walking due to the location.

Care and Treatment

Conventional Treatment

Most warts are harmless and resolve on their own (20% within 6 months, and 65% within 2 years), but some children are embarrassed about having them. Warts recur in up to 30% of cases. Standard treatments include topical medicines that contain ingredients such as salicylic acid. More aggressive measures include freezing off the warts with liquid nitrogen, employing a laser, and injecting medications. A podiatrist may have to surgically remove a painful plantar wart.

Home Treatment

Some people have used duct tape with success. Considered a less painful alternative to liquid nitrogen, a small piece of duct tape is placed on the wart for 6 days. Remove the tape, and soak the affected area and file down with an emory board. The following day the tape is reapplied for another six days. The process is repeated up till two months or until the wart has disappeared.

Homeopathic Medicines

The following is a small list of remedies that have been used to treat warts. If your child's symptoms match below, give the remedy in the 30C potency once a week for 4 weeks and wait a month.

Antimonium crudum is for warts that are horn-like and hard, especially on the hands and soles. In addition, it can also be used for smooth warts, callouses, and thickened nails. Child can have a tendency to chubbiness as they love to eat. They are worse from heat and the sun, and can be irritable. They love pickles and sour foods. *Antimonium crudum* is useful for warts on hands and plantar warts.

Causticum is for the child who is prone to endless warts. Especially common are warts on the hand and face, including the eyelids, brow, and nose. The warts can be large and jagged and bleed easily. The personality of the child is sensitive, excitable, and fearful. A strong keynote for *Causticum* is sensitivity to the suffering of others.

Dulcamara is recommended for large, flat, smooth warts. The child is worse in the damp or cold weather, and prone to thick yellow mucus.

Thuja is for warts and skin tags. The child may have multiple warts, large and small. They often look like cauliflower with a pedicle, and can be soft and bleed. They may also occur in the genital region. The child sweats when uncovered, and becomes chilly and shivers. The child is emotionally sensitive and responsive to kindness from others, often showing a sensitivity to music.

Gemmotherapy

Briar Rose, European Grape Vine, and **Fig Tree** are all indicated for warts and are helpful in strengthening a child's immune system.

WHOOPING COUGH

See *Cough*.

PART V

Natural Medicine Chest

Nature has given us the seeds of knowledge, not knowledge itself.

–Seneca

I NEVER CEASE TO BE AMAZED BY THE MYRIAD OF healing modalities that come from nature and simple home remedies. Although the body does the healing, there are times we need to employ medicines to direct the course. When possible, I prefer natural medicine and treatments to speed the healing process. In this section, I've listed some of the more commonly used medicines for everyday complaints in our household and in my office. Each medicine is presented with an in-depth description, including keynotes or the characteristic symptoms that can help you choose the right remedy.

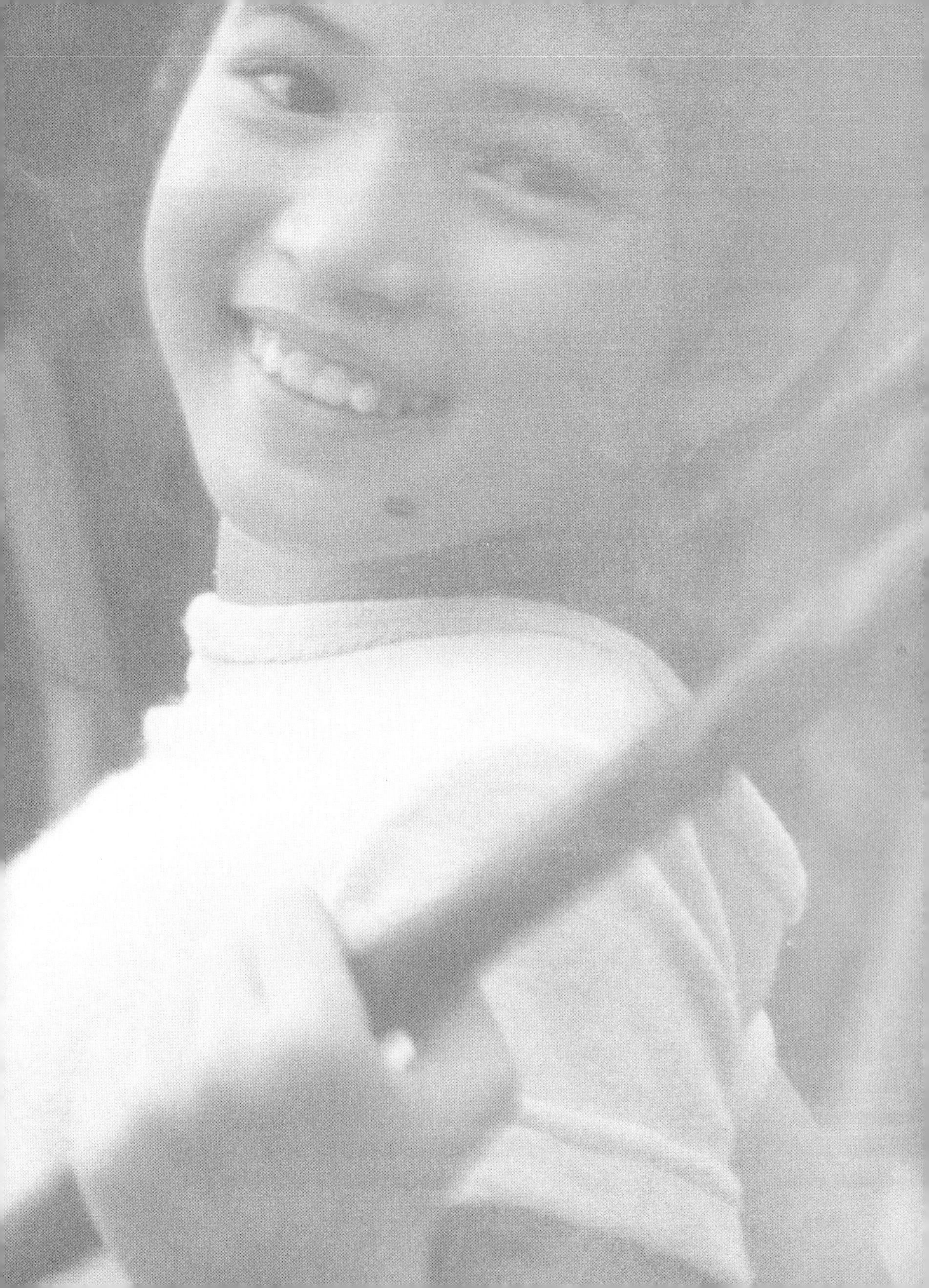

Homeopathic Medicines

Homeopathic medicines for home use are available in a variety of potencies from 6 (6X or 6C) to 30 (30X or 30C); 30C is my preference as it does not need to be repeated as frequently. For children and adults take three pellets (or quick dissolve tablets) up to three times a day dissolved under the tongue. In acute cases, take every hour until relieved, or as directed by your practitioner. If you see no improvement after three doses, discontinue the remedy. For infants, place three pellets in ½ glass of water. Let stand for five minutes. Stir ten times. If you are using the hard pellets, they will not dissolve, but the water becomes medicated. Give ¼ teaspoon (can be placed in a dropper) of the medicated liquid to equal one dose. Avoid eating or drinking 10 minutes before or after taking the remedy. When possible avoid touching the medicine. See "Administering Homeopathic Medicines" in Chapter 9 for more details.

Aconitum napellus (Aconite) — Monkshood

Aconite is also known as SOS, and is truly a rescue medication for a variety of symptoms. Children who benefit from *Aconite* look panicked and are constantly moving around. In January 1994, all of Los Angeles was abruptly awakened to the jolting of a very strong earthquake. Our own house was in complete disarray, but my husband quickly managed to find our homeopathic remedies in the dark. *Aconite* immediately helped calm our shaken nerves. During the week that followed all the local pharmacies and health food stores claimed to have sold out of this remedy.

In addition to first aid symptoms, it is useful in the treatment of illnesses that begin very suddenly. It is the first medicine I reach for when my sons wake up in the middle of the night with a fever or cough, especially after having played outside on a cool windy afternoon.

***Aconitum napellus* is useful for:**

Mind/Emotions:

- Anxiety and panic from accidents and frightening or shocking events
- Feelings of agitation, anxiety, and restlessness
- Forebodings and fears one will soon die
- Fears of crowds, airplanes, ghosts
- Claustrophobia

- Startles easily
- Sleeplessness and restlessness, with crying and complaining
- Nightmares and anxious dreams

Body:

- Early stages of illnesses that come on suddenly with intense pain (i.e. high fever, chills, flu, sore throat, earaches, coughs, croup, colds)
- Intolerable pains
- Complaints begin from becoming sweaty and chilled in dry, cold, windy weather
- Profuse sweating during sleep
- Chilly if uncovered
- Face is red, hot, and flushed. One cheek red, the other pale (similar to *Chamomilla*)
- Unquenchable thirst for cold drinks
- Hoarse, dry, croupy cough, worse at night and after midnight
- Pulse is full and strong

Symptoms improve: fresh air, with company
Symptoms worsen: at night and evening, in a warm room, lying on affected side, and with noise and light

Allium cepa — Red Onion

Allium cepa, made from the red onion, is well known for treating the classic watery, runny nose and irritated eyes resulting from allergies, hay fever, and common cold symptoms—similar complaints one would have when cutting up an onion.

***Allium cepa* is useful for**:
Mind/Emotions:

- Melancholy
- Fear that pain will become unbearable

Body:

- Watery, runny nose, "drips like water"
- Red, sore, and raw nose and upper lip

- Sneezing when coming into a warm room
- Burning, stinging, and tearing of the eyes
- Colds travel down into throat and chest
- Tickling in the throat with hoarseness
- Painful hacking cough
- Headache during runny nose
- Craving for onions

Symptoms improve: in open air, cold room
Symptoms worsen: in warm room, late afternoon and evening, when around flowers, when lying on the left side

Antimonium tartaricum — Tartar Emetic

Originally an invention of the alchemists, *Antimonium tartaricum* has been used since the 1800s by homeopaths for many conditions, especially those of the lungs. It treats mild chest colds, bronchitis, and pneumonia. For any severe condition that impedes breathing, seek immediate medical attention.

***Antimonium tartaricum* is useful for:**

Mind/Emotions:

- Becomes angry or cries if looked at
- Averse to being touched, wants to be alone
- Anxious expression
- Infant cries and cannot nurse
- Desire to be carried
- Drowsy, weak, and pale with cough

Body:

- Chest congestion, great rattling of mucus in the chest with each breath
- Wet cough, though unable to bring up much mucus
- Bends backwards while coughing
- Eyes sunken, surrounded by dark circles
- In severe illnesses, the child makes an effort to breathe
- Cold sweat on the face
- Blue lips (in severe cases)
- Coated, white tongue

- Gagging, nausea, and vomiting with the cough
- Craving for apples and sour foods

Symptoms improve: when sitting upright, being carried, in open air, with belching or expectoration
Symptoms worsen: in the evening, when lying down at night, from 3 A.M. to 4 A.M., with heat, in the winter, with sour food or milk

Apis mellifica — HONEY BEE

Think of *Apis* when your child's symptoms are similar to a bee sting—swelling, burning, and stinging. *Apis* can be an excellent remedy for hives, bladder infections, and sore throat.

***Apis mellifica* is useful for**:
MIND/EMOTIONS:

- Busy bee with tendency to be fidgety
- Jealous (like the Queen Bee)
- Suddenly cries out during sleep
- Difficulty concentrating

BODY:

- Complains of feeling swollen, sore, burning, stinging, sensitive to touch
- Constricted or tight feeling
- Skin is red, puffy, hot
- Craving for milk
- Lack of thirst

Symptoms improve: with cold applications and cold bathing, open air, uncovered
Symptoms worsen: with heat, touch, pressure, late afternoon, warm room, on right side

Arnica montana — LEOPARD'S BANE

Arnica is a plant that grows high up in mountain slopes where one could easily get injured in the steep terrain. Hence, *Arnica* is an excellent treatment for trauma.

It is the medicine needed most often in my active household, and it works without any side effects. *Arnica* is the only remedy that I use routinely during childbirth, as well as during the postpartum period. I also use it for newborns who are bruised after birth. *Arnica* has no contraindications, and is safe for newborns and nursing mothers. *Arnica* in strong potency (200C or 1M) is used for major injuries.

***Arnica montana* is useful for:**

Mind/Emotions:

- Restlessness
- Bed and chairs feel too hard; difficultly finding comfortable position
- Says there is nothing wrong, even when seriously ill
- Desires to be alone
- Irritable
- Body feels "beaten up"

Body:

- Bruises, swelling, and muscle soreness
- Sprains, strains, and concussions
- Injuries and bleeding from trauma and accidents
- Jet lag (with muscle soreness)
- Falls and blows
- After-surgery swelling (dental procedures, plastic surgery, caesarean section)
- Over exertion from lifting, sports or work

Symptoms improve: when alone, lying down outstretched or with the head low
Symptoms worsen: with touch, jarred, cold and damp weather, lying on injured part

Arsenicum album — Arsenic

Arsenicum is helpful for many complaints and usually comes with a cluster of symptoms that include exhaustion, burning pains, chilliness, restlessness, and a midnight aggravation. It is commonly used for food poisoning and traveler's diarrhea.

***Arsenicum album* is useful for:**

MIND/EMOTIONS:

- Anxious, cautious, and responsible
- Fears suffocation while lying down
- Stinginess
- Fear of poverty, health, death, robbers, germs
- Orderly and fastidious

BODY:

- Burning pains relieved with warmth
- Chilliness
- Exhaustion and weakness
- Restlessness, going from place to place
- Thin, watery, irritating runny nose
- Wheezing, worse at midnight
- Thirst, drinking in small quantities, but often
- Craves milk

Symptoms improve: with company, warmth and hot drinks, head elevated
Symptoms worsen: when alone, damp, cold applications, cold food and drinks, from midnight to 2 A.M., on right side, at the seashore

Belladonna — DEADLY NIGHTSHADE

Belladonna was known as the "herba bella donna," or beautiful lady, since the 1500s during the time of the Italian Renaissance in Venice, when it was used cosmetically to darken and widen the eyes (by dilating the pupil) and flush the cheeks. Prepared as a homeopathic remedy, *Belladonna* is nontoxic and safe. Keynotes for *Belladonna* are sudden onset of intense illness, heat, and redness.

***Belladonna* is useful for:**

MIND/EMOTIONS:

- Intense delirium (i.e. during a high fever)
- Hypersensitivity to surroundings (light, noise, touch)
- Biting, hitting, and moaning
- Hallucinations—sees monsters, ferocious animals, scary faces

BODY:

- Bright red face, dilated pupils, radiating heat
- Earaches with severe pain in right ear, causing a child to cry during sleep
- Red, throbbing sore throat
- High fevers, usually above 102° F; radiates heat
- Head hot, glassy eyes, limbs cold with fever
- Twitching in the sleep
- No thirst with high fever or intense thirst for cold water
- Craves lemonade
- Skin is dry and hot

Symptoms improve: when bending backward, in semi-erect position, leaning head against something, light covering
Symptoms worsen: with pressure, jarring, light, noise, cold, right side, draft, lying down, afternoon

Bryonia alba — WILD HOPS

Use *Bryonia* when your child is worse from motion, better from being still. *Bryonia* treats many conditions, including flu, cough, headache, sore throat, injuries, arthritis, and mastitis.

***Bryonia alba* is useful for:**
MIND/EMOTIONS:

- Irritable and cross
- Aversion to being carried or touched
- Desires to be left alone
- Wants something, but does not know what
- Wants to go home (even when at home)
- Concerned about school work or business

BODY:

- All symptoms are worse with motion
- Stitching, stabbing, tearing pains
- Dryness everywhere (mouth, cough, stools, etc.)
- Bursting, splitting headache (worse on left side)

- Painful, dry, hacking cough (hold the chest to prevent moving)
- Faint when sitting up
- Thirsty for large amounts
- Craves meat

Symptoms improve: with rest, being still, lying on painful side, pressure, splinting
Symptoms worsen: with motion, warmth, at around 9 P.M., eating, exertion, touch, cold weather, right side

Calcarea carbonica — CALCIUM CARBONATE

Calcarea carbonica, a well known remedy for a variety childhood conditions, is made from the inner shell of the oyster. *Calcarea carbonica* is found throughout nature in chalk, marble, plaster, mother of pearl, and shells. The mineral, calcium, is vital to the body for bone development, which provides stability, support, and protection. The child who benefits from *Calcarea carbonica* is reminiscent of the oyster in its shell, attempting to protect itself from the environment. The child enjoys the security of home as she has tendency to feel concerns about security. It is known for its characteristic symptoms—flabby, fearful, and fair—and is used for many conditions, including anxieties, late in walking, low thyroid, and constipation.

***Calcarea carbonica* is useful for:**
MIND/EMOTIONS:

- Cautious before beginning new task
- Serious and observant
- Responsible and overwhelmed by homework
- Concerned about security
- Full of fears, anxious about health, family, heights, rats, insects, dark
- Nightmares—wakes up screaming
- Slow in moving
- Can play well by herself
- Stubborn

BODY:

- Chubby pale baby with large tummy and head
- Perspires easily (head, hand, feet etc.), worse during sleep

- Sourness (breath, sweat, stools)
- Low energy, lack of endurance, and easily out of breath
- Chilled easily (less common in children)
- Catches cold easily
- Constipation
- Eats dirt and indigestibles (sand, chalk, pencils)
- Loves eggs, cheese, and sweets

Symptoms improve: dry warm weather, lying on painful side, constipation, on rising
Symptoms worsen: exertion, cold weather, full moon, sun

Calcarea phosphorica — Phosphate of Lime

As one of the twelve cells salts identified by Dr. Schüssler which are part of every tissue in the body, *Calcarea phosphorica* is vital for healthy bones, tissue, and growth in childhood. It is a well-known remedy for headaches, stomachaches, and growing pains.

***Calcarea phosphorica* is useful for:**
Mind/Emotions:

- Irritable, touchy, and whiny
- Wants to be center of attention
- Desires to be carried
- School-aged children are easily overwhelmed
- Forgetful, doesn't remember what she just read
- Easily bored
- Loves to travel

Body:

- Child is thin, lanky with flabby muscles
- Sweating of the head, worse at night
- Tendency toward enlarged glands, tonsils, and adenoids
- Late in learning to walk
- Delayed teething
- Weakness; baby is late in holding her head up

- Weak ankles with frequent falling
- Growing pains; child cries out during sleep
- Teething with diarrhea (green and slimy)
- Infant constantly wants to nurse
- Headaches in school-aged children, can also have diarrhea
- Stomachaches in school-aged children
- Craves smoked meats, bacon, and ham

Symptoms improve: with rest, lying down, summer, warm and dry weather
Symptoms worsen: in cold weather, drafts, exertion, teething

Cantharis — Spanish Fly

Cantharis is well known for treatment of bladder infections and mild skin burns. The keynotes are acute burning pains due to inflammation and irritation.

***Cantharis* is useful for:**
Mind/Emotions:

- Oversensitive to pains
- Anger and irritability
- Rapid onset of conditions
- Anxious and restless with the pains

Body:

- Burning pains
- Bladder infections with burning pains while urinating
- Frequent urination that is passed drop by drop with scalding feeling
- Skin is raw and burns; feels better with cold applications

Symptoms improve: with rubbing, warmth, rest
Symptoms worsen: while urinating, cold drinks, bright objects, sound of water

Chamomilla — German Chamomile

A child who is in a "*Chamomilla* state" is unhappy, uncomfortable, and finds her symptoms unbearable. *Chamomilla* is useful for the characteristic symptoms associated with fussiness, colic, teething, cough, cold, and ear infections.

***Chamomilla* is useful for:**

Mind/Emotions:

- Anger, irritable, impatient, and contrary
- Inconsolable, screaming, and arching the back
- Asks for something, then refuses it

Body:

- Pains are unbearable (even for seemingly minor conditions)
- Head is warm and sweaty
- One cheek is red, the other pale
- Has earaches that are sensitive to cold and noise, and feels better with warmth; pain makes the child frantic
- Colds characterized by a watery, hot, runny nose that is also stuffed; difficulty sleeping
- Fevers in which the child alternates between feeling chilled and overheated
- Dry, tickling cough and hoarseness; worse from 9 P.M. to midnight
- Colicky; also known as the "impossible cranky irritable" baby, who moves about in agony
- Green diarrhea, like chopped spinach
- Thirsty for cold drinks

Symptoms improve: when carried, rocked, in warm, wet weather
Symptoms worsen: at nighttime (especially 9 P.M.), heat, anger, open air, wind, touch

Colocynthis — Bitter Cucumber

Colocynthis is commonly used for abdominal cramps which are better with hard pressure, when bending forward, and with warmth. It can be used for conditions ranging from colic to menstrual cramps.

***Colocynthis* is useful for:**

Mind/Emotions:

- Irritable
- Easily offended

- Angry if contradicted
- Indignant

Body:

- Abdominal pain from anger
- Cramping, gripping, agonizing pain
- Pain comes in waves of contractions
- Pain, colic, and diarrhea, worse after eating and when emotional
- Infant colic, better lying on belly; baby screams when moved
- Belly feels as if squeezed between stones
- Child twists and turns in pain, great restlessness
- Pain relieved after stool

Symptoms improve: with hard pressure, when bending forward, with warmth
Symptoms worsen: when emotional, at night, in cold and drafts, when eating, drinking, and lying on painless side

Drosera Sundew

Drosera is a carnivorous plant that feeds on trapped insects. It is an excellent remedy for intense coughs, croup, and whooping cough (pertussis).

***Drosera* is useful for:**

Mind/Emotions:

- Feels trapped, harassed, and persecuted by others
- Suspicious of others
- Easily angered

Body:

- Spasmodic, dry, harassing cough
- Painful cough, holds chest when coughing
- Fits of coughing, sometimes hard to catch the breath
- Coughing with bloody nose
- Barking cough
- Choking, gagging, and vomiting with cough

- Tickling in the throat causing cough
- Hoarseness

Symptoms improve: with company, pressure, open air
Symptoms worsen: after midnight, lying down, when head touches the pillow, when warm in bed, and when drinking, talking, singing, laughing, eating cold food, stooping, or vomiting

Euphrasia officinalis EYEBRIGHT

Euphrasia has been used in folk medicine for generations and rightly deserves its name, eyebright. It is especially useful for eye complaints from hay fever, allergies, and conjunctivitis (pink eye). It can be used as eye drops (commercially prepared) or taken orally.

***Euphrasia* is useful for:**
MIND/EMOTIONS:

- Melancholy

BODY:

- Eyes water all the time
- Irritating tears and non-irritating runny nose (opposite of *Allium cepa)*
- Burning and swelling of the eyelids
- Blinking eyes
- Cough in the daytime

Symptoms improve: in open air, dark, cold washing
Symptoms worsen: in evening, indoors, warmth, light

Ferrum phosphoricum IRON PHOSPHATE

The symptoms that point to *Ferrum phosphoricum* are often easily confused with *Aconite* and *Belladonna*, as all three are used in the first stages of infections. Made from iron and found in red blood cells, *Ferrum phosphoricum* increases the supply of oxygen to the blood. *Ferrum phosphoricum* is well known as one of Dr.

Schüssler's twelve tissue salts (cell salts), which are an integral part of the composition of every tissue in the body.

***Ferrum phosphoricum* is useful for:**

MIND/EMOTIONS:

- Moody with anxiety and anger
- Sensitive to noise
- Fear of people, crowds, and death
- Inclined to lie down

BODY:

- First stages of colds, coughs, and fevers
- Gradual onset of symptoms, less intense than *Belladonna* and *Aconite*
- Anemic, pale, and weak
- High fever with no other clear cut symptoms
- Headaches, right-sided
- Bleeds easily—bloody nose, bruising, etc.
- Flushes of heat in the face
- Red cheeks or paleness
- Pains, worse from motion, and better with cold applications
- Right-sided complaints
- Aversion to meat and milk
- Desire for cold drinks, sour foods

Symptoms improve: with cold applications, lying down, gentle motion, rest, eating
Symptoms worsen: in heat of the sun, at night, from 4 to 6 A.M., with jarring, motion, touch, right side, noise, cold air, exertion

Gelsemium — YELLOW JASMINE

Gelsemium is well known as a flu remedy, with weakness as the particular keynote. In addition, this remedy is called for when someone lacks confidence before facing a challenge—for example, a child beginning a new school, a violinist before a performance, and even a soldier prior to combat. The symptoms of weakness, anxiety, trembling, and diarrhea all point to *Gelsemium.*

***Gelsemium* is useful for:**

Mind/Emotions:

- Fearful and frightened easily (crowds, falling, exams, heart will stop)
- Anticipatory anxiety
- Stage fright
- Cowardice
- Sluggishness
- Fear of falling
- Trembling

Body:

- Flu-like symptoms
- Great fatigue and exhaustion
- Heaviness of eyelids, limbs, and body
- Dizziness, muscle aches and weakness, trembling
- Chills up and down the spine
- Diarrhea from nerves, fright, bad news
- Headaches in the back of the head
- Difficulty sleeping before an event or from excitement

Symptoms improve: with stimulants, cold, open air, urination, sweating, bending forward, in the afternoon, lying down with head propped up

Symptoms worsen: with motion, damp weather, fright, bad news, excitement, around 10 A.M.

Hepar sulphuris calcareum — Calcium sulphide

Any condition that calls for *Hepar sulphuris* has the characteristic of hypersensitivity in body and emotions—from an infection of the nail bed, to a sore throat, to croup.

***Hepar sulphuris* is useful for:**

Mind/Emotions:

- Overly sensitive mood and emotions
- Easily irritated

- Angry, abusive, and impatient
- Hypochondriacal
- Fears the dentist, injuries, or seeing violent movies

Body:

- Overly sensitive to pain (reaction seems out of proportion)
- Inconsolable over pains
- Pain causes child to feel faint
- Pain described as jabbing, as from sharp sticks, splinters, or fish bones
- Inflammations with thick, yellow, acrid discharge (colds, boils, ulcers, etc.)
- Discharges smell sour or like old cheese
- Croupy cough
- Swollen, tender glands
- Chilliness, aggravated by the cold
- Perspires easily
- Desire for vinegar

Symptoms improve: with warmth, wrapping the head, when covered, in damp weather, after eating
Symptoms worsen: with exposure to cold, in a dry, cold wind, at night, in a draft, uncovered, when touched, when lying on painful side

Hypericum perforatum — St. John's wort

Homeopathically prepared, *Hypericum* is a remedy for injuries to the nerves and generally serves different purposes than its well-known herbal kin, the antidepressant, St. John's wort. Although *Hypericum* is indicated for depression following injuries, it is better known as "*Arnica* for the nerves."

***Hypericum perforatum* is useful for:**
Mind/Emotions:

- Melancholy
- Depression following shock or fright
- Drowsiness

Body:

- Crush injuries, puncture wounds, and lacerations
- Injuries to nerves, especially crushed fingers, nails, and toes
- Injury to tailbone (after a fall) and spinal cord
- Herniated disc
- Excessive pain with sharp, shooting sensations
- Painful, sore parts and tenderness
- Tingling, numbness, and burning
- Pain after operations
- Tetanus

Symptoms improve: when bending head backward, rubbing
Symptoms worsen: with touch, cold, exertion

Ignatia amara — St. Ignatius Bean

Ignatia is well known as a grief remedy for use following the loss of a person or object that was very dear. It is also extremely helpful for tearful new mothers in the postpartum period.

***Ignatia* is useful for:**
Mind/Emotions:

- Complaints from grief, fright, loss, and unrequited love
- Tendency toward sobbing, sadness, and sighing
- Suppression of grief
- Frequent yawning
- Aversion to being consoled
- Hysterical symptoms
- Oversensitive and anxious
- Alternating moods (hysterical crying to laughing)
- Dreams of water
- Startles easily

Body:

- Complaints of contradictory, erratic, changeable symptoms with grief
- Lump in the throat

- Numbness, twitches, and spasms
- Craves cheese

Symptoms improve: when eating, change of position, alone, deep breathing
Symptoms worsen: cold, touch

Ipecacuanha IPECAC ROOT

Ipecacuanha is prepared from ipecac root. Prepared as syrup of ipecac, it is used in orthodox medicine to induce vomiting after a child has ingested a poison. In homeopathy, ipecac is the most common remedy given for nausea and vomiting.

***Ipecacuanha* is useful for:**
MIND/EMOTIONS:

- Desire for many things, but child does not know exactly what she wants
- Unhappy expression of disgust on the account of extreme nausea
- Irritable
- Difficult to please

BODY:

- Extreme nausea and vomiting (nausea not relieved with vomiting)
- Shortness of breath with nausea
- Salivation increased, clean tongue
- Tendency to contract colds in warm, damp weather
- Overly sensitive to extremes of temperatures (hot or cold)
- Abdominal pain around the navel
- Aversion to food, lack of thirst
- Cough remedy (bronchitis, croup, whooping cough)
- Cough is continuous, hard, loose, and rattling with gagging and suffocative feeling
- Cough can be so intense that child becomes stiff and blue in the face
- Vomiting with the cough
- Bloody nose

Symptoms improve: open air, rest, pressure, closing eyes, cold drinks
Symptoms worsen: overeating, vomiting, motion, lying down, warmth, damp room

Kali bichromicum — POTASSIUM BICHROMATE

Kali bichromicum is the most common medicine given for acute sinus complaints with the characteristic thick, stringy, gluelike discharge. When indicated, it is also used for coughs, bronchitis, and croup.

***Kali bichromicum* is useful for:**

MIND/EMOTIONS:

- Indifferent
- Doesn't want to do homework
- Avoids people

BODY:

- Sinus infection and stuffed nose in children
- Colds with sneezing and stuffed nose (unable to breathe through the nose)
- Discharges from nose (and other orifices) are thick, ropy, stringy, and gluey
- Yellow-green discharge with formation of crusts and scabs (bleed when removed)
- Loss of smell and taste
- Sensation of hair on tongue
- Sinus headache, can point to exact point of pain
- Pressure at bridge of the nose
- Pains come and go
- Hoarse, metallic cough, worse in cold weather
- Tickling at the trachea with cough

Symptoms improve: with warmth
Symptoms worsen: with cold, damp, open air, undressing, morning, 2 to 3 A.M., stooping

Ledum palustre — MARSH TEA

Ledum palustre is a first aid remedy commonly used for insect bites and puncture wounds. The characteristic symptoms with *Ledum* are that the affected area is cold to touch and feels better with cold applications.

***Ledum palustre* is useful for:**

MIND/EMOTIONS:

- Angry
- Desire to be alone

BODY:

- Mosquito bites, insect bites, animal bites, puncture wounds
- Affected area is swollen, inflamed, bruised
- Black eye from a blow
- Affected area is cold, pale, puffy
- Numbness, redness, swelling
- Throbbing pain

Symptoms improve: with cold applications, cold air
Symptoms worsen: with warmth, night, motion, touch

Magnesia phosphorica — MAGNESIUM PHOSPHATE

Magnesia phosphorica is one of Schüssler's twelve tissue salts (cell salts) that are part of the composition of every tissue in the body. It is found in muscles, bones, teeth, nerves, brain, spinal cord, and blood and is important for the contraction of fibers. This makes *Magnesia phosphorica* an excellent remedy for menstrual cramps, with the keynote that pain is better from warmth and pressure.

***Magnesia phosphorica* is useful for:**

MIND/EMOTIONS:

- Anxious
- Irritable

Body:

- Cramps, spasms (menstrual cramps, writer's and player's cramp, and colic)
- Sharp, shooting pains
- Pains change places
- Toothache and headache worse at night and from cold drinks, and better with heat
- Hiccoughs
- Colic with gas and burping
- Abdomen is bloated (child prefers loose clothing around belly)
- Thirsty for cold drinks

Symptoms improve: with warmth, hot water bottle, firm pressure, rest, rubbing, bending double
Symptoms worsen: with cold, uncovered, with touch, at night, on right side, after having milk

Mercurius (Mercurius vivus or Mercurius solubilis) Mercury

Children who respond to *Mercurius* are like human barometers: they react to extremes of hot and cold temperature. *Mercurius* is a commonly used remedy for many types of ear, nose, and throat infections. If available, *Mercurius iodatus ruber* can be used for left-sided symptoms, and *Mercurius iodatus flavus* for the right side.

***Mercurius* is useful for:**
Mind/Emotions:

- Hurried and anxious
- Restless
- Violent impulses (which may not be overtly expressed)

Body:

- Infections with greenish-yellow pus
- Discharges are irritating to the skin (i.e. runny nose irritating the upper lip and nose)
- Sensitive to extremes of heat and cold (like a barometer)
- Tendency to perspire easily

- Raw, smarting burning pains in the throat with ear pain on swallowing
- Ulcers and pus on tonsils
- Inclined to swallow
- Profuse salivation (drooling)
- Swollen glands
- Offensive odors (i.e. foul breath, sweat, and discharges)
- Bleeding gums, tongue indented, with metallic taste in the mouth
- Tendency towards frequent infections
- Trembling and weakness with illness
- Craves bread and butter

Symptoms improve: with rest, moderate temperature
Symptoms worsen: at night, in warmth of the bed, sweating, lying on the right side, extremes of temperature, open air

Natrum muriaticum — Common Salt

Natrum muriaticum, homeopathic sodium chloride, is one of the Schüssler tissue salts, found in fluids and solids throughout the body. *Natrum muriaticum* is useful for many conditions, including headaches, cold sores, and allergies, and a common trait among sufferers is melancholy or sadness. It is reminiscent of our salty tears.

***Natrum muriaticum* is useful for:**
Mind/Emotions:

- Grief, loss, unrequited love
- Loneliness
- Sensitive, easily hurt feelings (which child doesn't reveal)
- Averse to company and consolation
- Desire for solitude
- Desire to cry when alone (but may be unable to cry)
- Child is mature, responsible with a serious disposition

Body:

- Dryness of mouth, throat, nose
- Dry, cracked lips (center lower lip)
- Allergies with egg white-like discharge

- Headaches, worse from sun, heat, light, noise, study
- Tearing of the eyes, worse in the wind
- Cold sores
- Thirsty for cold drinks
- Craving for salty foods, lemon, and chocolate

Symptoms improve: with fresh air
Symptoms worsen: sun, around 10 A.M.

Nux vomica — Quaker Buttons

Nux vomica is the best remedy for "too much"—too much food, birthday cake, or stimulation. But its powers extend beyond relieving indigestion after a Thanksgiving meal; it can also be used for the common cold, constipation, and the kind of insomnia brought on by doing—you guessed it—too much.

***Nux vomica* is useful for:**

Mind/Emotions:

- Hardworking personality (Type A kid)
- Competitive in sports, high achiever in school
- Irritability, impatience, and anger
- Easily frustrated

Body:

- Overeating (especially spicy or rich foods)
- Fullness, heartburn, indigestion, upset stomach, vomiting, bloating, gas
- Constipation, straining with incomplete sensation
- Infant colic with arching of the back
- Jetlag (with stomach upset)
- Insomnia (from doing too much)
- Stuffed nose with watery discharge and sneezing, plugged at night, runny during the day
- Extremely chilly
- Sensitive to stimuli (noise and light)
- Difficult sleeping, waking at 3 or 4 A.M.

Symptoms improve: with rest, in the evening
Symptoms worsen: in cold, dry weather, wind, in the early morning, outdoors

Oscillococcinum

Oscillococcinum is a popular homeopathic flu medicine originally from France and used in more than 40 countries around the world. *Oscillo* helps reduce the duration and severity of flu symptoms, as evidenced by four clinical studies. It works best when taken at the first sign of flu symptoms.

***Oscillococcinum* is useful for:**
MIND/EMOTIONS:

- Fear of catching germs or illness
- Desire to wash the hands

BODY:

- Flu symptoms with muscle aches, fever, and chills
- Stuffed nose and eye discharge
- Bronchial congestion and painful cough
- Sensitive to barometric weather changes
- Bursting throbbing headache
- Earache and ear congestion

Symptoms improve: with heat, rest
Symptoms worsen: after drinking milk, eating eggs

Pulsatilla nigricans — PASQUE FLOWER

Pulsatilla is rich in history and medicinal uses. The pasque flower blooms at Easter and once was used to color Easter eggs. Since ancient times, it has been valued for its effectiveness in treating conditions of the eye. According to legend, the flower sprang from the tears of Venus. *Pulsatilla* is a windflower, one that sways in the wind. Hence, the child who responds to *Pulsatilla* has changeable symptoms, and is easily moved to tears.

***Pulsatilla* is useful for:**

MIND/EMOTIONS:

- Emotional
- Easily moved to tears and laughter
- Desire for consolation, sympathy, and affection
- Timid, gentle, and clingy personality
- Easily irritated, touchy
- Fears being alone and in the dark

BODY:

- Warm-blooded and worse in the heat
- Infections with bland, yellow-green discharge (ear, eye, nose, sinus, etc.)
- Cough, which is worse at night, when lying down, and with emotions
- Craves ice cream, butter, pastries (despite causing indigestion)
- Lack of thirst even though has a dry mouth
- Painful and irregular periods (for girls)

Symptoms improve: in open air, breezes, slow walks outside, cool and crisp weather, cold applications
Symptoms worsen: alone, in the heat, in a warm and stuffy room, in the evenings and at night, with greasy, rich foods

Rhus toxicodendron — POISON IVY

Rhus toxicodendron (poison ivy) and *Rhus diversiloba* (poison oak) are both members of the sumac plant family. As plants, they cause similar skin reactions in your child following exposure; as remedies, they are useful in treating and alleviating many conditions, including chickenpox, flu, sore throat, sprains and injuries, and even attention deficit disorder. Fidgetiness is the guiding symptom that will lead you to *Rhus toxicodendron.* Interestingly, the plant itself is considered restless, as it grows all over the countryside. The *Rhus toxicodendron* profile is a child who feels relief when moving.

***Rhus toxicodendron* is useful for:**

Mind/Emotions:

- Restless of mind, jumps from subject to subject
- Active child
- Cheerful and joking

Body:

- Body aches, worse with damp and cold
- Morning stiffness when beginning to move, better with continued motion (like a rusty gate)
- Stiffness and aches following a day of sports, lifting, and overexertion
- Changes positions frequently, since remaining still is uncomfortable
- Tendency to skin conditions, blisters with extreme itching; symptoms are better with scalding hot water
- Tongue has a red triangular tip
- Craves cold milk and cheese

Symptoms improve: with warmth, exercise, motion
Symptoms worsen: with cold, getting wet, cold and wet weather, drafts, when uncovered, in the morning

Ruta graveolens — Rue

Ruta is a well known treatment for injuries such as sprains and strains.

***Ruta graveolens* is useful for:**

Mind/Emotions:

- Anxious and contradictory
- Rigid thinking
- Feels weak

Body:

- Injuries to joints, tendons, and bruised bones
- Stiffness with sore, bruised feeling
- Lower back pain that is better when lying down
- Sprains, strains, and twisting joints (e.g., sprained ankle)

- Restlessness with the pain
- Eyestrain from reading (red, hot, and tearing)
- Headache from eyestrain

Symptoms improve: with warmth, motion, and rubbing
Symptoms worsen: with exertion, in the cold and damp, from overuse and lifting heavy weights

Spongia tosta — Roasted Sponge

Among families who use homeopathy, *Spongia* is well known as a remedy for dry coughs, especially intense coughs, croup, and whooping cough. Medicinally, this saltwater animal has been used for centuries for thyroid conditions.

***Spongia tosta* is useful for:**
Mind/Emotions:

- Anxiety with cough and difficulty breathing
- Awakens frightened, fear of suffocating

Body:

- Coughs sound as if a saw is being driven through a board or like a seal bark
- Dry cough, barking
- Croupy cough
- Feeling as if breathing through a dry sponge
- Constriction, dry tickling in the throat
- Hoarseness
- Clears throat
- Cough, worse before midnight (sometimes after, too)
- Excessive thirst

Symptoms improve: with eating, drinking, swallowing, warm foods, with lying with head low, and when resting
Symptoms worsen: when talking, with exertion, in dry, cold winds or a warm room

Gemmotherapy

The dosage for infants is 5 to 8 drops. Give children ages 2 to 8 years old 12 to 15 drops, and older children and adults, 25 drops. The remedies can be used as often as 2 to 3 times per day during acute illness. Give the drops mixed in water or juice. See Chapter 9 "Administering Gemmotherapy" for more details.

Black Currant (Ribes nigrum)

This is an excellent remedy for strengthening the constitution especially when depleted from stress and fatigue. I use this remedy before and after vaccinations to strengthen the child and minimize vaccine side effects. It is also good for adults. Use in the morning, and, if needed, in the afternoon. Avoid taking it before going to bed as it increases energy.

Black Currant is useful for:

- Allergies
- Asthma
- Adrenal support (for a child on steroids, prednisone, and other medications)
- Anti-inflammatory (respiratory, digestive, or urinary)
- Autoimmune diseases
- Fatigue
- Vaccination safety (Use Black Currant alternating days with Briar Rose 7 days before and after the shots)

Black Honeysuckle (Lonicera nigra)

Black Honeysuckle is helpful for infections, and especially bladder infections when used in conjuction with *Wineberry*.

Black Honeysuckle is useful for:

- Bladder infections
- Infections in general

Briar Rose (Rosa canina)

Briar Rose fortifies a child's immune system and is especially helpful during the school year. I use this as a preventative 2 to 3 times a week during cold and flu season. For illness, use twice a day.

Briar Rose is useful for:

- Children's remedy: general and immune strengthener
- Earaches and ear infections
- Runny nose and congestion
- Sore throat
- Sinus infections
- Headaches, migraines caused by allergies
- Warts

Common Birch (Betula pubescens)

Common Birch targets the cleansing of the liver and other organ systems. It is known as the universal drainer and is an excellent general remedy for strengthening the immune system. As Black Currant is for the adrenals, Common Birch is for the immune system.

Common Birch is useful for:

- Infections of the ear, nose, and throat
- Allergies
- Adrenal gland
- Fatigue

English Elm (Ulmus campestre)

English Elm is specific for the treatment of skin conditions. In conjunction with Briar Rose and Hedge Maple, it is useful for herpes infections (cold sores).

English Elm is useful for:

- Herpes infections (cold sores)
- Weeping eczema
- Acne
- Psoriasis

European Alder (Alnus glutinosa)

This remedy is useful at the early onset of infections and inflammation.

European Alder is useful for:

- Early onset of infections of ear, nose, throat and sinus
- Beginning of inflammation of digestive tract (gastritis, gallbladder, colitis), and urinary tract (cystitis)

European Grapevine (Vitis vinifera)

Helpful in strengthening the immune system, and in the treatment of warts, along with Briar Rose and Fig Tree.

European Grapevine is useful for:

- Warts
- Painful, arthritic small joints, especially fingers and toes—including deforming rheumatoid arthritis

European Hornbean (Carpinus betulus)

European Hornbeam is known for treatment in ear, nose and throat infections. It is also indicated for sinus inflammation and nasal allergies.

European Hornbean is useful for:

- Sinus infections
- Chronic sinusitis
- Ear, nose, throat infections
- Mucous membrane of lung
- Coughs
- Bronchitis

European Walnut (Juglans regia)

European Walnut is indicated for deep-seated infections, from the skin to organs such as the gallbladder.

European Walnut is useful for:

- Boils and abscesses
- Impetigo
- Sinus infections
- Dental abscess and infection

Fig Tree (Ficus carica)

Fig Tree balances the acid secretions in the stomach and aids in healing the lining of the stomach. Hence, Fig Tree is indicated for conditions mainly of the stomach. It is also used in conjunction with Briar Rose and European Grapevine in strengthening a child's immune system in the treatment of warts.

Fig Tree is useful for:

- Stomach pain
- Gastritis
- Warts

Hedge Maple (Acer campestre)

Hedge Maple is indicated in the treatment of viruses such as herpes, and not for the common cold or flu.

Hedge Maple is useful for:

- Herpes virus: cold sores, chickenpox, shingles, genital herpes
- Epstein-Barr virus

Lemon Bark (Citrus limonum)

Lemon Bark is an excellent remedy for headaches, especially migraines. It is useful for treating spasmodic conditions such as strong coughs and hiccoughs. It works well with Briar Rose.

Lemon Bark useful for:

- Migraines and tension headaches
- Spasmodic cough
- Hiccoughs

Lime Tree (Tilia tomentosa)

Lime Tree is known for its calming effects and can be used for anxiety as well as insomnia. My boys use "dream drops" occasionally if they are having a difficult time falling asleep.

Lime Tree is useful for:

- Calms the nerves
- Calms the pain (i.e. intense menstrual cramps)
- Insomnia

Lithy Tree (Viburnum lantana)

This drainage remedy targets the lungs and aids in restoring pulmonary function.

Lithy Tree is useful for:

- Cough (including spasmodic fits of coughing)
- Bronchial spasms
- Bronchitis

Oriental Plane Tree (Platanus orientalis)

The treatment of acne responds well to constitutional homeopathy and other forms of alternative medicine. I have found that simple pimples and skin breakouts during puberty respond well to Oriental Plane Tree used daily as needed.

Oriental Plane Tree is useful for:

- Pimples and mild acne

Prim Wort (Ligustrum vulgare)

As a drainage remedy for the skin and mucous membrane, Prim Wort, is indicated for mouth sores.

Prim Wort is useful for:

- Mouth sores
- Canker sores
- Thrush
- Intestinal conditions (i.e. colitis, candida)

Raspberry (Rubus idaeus)

Raspberry has an affinity for the female pelvic organs and is helpful in alleviating painful periods that are common among adolescent girls. Take 3 times daily at the onset of the period. Raspberry can also be used once daily throughout the month.

Raspberry is useful for:

- Irregular periods
- Painful periods
- Ovarian cysts
- Endometriosis

Red Spruce (Abies pectinata)

Red Spruce targets the tonsils, throat, and nose. It has positive effects on calcium absorption in bones, and is an important for growth problems.

Red Spruce is useful for:

- Tonsilitis
- Sore throat
- Deficient growth conditions in children (which include frequent infections of the ear, nose, and throat, poor appetite, and fatigue)

Rosemary (Rosmarinus officinalis)

Rosemary is the consummate remedy for draining and cleansing the liver and gallbladder. As a vital organ, the liver plays many important roles essential for health, some of which include cleansing the blood of toxins, regulating metabolism, and aiding digestion. The dosage for Rosemary is up to 15 drops per day. Avoid using for more than 3 weeks in a row. Rosemary should not be taken by anyone with a history of seizures.

Rosemary is useful for:

- Cleansing the liver of side effects from medications such as the birth control pill
- Hepatitis
- Jaundice

- Gallbladder conditions
- Constipation

Wineberry (Vaccinum vitis idaea)

Wineberry restores the intestines from inflammation from colitis and diarrhea. With vaginal yeast infections, Wineberry is used with European Walnut.

Wineberry is useful for:

- Colitis
- Parasites with diarrhea
- Diarrhea
- Vaginal yeast infections
- Urinary tract infections

Natural Essentials

In addition to homeopathic medicines and gemmos, I have compiled a list of additional remedies and natural essentials that we use on a regular basis.

Calendula officinalis (Marigold)

Known as both an herb and homeopathic medicine, *Calendula* is used topically as an antiseptic, astringent, and pain reliever. As nature would have it, *Calendula* comes from the same plant family as some other popular trauma medicine *Arnica*. *Calendula* is available as a cream, gel, tincture, spray, or ointment.

***Calendula* is useful for:**

- Rapid healing in wounds
- Prevents infection
- Diaper rash
- Lacerations, bruises, open wounds, sores, fissures, burns, sunburns, scratches, and rashes
- Mouthwash for conditions of the teeth and mouth

Dosage: To use *Calendula* tincture, dilute 1:4 dilution with water and apply to affected area. As a mouthwash, dilute 1 tablespoon tincture in ½ cup warm water.

For older children, use as a mouthwash; for younger children, spot dab with a cotton swab.

Hot Water Bottle

Used by our grandparents and their parents before, the hot water bottle is an essential part of every family's medicine chest. As a symbol of warmth and security, its uses vary from warming up a cold bed to soothing physical aches and comforting mental anguish. Keep several of them in the home. In my experience, my sons enjoy having two at a time. Do not use an electric heating pad, as studies have linked exposure to low level electromagnetic radiation from these devices to cancer and other health conditions.

Use: To avoid burns, follow manufacturer's instructions when using. While holding the neck of the bottle, carefully pour the hot water up to half full. Expel remaining air by folding over the empty top half, and screw cap tightly. Wrap with a soft protective cloth before use.

Hydrogen Peroxide

Hydrogen peroxide, known for its germicidal and antiseptic properties, is considered a safe and natural cleanser. It is made of water and oxygen (H_20_2) and kills organisms through oxidation. In addition to having a multitude of household uses, hydrogen peroxide has been shown to be effective in aiding the prevention and treatment of colds, flu, and ear infections. In 1928, Dr. Richard Simmons presented his theory that viruses enter the body through the ear canal, which contradicted the current thinking that illness entered through the mouth and nose. Although his work was not accepted by the standard medical community, many people have experienced excellent results when placing several drops of hydrogen peroxide in the ear at the onset of the common cold or flu. Use the 3% hydrogen peroxide.

Hydrogen peroxide is useful for:

- Onset of cold and flu symptoms
- Wounds, cuts and sores
- Ear wax removal. Hydrogen peroxide first, followed by olive oil (place each solution in affected ear for a few minutes each side)

- Household cleanser (see "Creating a Nontoxic Environment for Your Baby" in Chapter 10)

Dosage: At the onset of cold or flu symptoms, place four drops of hydrogen peroxide (3%) into both ears. The solution will bubble and there may be a little stinging. Within a couple minutes, the liquid will drain out. This treatment is considered safe for infants. Avoid the eyes (if so, flush immediately with water). Avoid any ear drops if there is fluid coming out of the ear (rupture of the eardrum). It is best to use hydrogen peroxide within the first 12 to 24 hours of illness.

Lavender

Lavender has wide applications in herbal medicine and aromatherapy and was once a staple in every family's medicine chest. A symbol of cleanliness, its name derives from the Latin root *lavare*, which means to wash. Lavender is also known for its calming effects and antibacterial, antiseptic, and antidepressant properties. Throughout the centuries, lavender has been used to soothe the nerves, to treat insomnia, infections, and skin conditions, as a disinfectant, to alleviate muscle soreness, and for fragrance. Lavender is available commercially for children in lotion, soap, shampoos, and bathing oils.

Note on aromatherapy and essential oils: Essential oils, such as lavender, chamomile, and tea tree, are highly concentrated. Do not apply undiluted essential oils on your child's sensitive skin. To use, place a quarter size amount of preblended oil in the palm of your hand. Rub your hands together to warm the oil and massage into skin as needed. Avoid applying on the delicate areas of the face, ears and bottom. Essential oils are not to be taken internally. See Chapter 9, "Administering Essential Oils" for more details.

Dosage: Use topically. Oral use is not recommended in children.

Mullein-Garlic Ear Drops

Mullein oil (Verbascum thapsus) is useful for relieving earaches due to local irritation and ear infections. I use the commercially prepared infusion of Mullein-Garlic ear drops in conjunction with remedies to treat ear infections. Mullein is known for its anti-bacterial properties and garlic (Allium sativum) is used for its broad spectrum anti-microbial and anti-inflammatory activity.

Dosages. Place three drops in the affected ear three times daily. Use cotton if needed. Avoid any ear drops if there is fluid coming out of the ear (rupture of the eardrum). (See *Ear Infections* in Part IV.)

Your Natural First Aid Kit

The Natural First Aid Kit contains the list of equipment, natural essentials and medicines that we use on a regular basis.

Equipment

Ace bandage ✿ Adhesive bandages (Band-Aids) ✿ Cloth (for compresses and poultices) ✿ Dropper ✿ Gauze pads ✿ Hot water bottles (2) ✿ Ice bag ✿ Safety pins ✿ Scissors ✿ Tape ✿ Thermometer ✿ Tweezers ✿ Wool scarves (for sore throats and calf wraps)

Natural Essentials Plus

Calendula tincture and ointment ✿ Chamomile tea ✿ Hydrogen peroxide ✿ Juice Plus+ ✿ Lavender ✿ Mullein-Garlic Ear Drops ✿ Rescue Remedy

Homeopathic Medicines

Aconite ✿ *Allium cepa* ✿ *Apis* ✿ *Arnica* ✿ *Arsenicum album* ✿ *Belladonna* ✿ *Bryonia* ✿ *Cantharis* ✿ *Chamomilla* ✿ *Colocynthis* ✿ *Drosera* ✿ *Euphrasia* ✿ *Ferrum phosphoricum* ✿ *Gelsemium* ✿ *Hepar sulphuris* ✿ *Hypericum* ✿ *Ignatia* ✿ *Ipecacuanha* ✿ *Kali bichromicum* ✿ *Ledum* ✿ *Magnesia phosphorica* ✿ *Mercurius* ✿ *Nux vomica* ✿ *Oscillococcinum®* ✿ *Pulsatilla* ✿ *Rhus toxicodendron* ✿ *Ruta* ✿ *Spongia tosta*

Gemmotherapy

Black Currant ✿ Briar Rose ✿ European Hornbean ✿ Lime Tree ✿ Lithy Tree

CASE-TAKING WITH THE SOAP CHART

As we learned in Chapter 9, case-taking and record keeping are important skills for you to learn as a parent practitioner. Here is a blank SOAP chart for you to use when observing and assessing your child's health.

Name: **Date:** **Age:**

SUBJECTIVE

OBJECTIVE

ASSESSMENT

PLAN

GUIDE TO COMMON SYMPTOMS AND REMEDIES

COMMON SYMPTOMS AND REMEDIES

Symptom	Possible Condition	Potential Treatment	When to Call the Doctor
Abdominal pain	Colic, constipation, emotional upset, gas pains, indigestion, menstrual cramps, overeating	Abdominal massage, peppermint or chamomile tea, hot water bottle, *Arsenicum album, Bryonia, Calcarea phosphorica, Carbo vegetabilis, Colocynthis, Lycopodium, Magnesia phosphorica, Nux vomica, Pulsatilla, Sulphur,* Gripe Water, Fig Tree, Wineberry	If you suspect appendicitis, abdominal pain that lasts more than 2 days
Anxiety	Anticipation, phobias, separation anxiety, traumatic events	*Aconite, Argentum nitricum, Arsenicum album, Gelsemium, Ignatia, Kali phosphoricum, Silica,* Lime Tree, Rescue Remedy	Severe anxiety or panic attacks
Bruises, musculoskeletal pain and soreness	Injuries, sprains, strains	Ice, *Arnica, Bellis perennis, Bryonia, Hypericum, Ledum, Rhus toxicodendron, Ruta, Symphytum,* Rescue Remedy	Broken bone, head injury limping severe swelling
Chills	Common cold, fever, flu	Hot water bottle, *Aconite, Arsenicum album, Gelsemium, Hepar sulphuris, Oscillococcinum, Phosphorus,* Briar Rose	Fever of 103°F (39.4°C) for more than three days
Cough	Allergies, asthma, bronchitis, common cold, croup, whooping cough	Onion, lemon, or potato applications, hot water bottle, *Aconite, Allium cepa, Antimonium tartaricum, Bryonia, Chamomilla, Coccus cacti, Cuprum, Drosera, Hepar sulphuris, Ipecacuanha, Pulsatilla, Spongia tosta,* Briar Rose, European Hornbean, Lemon Bark, Lithy Tree	Severe cough, difficulty breathing, wheezing, fever higher than 103°F (39.4°C) for over 3 days, chest pain

COMMON SYMPTOMS AND REMEDIES, Continued

Symptom	**Possible Condition**	**Potential Treatment**	**When to Call the Doctor**
Constipation	Diet, stress	*Alumina, Bryonia, Calcarea carbonica, Nux vomica, Silica,* Wineberry, Rosemary	Chronic constipation, painful elimination, blood in stool
Diarrhea	Food allergy, food poisoning, nervous stomach, parasites, teething	Rehydration electrolyte fluids, *Arsenicum album, Chamomilla, Croton tiglium, Gelsemium, Podophyllum, Sulphur, Veratrum album,* European Walnut, Wineberry	10 or more loose stools in a 24-hour period, dehydration, bloody stool, lack of thirst, severe abdominal pain
Earache	Common cold, ear infection, sinus infection	Breastmilk ear drops, hydrogen peroxide, onion poultice, *Aconite, Belladonna, Chamomilla, Mercurius, Oscillococcinum, Pulsatilla,* Briar Rose, Mullein-Garlic ear drops	Prolonged or high fever, fluid or blood leaking from ear, swelling, pain, redness or tenderness behind ear, hearing loss
Eye inflammation or redness	Allergies, blocked tear duct, common cold, conjunctivitis, (pink eye)	Breastmilk, chamomile compress, Euphrasia eyedrops, *Apis, Argentum nitricum, Belladonna, Calcarea carbonica, Pulsatilla, Silica,* Briar Rose	Trauma and scratches to the eye; eye conditions with no improvement after 5 days
Fatigue, Weakness	Common cold, depression, flu, viral infection	*Arsenicum album, Ferrum phosphoricum, Gelsemium, Mercurius, Phosphoricum acidum,* Black Currant, Hedge Maple	Prolonged fatigue and weakness

COMMON SYMPTOMS AND REMEDIES, Continued

Symptom	**Possible Condition**	**Potential Treatment**	**When to Call the Doctor**
Fever	Common cold, flu	Lemon compress, sponge bath, *Aconite, Belladonna, Chamomilla, Ferrum phosphoricum, Gelsemium, Phosphorus*	Fever 104°F (40°C) and higher; fever 103°F (39.4°C) that lasts more than 3 days, febrile seizure, stiff or painful neck
Grief, melancholy	Depression, loss	*Ignatia amara, Natrum muriaticum, Phosphoricum acidum,* Star of Bethlehem, Rescue Remedy	Persistent symptoms, hallucinations, anxiety attacks
Headache	Allergies, common cold, emotional upset, flu, sinus infection	Ginger or peppermint tea, cold compress, *Allium cepa, Belladonna, Bryonia, Calcarea phosphorica, Ferrum phosphoricum, Gelsemium, Iris, Natrum muriaticum, Sanguinaria, Spigelia,* Briar Rose, Lemon Bark	Severe, unexplained, or recurrent headache
Itching	Chickenpox, hives, insect bites lice, pin-worm, poison ivy	Oatmeal bath, *Anacardium, Apis, Cina, Croton tiglium, Graphites, Ledum, Nux vomica, Rhus toxicodendron, Sulphur, Urtica urens,* Black Currant, Rescue Remedy	If you suspect lice, allergic reactions with difficulty breathing, severe itching
Mouth sores and pain	Canker sores, cold sores, hand-foot-mouth disease, thrush	Hydrogen peroxide, Calendula mouthwash, black tea, *Borax, Calcarea carbonica, Mercurius, Natrum muriaticum, Rhus toxicodendron, Sepia,* Briar Rose, English Elm, Hedge Maple, Prim Wort	Persists more than 2 weeks, difficulty eating

COMMON SYMPTOMS AND REMEDIES, Continued

Symptom	**Possible Condition**	**Potential Treatment**	**When to Call the Doctor**
Nose, stuffed or runny nose	Allergies, common cold, sinus infection	*Allium cepa, Chamomilla, Dulcamara, Hepar sulphuris, Kali bichromicum, Lycopodium, Mercurius, Nux vomica, Pulsatilla, Sambucas nigra,* Briar Rose, European Hornbean	Continual nasal discharge for more than ten days, chronic nasal stuffiness
Rash	Cradle cap, diaper rash, yeast infection	*Calcarea carbonica, Graphites, Hepar sulphuris, Mercurius, Sulphur, Viola tricolor,* Acidophilus, Grapefruit seed extract, *Calendula*	Serious infection, extreme redness or irritation
Sore throat	Common cold, flu, strep throat	Potato poultice, lemon compress, warm salt water and Calendula gargle, *Aconite, Apis, Belladonna, Hepar sulphuris, Lachesis, Lycopodium, Mercurius, Phytolacca,* Briar Rose, Red Spruce	Strep throat, severe pain, extreme difficulty swallowing
Urination, frequent or painful	Bladder infection	Cranberry juice, D-Mannose, *Cantharis, Sarsparilla, Staphysagria,* Black Honeysuckle, Wineberry, European Alder	Fever, pain, strong-smelling urine
Vomiting, nausea	Emotional upset, food poisoning, stomach flu, motion sickness	Ginger, peppermint, or chamomile tea, rehydration electrolyte fluids, *Arsenicum album, Calcarea carbonica, Cocculus, Ipecacuanha, Nux vomica, Petroleum, Sepia, Tabacum*	Dehydration, blood in vomit, vomiting longer than 8 to 12 hours

RESOURCES AND FURTHER READINGS

For almost every condition or philosophy, there is at least one organization devoted to providing information, useful products, and connections to a community of practitioners and like-minded patients. The following is but a selected list of organizations and books or other resources where you can find more information about the topics and products discussed in this book.

In addition, I've listed some commonly used brands of natural products and homeopathic medicines but there are many high quality brands available in health food stores and in homeopathic pharmacies.

www.drfeder.com

DrFeder.com is a resource on homeopathy, osteopathy, holistic medicine, and natural parenting. The website also features a family of experts in the fields of pregnancy, natural childbirth, naturopathic medicine, nutrition, massage, feng shui, philosophy, and animal health. For your convenience, DrFeder.com also carries a comprehensive line of homeopathic medicines, homeopathic kits, gemmotherapy, and other products mentioned in this book.

How to Find Holistic Practitioners

Organizations

American Academy of Osteopathy
3500 DePauw Blvd., Suite 1100
Indianapolis, Indiana 46268
(317) 879-1881
www.academyofosteopathy.org

American Association of Naturopathic Physicians
818 18th St NW, Suite 250
Washington, DC 20006
(202) 237-8150
www.naturopathic.org

International Academy of Oral Medicine & Toxicology
8297 Champions Gate Blvd, #193
Champions Gate, FL 33896
(863) 420-6373
www.iaomt.org
Dentists who promote mercury-free treatments.

National Center for Homeopathy
7918 Jones Branch Drive
Suite 300
McLean, VA 22102
www.homeopathycenter.org

National Center for Homeopathy
801 N. Fairfax Street, Suite 306
Alexandria, Virginia 22314
(877) 624-0613
www.homeopathic.org

First Aid and Safety

Organizations

American Heart Association
National Center
7272 Greenville Avenue
Dallas, TX 75231
(800) 242-8721
www.americanheart.org
Courses on cardiopulmonary resuscitation

American Red Cross National Headquarters
430 18th St NW
Washington, DC 20006
1-800-RED-CROSS
www.redcross.org/ux/take-a-class
Courses on cardiopulmonary resuscitation and first aid

United States Consumer Product Safety Commission
Washington, D.C. 20207-0001
(800) 638-2772
www.cpsc.gov
information about safety standards and ratings of commonly used products and furniture for children.

Books, Magazines, and Newsletters

Home Safe Home: Protecting Yourself and Your Family from Everyday Toxics and Harmful Household Products by Debra Lynn Dadd (Tarcher, 1997)

Homeopathy

Books, Magazines, and Newsletters

Everybody's Guide to Homeopathic Medicines by Stephen Cummings, M.D., and Dana Ullman, M.P.H. (Tarcher, 1997)

Homeopathic Self-Care: The Quick & Easy Guide for the Whole Family, Revised 3rd Edition by Robert Ullman, N.D., and Judyth Reichenberg Ullman, N.D. (Three Rivers Press, 1997)

Homeopathy Today Magazine
National Center for Homeopathy
7918 Jones Branch Drive, Suite 300
McLean, VA 22102
www.homeopathycenter.org/homeopathy-today-magazine

Impossible Cure: The Promise of Homeopathy by Amy L. Lansky, Ph.D. (R L Ranch Press, 2003)

The Patient's Guide to Homeopathic Medicine by Robert Ullman, N.D., and Judyth Reichenberg Ullman, N.D. (Picnic Point Press, 2000)

Ritalin-Free Kids: Safe and Effective Homeopathic Medicine for ADHD and Other Behavioral and Learning Problems, Revised 3rd Edition by Judyth Reichenberg-Ullman, N.D. M.S.W. and Robert Ullman, N.D. (Three Rivers Press, 2000)

Products

Boiron
6 Campus Boulevard
Building A
Newtown Square, PA 19073
(800) BLU-TUBE
www.boironusa.com
Boiron offers an extensive line of homeopathic medicines, including Oscillococcinum, and gemmotherapy.

Hyland's and Standard Homeopathic Company
210 W 131st St
PO Box 61067
Los Angeles, CA 90061
(800) 624-9659
www.hylands.com
Hyland's and Standard Homeopathic Company, makers of Hyland's Teething tablets, offer an extensive line of homeopathic medicines.

Nelson Bach USA Ltd
21 High Street, Suite 302
North Andover, MA 01845
(800) 319-9151
www.iherb.com/nelson-bach-usa
Nelson Bach is the supplier for Rescue Remedy and other Bach Flower Essences.

Herbal Remedies and Gemmotherapy

Books, Magazines, and Newsletters

Gemmotherapy and Oligotherapy Regenerators of Dying Intoxicated Cells by Marcus Greaves, M.D., N.M.D. (Xlibris Corporation, 2003)

Products

Boiron
6 Campus Boulevard
Building A
Newtown Square, PA 19073
(800) BLU-TUBE
www.boiron.usa.com
Boiron offers a complete line of gemmotherapy.

ChildLife Essentials
8690 Hayden Place
Culver City, CA 90232
(800) 993-0332
www.childlife.net
ChildLife carries a line of immune support products including First Defense, a natural formula of herbs and minerals known for its effective immune response properties.

Eclectic Institute
12960 Ten Eyck Rd
Sandy, OR 97055
(800) 332-4372
www.eclecticherb.com
Eclectic Institute offers a complete line of high quality herbal products including Eclectic Kids Ear Drops made with garlic and mullein.

Traditional Medicinals
4515 Ross Road
Sebastopol, CA 95472
(800) 543-4372
www.traditionalmedicinals.com
Traditional Medicinals offers a Just for Kids line of organic herbal teas which include Throat Coat®, Tummy Comfort™, Nighty Night®, and Cold Care®.

Natural Parenting Basics

Organizations

Doulas of North America (DONA)
DONA International
35 E. Wacker Dr., Ste. 850
Chicago, IL 60601-2106
(888) 788-DONA (3662)
www.dona.org

Holistic Moms Network National Office
PO Box 408
Caldwell, NJ 07006
(877) HOL-MOMS
973-228-2110
www.holisticmoms.org

National Organization of Circumcision Resource Centers (NOCIRC)
PO Box 2512
San Anselmo
CA 94979-2512
(415) 488-9883
www.nocirc.org

Books, Magazines, and Newsletters

The Baby Book, Revised Edition: Everything You Need to Know About Your Baby from Birth to Age Two by William Sears, M.D. and Martha Sears, R.N. (Little, Brown, 2003)

The Complete Teething Guide: From Birth to Adolescence by Kathy Arnos (Spirit Dance Publishing, 2003)

The Happiest Baby on the Block: The New Way to Calm Crying and Help Your Newborn Baby Sleep Longer by Harvey Karp, M.D. (Bantam, 2003)

The Happiest Toddler on the Block: The New Way to Stop the Daily Battle of Wills and Raise a Secure and Well-Behaved One to Four-Year-Old by Harvey Karp, M.D. (Bantam, 2004)

How to Raise a Healthy Child in Spite of Your Doctor by Robert S. Mendelsohn, M.D. (Ballantine Books, 1987)

Natural Family Living: The Mothering Magazine Guide to Parenting by Peggy O'Mara (Atria, 2000)

Natural Pregnancy: Practical Medical Advice and Holistic Wisdom for a Healthy Pregnancy and Childbirth by Lauren Feder, M.D. (Hatherleigh Press, 2014)

Natural Pregnancy Cookbook: Over 125 Nutritious Recipes for a Healthy Pregnancy by Sonali Ruder, D.O. (Hatherleigh, 2016)

Natural Baby Food: Over 150 Wholesome, Nutritious Recipes For Your Baby and Toddler by Sonali Ruder, D.O. (Hatherleigh, 2016)

The Parents' Concise Guide to Childhood Vaccinations, Second Edition: From Newborns to Teens, Practical Medical and Natural Ways to Protect Your Child by Lauren Feder, M.D. and LeTrinh Hoang, D.O. (Hatherleigh, 2017)

Smart Medicine for a Healthier Child: A Practical A-to-Z Reference to Natural and Conventional Treatments for Infants and Children by Janet Zand N.D., L.AC., Robert Rountree, M.D., and Rachel Walton, M.S.N., C.R.N.P. (Avery, 2004).
A comprehensive reference guide that provides a multi-faceted approach to health care including conventional treatment, diet, supplements, herbs, homeopathy, acupressure and more.

Products

California Baby
5933 Bowcroft Street
Los Angeles, CA 90016
(310) 815-8201
www.californiababy.com
California Baby offers natural and organic products for skin, hair, diaper, bath, aromatherapy, sun care, and insect repellents for babies, kids, and sensitive adults.

Tom's of Maine
Consumer Dialogue Department
302 Lafayette Center Kennebunk, ME 04043
(800) 367-8667
www.tomsofmaine.com
Tom's of Maine carries Natural Care for Kids fluoride-free toothpastes and other natural body care products.

Weleda, Inc.
Customer Care
1 Bridge St, Suite 42,
Irvington, NY 10533
(800) 241-1030
www.usa.weleda.com
Weleda carries many natural mother and baby care products, including Calendula diaper creams.

Sleep

Books, Magazines, and Newsletters

Family Bed by Tine Thevenin (Perigee, 1987)

Good Nights: The Happy Parents' Guide to the Family Bed (and a Peaceful Night's Sleep!) by Jay Gordon, M.D., and Maria Goodavage (St. Martin's Griffin, 2002)

Sweet Dreams: A Pediatrician's Secrets for Baby's Good Night's Sleep by Paul M. Fleiss, M.D. (McGraw-Hill, 2000)

Products

Arm's Reach® Concepts, Inc.
2081 N Oxnard Blvd. PMB #187
Oxnard, CA 93030
(800) 954-9353
www.armsreach.com
Arm's Reach® makes co-sleeping and bedding accessories.

Breastfeeding

Organizations

La Leche League International
110 Horizon Drive, Suite 210
Raleigh, NC 27615
(800) LALECHE
www.llli.org

Medela, Inc.
Medela, Inc.
1101 Corporate Dr.
McHenry, IL 60050
(800) 435.8316
Breastpumps and breastfeeding accessories for nursing mothers

Books, Magazines, and Newsletters

The Breastfeeding Book : Everything You Need to Know About Nursing Your Child from Birth Through Weaning by Martha Sears, R.N., and William Sears, M.D. (Little, Brown, 2000)

The Womanly Art of Breastfeeding: Completely Revised and Updated 8th Edition by Gwen Gotsch and Judy Torgus (Plume, 1997)

Products

Traditional Medicinals
4515 Ross Road
Sebastopol, CA 95472
(800) 543-4372
www.traditionalmedicinals.com
Traditional Medicinals' Organic Mother's Milk Tea promotes healthy lactation.

Healthy Nutrition

Organizations

The Weston A. Price Foundation
PMB 106-380
4200 Wisconsin Ave. NW
Washington, DC 20016
(202) 363-4394
www.westonaprice.org

Books, Magazines, and Newsletters

Dr. Mercola's Natural Health Newsletter
www.mercola.com
Named as one of the top 10 health sites on the Internet

Nourishing Traditions by Sally Fallon (NewTrends Publishing, Inc., 1999)

Super Baby Food, 3rd Edition by Ruth Yaron (F. J. Roberts Publishing Company, 1998)

Raising Vegan Children in a Non-Vegan World: A Complete Guide for Parents by Erin Pavlina (VegFamily, 2003)

Wholesome Baby Food.com
www.wholesomebabyfood.com
Information about how to prepare your own nutritious baby food.

Products

ChildLife Essentials
Nutritional Supplements for Infants and Children
8690 Hayden Place
Culver City, CA 90232
(800) 993-0332
www.childlife.net
ChildLife carries a line of nutritional formulas including Essential Fatty Acids made of vegetable based Omega 3 and 6 fatty acids.

J.R. Carlson Laboratories, Inc.
15 College Drive
Arlington Heights, IL
60004-1985
(888) 234-5656
www.carlsonlabs.com
Carlson offers a line of Carlson Kids Cod Liver Oil and Very Finest Fish Oil.

Vaccinations

Organizations

Center for Disease Control
National Immunization Program
NIP Public Inquiries
Mailstop E-05
1600 Clifton Rd., NE
Atlanta, GA 30333
(800) 232-4636
www.cdc.gov/nip

National Vaccine Information Center (NVIC)
21525 Ridgetop Circle, Suite 100
Sterling VA 20166
(703) 938-0342
www.nvic.org

National Vaccine Injury Compensation Program
Parklawn Building, Room 8A-35
5600 Fishers Lane
Rockville, Maryland 20857
(800) 338-2382
https://www.hrsa.gov/vaccinecompensation/

Vaccine Adverse Event Reporting System (VAERS)
P.O. Box 1100
Rockville, MD 20849-1100
(800) 822-7967
www.vaers.hhs.gov

Books, Magazines, and Newsletters

What Your Doctor May Not Tell You About Children's Vaccinations by Stephanie Cave, M.D., F.A.A.F.P., with Deborah Mitchell (Warner Books, 2001)

The Vaccine Guide: Risks and Benefits for Children and Adults by Randall Newstaedter, O.M.D. (North Atlantic Books, 2002)

Vaccinations: A Thoughtful Parent's Guide: How to Make Safe, Sensible Decisions about the Risks, Benefits, and Alternatives by Aviva Jill Romm (Healing Arts Press, 2001)

Bonding, Mind, Spirit, and Education

Organizations

Attachment Parenting International
P.O. Box 4615
Alpharetta, GA 30023
(800) 850-8230
www.attachmentparenting.org

Association Montessori Internationale of the United States of America
206 N. Washington St., Ste. 330
Alexandria, VA 22314
(703) 746-9919
amiusa.org

Association of Waldorf Schools of North America
515 Kimbark, Suite 106
Longmont, CO 80501
(612) 870-8310
www.waldorfeducation.org

Homeschool.com, Inc.
12210 Herdal Drive Suite #11
Auburn, CA 95603
www.homeschool.com

Resources for Infant Educarers (RIE)™
6720 Melrose Avenue
Los Angeles, CA 90038
(323) 663-5330
www.rie.org

Books, Magazines, and Newsletters

A Treasury of Children's Literature edited by Armand Eisen (Houghton Mifflin, 1992)

The Theory of Celestial Influence by Rodney Collin (Mercury Publications, 2006)

INDEX

A

abdominal pain, 22, 69, 295–297, 324, 335, 349, 359, 434, 435, 470, 476, 499, 500
Abies pectinata. See Red Spruce
Abrotanum, 418
Acer campestre. *See* Hedge Maple
acidophilus, 423, 446, 502
acne, 129, 143, 130, 142, 320, 487, 490, 515, 523
Aconitum napellus (*Aconite*), xiv, 4,322, 340, 351, 366, 369, 390, 397, 400, 407, 432, 459,
acupuncture, xi, 2, 14, 25, 32, 34
acute illnesses, 18, 29, 371
adoption, xii, 315, 317
adoptive nursing, xii, 217, 231
advertising, impact of, 53, 135-136, 228
Aethusa, 336, 452
allegory, 309
allergenic preservatives, 271
allergies, 314, 379–381
allergies, food. *See also* allergies
common allergenic foods, 261, 263, 277, 365
elimination diet, 262, 263
preventing and discovering, 261
symptoms, 301, 288-289, 291-297
Allium cepa, xiv, 27, 340, 381, 490, 471, 495, 499, 501, 502
Allium sativum. *See* Garlic allopathic medicine, 365, 494
Alnus glutinosa. *See* European Alder aloe vera, 331
Alumina, 346, 401, 500
anabolic steroids, 130, 143
Anacardium, 425, 501
anemia, 68, 131, 204, 243-248, 420-421
anise, 374, 403, 438
anthrax, 296
anthroposophical medicine, xi, 34
antibiotic usage, 19
antihistamine, 2, 12, 27, 338, 351, 380, 385, 386, 395, 413, 424
Antimonium crudum, 332, 452, 454
Antimonium tartaricum, xiv, 333, 352, 461, 499
anxiety, xiii, 320-322, 367, 369, 375, 382, 390, 397, 409, 439, 459, 472-473, 485, 490, 499, 501
Apgar Score, xi, 44, 64
Apis mellifica, xiv, 27, 325, 330, 344, 386, 396, 407, 432, 462
appendicitis, xii, 158, 323, 435, 499
Argentum nitricum, 322, 344, 499, 500
Arnica montana, xiv, 51, 390, 399, 400, 434, 440, 462-463
aromatherapy, xi, 31-32, 153, 156, 188, 372, 397, 494, 510
Arsenicum album, xiv, 16, 149, 322, 340, 361, 362, 398, 436, 452, 463-464, 495, 499-500
artificial sweeteners, 72, 89, 273-274, 277
Asperger's syndrome, 103-104. *See also* Autism Spectrum Disorder
assisted reproduction technology (ART), xii, 315, 317, 317
asthma, xii, 13, 18, 20, 21, 22, 27, 65, 147, 171, 260, 261, 285, 318, 323, 347, 348, 379, 450, 486, 499
attachment parenting, xi, 61, 62, 65, 193, 514,
Deficit Attention Disorder (ADD), 103. *See also* Attention Deficit Hyperactivity Disorder
Attention Deficit Hyperactivity Disorder (ADHD), 18, 28, 103, 111, 121, 397, 401, *See also* Attention Deficit Disorder
Auditory Processing Disorder (APD), 103,

Augmentin, 21,
Autism Spectrum Disorder, 104,
Ayurveda, 14,

B

Babinski reflex, 41,
baby powders, 56, 57,
babyproofing,– xii, 94, 95, 107,

babywearing and carrying, xi, 59, 65,
Bach Flower Essences, xi, 31, 153, 323, 376, 506,
Bach, Edward, 31
baking soda rinse, 416
baths, 27, 154, 155, 156, 159, 167, 179, 188, 189, 197, 325, 386, 425, *See also* family bath *and* oatmeal baths
bedtime rituals, 188, 189, 197, . *See also* sleep bedwetting
bee stings, xiii, 27, 324, 392, 393, 396,
Belladonna, xiv, 29, 340, 344, 366, 369, 405, 407, 410, 418, 420, 432, 433, 442, 464, 471, 472, 495, 500, 501, 502
Bellis perennis, 391, 440, 499,
Betula pubescens.487, *See* Common Birch bili lights
biotin (vitamin H, vitamin B7), 244,
birth control pill, 128, 129, 409, 491
birth order, xii, 104, 105, 108,
Bisphenol A (BPA), 169,
Black Currant (Ribes nigrum), 486,
Black Honeysuckle (Lonicera nigra), 486,
black tea, 501,
bladder infections, xiii, 20, 161, 203, 324, 325, 326, 339, 462, 468, 486,
bloodletting, 28,
boils, xiii, 161, 162, 326, 327, 328, 355, 406, 474, 489,
bonding with your baby, 64,
Borax, 501,
botanical medicine, 30,
Brady, Mervyn, v, ix, 305
adoptive nursing, xiii, 217, 231,
augmentation, after, xiii, 212, 214, 231
benefits of, xiii, 16, 22, 47, 70, 73, 172, 193, 202, 230, 238, 267, 283, 297, 302,
best diet for nursing mothers, 199–200
cesarean birth, after, 204, 206, 210
challenges, 209–211
clutch hold, 204
colostrum, 194
components of breastmilk, 194–196

cradle hold, 209, 210. 230,
cross-cradle hold, 210,
donor milk, xiii, 213, 217, 218, 231,
engorgement, 215, 216, 223, 231, 404, 406,
hand expression, 220, 231,
La Leche League, 199, 207, 217, 222, 511,
Marmet Technique, 220,
mastitis, 215
nipple confusion, 79, 89, 215, 216, 231, 411,
overview 26, 36
positions, 211, 214,
precautions 173, 181, 182, 195, 223, 240,
premature baby, breastfeeding the, xiii, 212, 217, 231
public breastfeeding, 221
pumping, xiii, 102, 108, 204, 214, 216, 218, 219, 220, 221, 231, 404, 412,
relactation, xiii, 217, 231,
side lying position, 211, 212, 230,
storing milk, xiii, 218, 231,
supplemental nursing system, 217
supporting the breast, 211
techniques, 4, 13, 163, 164,
thrush, 21, 215, 446,
transitional milk, 200-201, 229
twins, xiii, 212, 213, 214, 231,
weaning, xiii, 79, 80, 193, 222, 223, 224, 232, 406, 511,
Briar Rose (Rosa canina), xiv, 31, 328, 333, 335, 342, 345, 353, 367, 370, 374, 378,

382, 385, 408, 417, 419, 430, 434, 439, 443, 448, 455, 486, 487, 488, 489, 495, 499, 500, 501, 502,
broken bones. *See* Injuries xii, 328, 387-388, 392
bronchiolitis, 347-348
bronchitis, xiii, 158, 159, 160, 290, 328, 333, 342, 347, 348, 349, 351, 354, 439, 461, 476, 477, 488, 490, 499, *See* Cough
bruises, 144, 387, 390, 440, 463, 492, 499, *See* Injuries
Bryonia alba (*Bryonia*) xiv, 465
burns, 329, 330, 331, 386, 387, 391, 396, 425, 492, 493,

C

cage-free eggs, 252, 268
Calcarea carbonica, xiv, 113, 344, 346, 354, 417, 442, 443, 452, 466, 500, 501, 502,
Calcarea phosphorica, xiv, 378, 384, 437, 443, 467, 44
467, 499, 501,
calcium, 201, 225, 227, 266, 267, 275, 466,
Calendula officinalis (*Calendula*), xiv, 331-332, 391, 395, 444, 492
Candida albicans, 356
canker sores, xiii, 331, 334, 414, 415, 447, 490, 501, *See also* Mouth sores
Cantharis, 502
Carbo vegetabilis, 418, 437, 499
carbohydrates, 200-201, 225, 229, 234-238, 242-245, 269, 272, 276, 365, 436, 451, 517
Carbolic acid, 386, 396
caregivers, selecting, 84, 102, 255, 311, 317
Carpinus betulus 488, *See* European Hornbean
case-taking, xii, xiv, 147, 166, 318, 497
Castor equi, 405
Causticum, 112, 401
cavities, 73-74, 194-195, 203, 247, 428
cell phones, xii, 136-137, 143
cesarean birth, breastfeeding after, xiii, 212, 231
See also breastfeeding
chamomile, 153, 155, 158, 167, 438, 494
chamomile tea, 11, 154, 327, 397, 435, 451, 495, 499, 502
Chamomilla, 20, 499, 500-502
charting your child, 23, 36, 115, 147-149, 497
Chelidonium maius, 400
chemicals, additives, and preservatives, 269, 277,
chickenpox (varicella), 286, 294, 303, 332,
chills, 156, 288, 326, 340, 348, 349, 368, 370, 372-373, 404, 418, 431, 460, 473, 482, 499
China officinalis (*Cinchona officinalis*), 420
Chinese medicine, xi, 14, 34, 104, 252, 316, 317, 399, 407, 412, 418
chiropractic medicine, 14
choking hazards, 107, 254, 258, 442
choosing conventional and holistic practitioners, xi, 22
chronic illness, 13, 18-20, 28, 203
Cina, xiii, xiv, 1, 3, 5, 24, 34, 81-83, 157-159, 169, 278-280, 282-289, 293, 296-304, 312, 317, 331, 332, 340, 350, 375, 391, 392, 395, 407, 420, 423, 427, 443-444, 448, 464, 471, 482, 485-486, 491-493, 501, 507, 509, 511, 513
Cinchona officinalis. See China officinalis 420
circumcision, 50. *See* Surgery
Citrus limonum. 489, *See* Lemon Bark
clutch hold, 210, 214, 230
Cocculus indicus, 414
Coccus cacti, 352, 499
Coffea cruda, 398
cold sores, 334, 414, 480, 489, 501
colds, 2, 12, 18, 20, 21, 28, 29, 101, 108, 156-157, 160-161, 163, 167, 179, 203, 334, 338-339, 340-342, 345, 347, 366, 439, 460, 461, 469, 472, 474, 476, 477, 493
colic, 33, 89, 163, 197, 336, 361, 398, 423, 438, 468, 470, 499
Collin, Rodney, 115, 307, 514
Colocynthis, xiv, 150, 337, 410, 469, 495, 499

colostrum, 47, 200-201, 229
Common Birch (Betula pubescens), 487
competitive sports, participation in, xii, 116, 129, 143
complementary and alternative medicine (CAM), 25
compresses, 31, 34, 154-155, 167, 216, 327
conjunctivitis, xiii, 45, 342-344, 373, 422, 431, 471, 500
constipation, xiii, 12, 22, 48, 68-69, 78, 89, 111, 121, 131, 158, 163, 225, 238, 260, 324, 335, 337, 344-345, 346-347, 354, 368, 397-398, 401, 423, 434-435, 438, 439, 442, 466, 481, 492, 499-500
co-sleeping, 83, 185, 192-198, 213, 510
cough, xiii, 4, 12, 20, 45, 57, 85, 97, 101, 108, 144, 148-149, 157-160, 162, 165, 260, 281, 283, 285, 288-289, 290, 292-293, 295-296, 323, 328, 333, 338-339, 340, 342, 347-355, 363, 370, 372-373, 379, 383, 406-408, 420, 424, 427-428, 430-431, 439, 449-450, 452, 455, 459-462, 465-479, 482-490, 499
Coxsackie virus, 415, 430-431
cradle cap, xiii, 354-355, 502
cradle hold, 209-210, 230
cramps. *See* Menstrual cramps
Craniosacral therapy, xi, 33
crawling, xii, 68-70, 88-91, 402, 423
cribs, playpens, and walkers, xii, 80, 89, 196
cross-cradle hold, 210
Crotalus horridus, 420
Croton tiglium, 361, 425, 500-501
croup, xiii, 347, 349, 351-355, 408, 439, 460, 470, 473-477, 485, 499
Cuprum metallicum, 352
cyanocobalamin (vitamin B12), 245

D

D-Mannose, 325, 502
dairy, 253, 258, 262, 275, 334, 366, 369, 385, 423
daycare and preschool, xii, 84, 100, 108
selecting, 84, 102, 255, 311, 317
germs, xiii, 15, 85, 100, 108, 200, 226, 280-282, 302, 321, 371, 446, 464, 482
decorating your baby's room, 170
developmental milestones children (ages 5 to 10), xi, xii, 5, 40, 63, 66, 88, 91, 106, 109, 118, 121, 123, 142,
infants (one month to one year), xii, 66, 67, 69, 71, 73, 75, 77, 79, 81, 83, 85, 87, 89
newborns (birth to one month), xi, 39, 41, 43, 45, 47, 49, 51, 53, 55, 57, 59, 61, 63, 65
preteens (ages 11 to 13), xii, 123, 125, 127, 129, 131, 133, 135, 137, 139, 141, 143
toddlers (ages 1 to 4), xii, 91, 93, 95, 99, 101, 103, 105, 107
diapers changing, 54-55, 67, 176, 182, 191, 295, 357, 396
cloth, xi, xii, 50, 52-58, 65, 72, 76, 92, 100, 135, 154-155, 159-162, 167-169, 171-182, 222, 275, 312, 327, 330, 337, 339, 343, 357, 384, 393-395, 401-406, 410, 413, 424-425, 437, 442, 450, 453, 479, 493, 495
disposable, xi, 52-56, 65, 100, 356-357
selecting, 84, 102, 255, 311, 317
diaper creams, 56, 168, 510
diaper rash, xiii, 5, 21, 28, 31, 53-57, 65, 216, 356-358, 426, 445, 447, 492, 502
diarrhea, xiiii, 12, 16, 21-22, 69, 71, 78, 89, 100-101, 108, 130, 132, 144, 158, 203, 225, 227, 229, 243, 244, 246, 259, 260, 266, 270, 273, 277, 287, 291, 295,-296, 322, 324, 335, 337, 349, 355, 356, 358-359, 360-362, 368, 374, 408, 410-411, 415, 420, 425, 434-438, 441, 446-447, 450-453, 463, 468-470, 472, 473, 492, 500
digital addiction, 7, 140,
dilutions, 28, 153
diptheria, 284, 288
donor milk, xiii, 213, 217-218, 231
dosages, 152, 153, 166, 319, 341, 486, 491-492, 494-495
doulas, xi, 43, 64, 207, 508
dressing your child, xii, 157, 172, 174, 182

Drosera, xiv, 352, 470, 495, 499
DTaP (diphtheria, tetanus, and pertussis) vaccine, 82, 83, 278, 286, 288-289, 290-291, 298, 303, 350, 443
Dulcamara, 439, 454, 502
dyslexia, 70, 103

E

ear infections (otitis media), xiii, 6, 18, 20-21, 33, 79, 89, 147, 202-203, 226, 274, 285, 290-292, 295, 301, 302, 304, 318, 324, 338, 362, 363, 364-367, 407, 468, 487, 493-495
eating disorders, xii, 130-131, 143
echinacea, 30, 341, 367, 374
EHS (electrohypersensitive syndrome), 6
Electroacupuncture, 34
Electromagnetic field, 6, 138, 190
Electromagnetic hypersensitive syndrome, 6, 168, 157, 190, 493
Electropollution, 34, 137
emotional plane, 15
energy medicine, 15
English Elm (Ulmus campestre), xiv, 333, 335, 487, 501
engorgement, 215-216, 223, 231, 404, 406
ephedra, 130, 143
Epstein-Barr virus, 430, 489
essence, 28, 31, 58, 153, 323, 376, 387, 392, 412, 506
essential oils, xii, 31-32, 57, 153-154, 166, 392, 403, 494
Eupatorium perfoliatum, 373
Euphrasia officinalis (*Euphrasia*), xiv, 471
European Alder (Alnus glutinosa), xiv, 342, 387, 488, 502
European Grapevine (Vitis vinifera), xiv, 488-489
European Hornbean (Carpinus betulus), xiv, 354, 367, 382, 430, 439, 488, 495, 499, 502
European Walnut (Juglans regia), xiv, 320, 328, 362, 406, 488-489, 492, 500
Eustachian, 6, 226, 363-364
exercise, xii, 26, 33, 96. 109, 115-117, 122, 129, 189, 253, 280, 346, 377, 384, 385, 410, 414, 484
external healing applications, xii, 154, 167
extracurricular activities, 314
eye drops for newborns, xi, 45

F

fable, 309
fairy tales, role of, xiii, 120, 309-310, 316
family activities, 116, 314, 317
family bath, xii, 176-177, 182. *See also* baths *and* oatmeal baths
family bed. *See* co-sleeping
fatigue, 96-97, 154-156, 159-160, 223-224, 248, 261, 287, 293, 295-296, 322, 334, 342, 348-349, 373-374, 378, 384, 401, 411, 417, 426-428, 430, 473, 486-487, 491, 500
fats and lipids, 238, 276
Feng Shui, 171, 182, 403
Ferrum phosphoricum, xiv, 340, 373, 421, 471-472, 495, 500-501
fever, xii, xiii, 4, 11, 17, 19-20, 27, 28, 31, 71, 89, 100-101, 113, 144, 149, 154-156, 158-159, 163,166, 175, 261, 281, 288-289, 290-297, 299, 320, 324, 326-327, 332, 334, 338-340, 347-349, 351-352, 359-360, 363-364, 366-370, 372-374, 378-381, 393, 396, 404, 405-408, 414-415, 417-420, 422-423, 426-431, 433-435, 441-442, 448-450, 459-460, 464-465, 469, 471-472, 482, 499, 500-502
Ficus carica. See Fig Tree, 489
fifth disease, xii, 370, 426-427. *See* Roseola Fig Tree (Ficus carica),
flat warts, 453
Fleming, Sir Alexander, 20
flu (influenza), 284, 286, 290, 294, 303
fluoride, 72-74, 89, 170, 247, 510
folic acid (vitamin B9), 128, 245, 267, 409, 415
fontanelles, 42

food poisoning, xiii, 16, 358, 360-361, 374, 434, 436, 449, 450, 463, 500, 502
food temperature, 252
food storage, 125, 253,
formula feeding business of, xiii, 204, 224, 228, 232
feeding guidelines, 221–222
hypoallergenic formula, 226-227
lactose-free formula, 227
selecting, 84, 102, 311, 317
soy-based formula, 226-227, 232
transitional baby milks, 225
forty-day period, xii, 42, 64
fungal superinfections, 21

G

Galactosemia, 47-48, 215, 231
garlic (Allium sativum), 365, 494
gas, 66, 69, 78, 89, 150, 163, 225, 259-260, 266, 277, 335-337, 345, 362, 400, 434-438, 479, 481, 499
gastroesophageal reflux, xiii, 374, 450. *See*Vomiting
Gelsemium, xiv, 322, 370, 373, 408, 472-473, 495, 499-501
gemmotherapy, 408, 411, 417, 419, 430, 434, 438-439, 443, 447, 445, 486, 495, 503, 506-507
generalized anxiety, 321
genetically modified organisms (GMO), 268, 277
genital warts, 453
germ theory, 280
German measles 293, *See* rubella ginger
glycemic index (GI), 272
goldenseal, 30, 49, 64, 367
grapefruit seed extract (GSE), 57, 65, 357, 447, 502
Graphites, 355, 358,425, 501-502
grief and sorrow, xiii, 367, 375
gripe water, 377, 438, 499
grocery shopping, 250
growing pains, xii, xiii, 110-111, 121, 190, 197, 376, 377-378, 421, 428, 467-498
Guillain-Barre syndrome (GBS), 288-289, 291, 293-295, 301

H

Haemophilus Influenza Type B (HIB), 290
Hahnemann, Dr. Samuel, 28, 372
Hamamelis, 421
hand expression, 220, 231. *See also* breast-feeding
hand-foot-mouth disease, xiii, 378, 415, 417
hay fever, xiii, 27, 261, 320, 340, 374, 378-381, 429, 460, 471
headaches, xiii, 22, 97, 114, 127, 128, 139, 154, 163, 243, 339, 372, 378, 382-385, 401, 409, 437, 467-468, 472-473, 480-481, 487, 489
heartburn, 368, 389, 434-435, 452, 481
Hedge Maple (Acer campestre), 489
Hepar sulphuris, xiv, 327, 341, 352-353, 358, 429, 433, 473, 495, 499. 502
Hepatitis A, 295, 299
Hepatitis B, 242, 278, 284, 286-287, 291, 295, 298, 303
herbal medicine, xi, 30, 34-35, 494
herbs, use of, 14, 30, 34-35, 50, 57, 102, 108, 151, 154-155, 269, 365, 411-412, 440, 507, 509
herpangina, 414-417, 431
hives, xiii, 21, 27, 260, 277, 300, 320, 324, 332, 362, 374, 385-387, 396, 422, 425-426, 462, 501
holistic medicine, integration of, v, xi, 8, 12, 14-15, 19, 21-22, 25-27, 29, 129, 142, 279-280, 302, 304, 359, 503
home schooling, 120-122
homeopathic medicines administering, xii, 152, 166, 319, 459,
buying, 166, 174, 178, 250, 312, 317
storing, xiii, 125, 152, 218, 220, 231, 253-254, 490, 516
homeopathic vaccines (nosodes), 299
homeopathy, v, vii, xi, 2-3, 6, 14-16, 18, 20, 22-23, 26-29, 32, 34, 97, 104, 112, 129, 131, 144, 147, 187, 302, 316-317, 320,

323, 336, 348, 358, 361, 368, 370, 372, 374, 393, 407, 418, 432, 442, 476, 485, 490, 503-504
homeostasis, 15
hot water bottle, xiv, 149-151, 157-159, 162, 167, 325, 336, 339, 369, 372, 377, 397, 404, 409, 435, 437, 451, 479, 493, 495, 499
humoral or adaptive immune system, 281
hydrogen peroxide, xiv, 169-170, 339, 366, 372, 416, 493-495, 500-501
hydrogenated fats, 241
hydrotherapy, 32
Hypericum perforatum, xiv, 331, 391, 441, 444, 474

I

Ignatia amara, xiv, 322, 475, 501
imagination, role of, 94, 110, 120, 141, 195, 271, 305-307, 309, 311-312, 316-317
imbalance, state of, 17, 34, 127, 131, 201, 263, 284, 303, 444-445, 449
immune system, xiii, 12, 13, 17, 20-21, 29-30, 49, 75, 89, 102, 114, 127, 132, 163, 167, 173, 184, 200, 202, 241, 245-246, 248, 251, 259-260, 263, 269, 271, 274, 277, 280-282, 284-285, 291, 294-295, 298, 301-303, 328, 333-335, 338, 341-342, 353, 364-365, 367-368, 370-371, 374, 379, 402, 408, 415, 419, 428, 432, 434, 445, 453, 455, 487-489
ImmunoCAP®, 262, 380
improving symptoms, 152
indigestion. *See* Stomachache infants
bathing, 15, 50, 64, 168-169, 171, 173, 175, 177-179, 181, 328, 333, 335, 358, 426, 462, 494
caregivers, selecting, xii, 41, 43, 59, 83-86, 90, 102, 163, 191
cavities, 73-74
colic, 197, 263, 335-337, 340, 361, 398, 423, 434, 438-439, 441, 447, 450, 468-470, 479, 481, 499
crawling, xii, 68-70, 88-89, 91, 402, 423
cribs, playpens, and walkers, xii, 80, 89, 196
decorating your baby's room, 170
developmental milestones, xi, xii, 5, 40, 63, 66, 88, 91, 106, 109, 118, 121, 123, 142
dressing your child, xii, 157, 172, 174, 182
Feng Shui, 171, 182, 503
fluoride, 72-74
massage, xii, 25, 33, 35, 43, 48, 61, 69, 89, 110, 121, 150, 153, 158, 162-167, 188-189, 197, 336-337, 344, 346, 376-377, 384, 390, 404-405, 435, 494, 499, 503
meal planning, 254, 277
oral hygeine, 72
pacifiers, use of, 168-169, 446
Resource for Infant Educators (RIE), 87
solids, introduction of, 92, 223, 255, 261, 346, 371, 451
Sudden Infant Death Syndrome (SIDS), xii, 81, 90
sun safety, 329
teething, xiii, 12, 67, 69, 71-72
thumbsucking, xii, 79–80, 89
working parents, xii, 83, 85, 90, 100, 102, 229
influenza. See flu inhalation, 294
injuries, 328-329, 331, 377-378, 387-392, 415, 434, 440, 443-444, 453, 436, 465, 474-475, 483-484, 499
innate immune system, 281, 284
inner world, importance of the, 305-306, 308-309, 313
insect bites and stings, xiii, 324, 391-392, 395, 418
insomnia, xiii, 75, 134, 156, 183, 244, 396-398, 481, 490, 494
Internet, xii, 23, 81, 83, 133, 135-138, 140, 143, 151, 511
intestinal microflora, 20
Ipecacuanha, x, 353, 452, 476, 495, 499, 502
Iris versicolor, 378
iron, 68-69, 225, 227, 415
iron cookware, 170, 182, 249
itching, 243, 328, 331, 333-334, 355, 362, 379, 381-382, 386-387, 393, 395-396, 402, 405, 422-426, 445, 447, 465, 484, 501

J

jaundice, xi, xiii, 51-52, 64, 200, 287, 295, 399-400, 491
Juglans regia. *See* European Walnut Juice Plus+, 488
junk food, xii, 115, 122, 124, 131-132, 135, 143, 205, 273, 311, 313, 451

K

Kali bichromicum, xiv, 429, 477, 495, 502
Kali phosphoricum, 323, 398, 499
kangaroo care, 213
Kapha, 35
kindergarten readiness, 118-119

L

Lac defloratum, 411
Lachesis mutus, 410, 421, 433
La Leche League, 199, 207, 217, 222, 511
lanolin, 56-57, 65, 275
laryngotracheobronchitis, 349
lavender, xiv, 153, 155, 157, 188, 372, 397, 403, 494, 495
law of similars, 27
leaching, 28
lead poisoning, xiii, 400-401
learning disabilities, xii, 33, 103, 108, 169, 291, 313, 401
Ledum palustre, xiv, 48, 391, 441, 444, 448, 478
lemon, xiv, 154-160, 167, 246, 269, 339, 351, 354, 366, 369, 372, 376, 381, 385, 394, 403, 432, 433, 465, 481, 489, 499, 501-502
Lemon Bark (Citrus limonum), 489
lice (Pediculus Capitis), xiii, 402-403
light therapy, 51, 399
Ligustrum vulgare. *See* Prim Wort Lime Tree (Tilia tomentosa), 490
Lithy Tree (Viburnum lantana), 490, 495, 499
Lycopodium clavatum, 337, 400, 433, 437, 439
Lyme disease. *See* Insect bites and stings lympathic work, xiii, 393, 404

M

Magnesia phosphorica, xiv, 337, 378, 410, 478, 495, 499
marigold. *See Calendula officinalis, 492*
Marmet Technique, 220
massage, infant and child, xii, 162, 167, 189, 336, 346, 435
mastitis, xiii, 215-216, 231, 404-405, 465
meal planning, 254, 277
birth to six months, 32, 185, 197, 254
nine to twelve months, 257
one and a half to two years, 258
seven to nine months, 256, 277
six months, 32, 40-42, 61, 64, 67-68, 74-77, 82-83, 88-89, 93, 178, 181-182, 185-186, 191, 197, 199, 215, 221, 229, 254, 255-256, 277, 298, 343, 359, 364, 426, 441
twelve to eighteen months, 242, 257
measles (rubeola), 292, 426
Melaleuca alternifolia. *See* tea tree oil menstrual cramps, 392
menstruation, xii, 124, 126-127, 142, 383, 408-409
Mercurius, xiv, 327, 335, 341, 385, 367, 417-418, 429, 433, 447, 479, 495, 500-502
mercury posioning, 28
metaphors, 110, 310
midwifery, 32
migraine headaches, 128, 382, 409
milk supply, xiii, 215, 217, 219, 223, 229, 411-412
milk, warm, 189, 221, 226, 361, 397
MMR (measles, mumps, and rubella) vaccine, 286, 292, 293-294, 303, 407
mononucleosis, 378, 430,
monosodium glutamate (MSG), 270
Montessori, 119, 122, 514
Moro reflex, 41
mother's milk tea, 412
motion sickness, xiii, 384, 412-414, 419, 435, 438, 447, 449, 451, 453, 502
mouth sores, xiii, 331, 378, 414-415, 417, 447, 490, 501

Mullein (Verbascum thapsus), 365
Mullein-Garlic ear drops, xiv, 29, 365, 494-495, 500
mumps, xiii, 283-284, 286, 292-294, 303, 407, 417-418
music, role of, 34, 67, 69, 88, 124, 135, 137, 164, 187-188, 193, 309-311, 314, 316-317, 453-454
myofascial release, 33
MyPlate, 235, 275

N

napping, 12, 187, 196-197. *See also* sleep
Natrum muriaticum, xiv, 341, 375, 381, 384, 417, 480, 501
natural first aid kit, 495
natural food, preparing, 276
natural medicine, 280, 323, 348, 375, 456
natural parenting, v, xi, xii, 1, 3, 4, 9, 16, 44, 62, 83, 117, 119, 122, 144, 191, 193, 197, 202, 279, 503, 508
nature-deficit disorder, 313-314
naturopathy, xi, 14, 32, 34, 104, 316-317, 393, 407, 418
nausea, xiii, 16, 100-101, 125, 127, 130, 148, 241, 243, 270, 287-288, 291, 295-296, 324, 334, 353, 359, 360, 363, 382-383, 384, 409, 412-414, 419, 428, 431, 434-435, 441, 449-452, 462, 476, 502. *See* Motion sickness newborns
Apgar Score, xi, 44, 64
attachment parenting, xi, 61-62, 65, 193, 514
Babinski reflex, 41
babywearing and carrying, xi, 59, 65
bonding with your baby, 64
circumcision, xiii, 49
developmental milestones, 63, 66, 88, 91, 106, 109, 118, 121, 123, 142
diapers changing, 54–55, 67, 176, 182, 191, 295, 357, 396
cloth, 50, 52-56, 58, 65, 72, 76, 92, 100, 135, 154-155, 159-162, 167-169, 171-182, 222, 275, 312, 327, 330, 337, 339, 343, 357, 384, 393-395, 401, 403-404, 406, 410, 413, 424-425, 437, 442, 450, 453, 479, 493, 495
disposable, 52-56
selecting, 84, 102, 255, 311, 317
doulas, xi, 43, 64, 207, 508
eye drops for newborns, xi, 45
fontanelles, 42
forty-day period, xi, 42, 64
jaundice, xi, xiii, 51-52, 64, 200, 287, 295, 399, 400, 491
Moro reflex, 41
opthalmia neonatorum, 45, 343
overview, 36, 63, 280,
palmar grasping reflex, 41
phenylketonuria (PKU) blood test, 47
righting reflex, 41
rooting reflex, 41, 254
swaddling, 57-59, 65, 69, 263, 336
test and procedures following birth, 247
tongue-thrust reflex, 41, 75, 255
tonic neck reflex, 41
umbilical cord care, xi, 48, 64
vitamin K, xi, 46-47, 63-64, 241, 247
walking or stepping reflex, 41
niacin (vitamin B3), 243
night terrors, 111-113, 121, 190, 423
nightmares, 111-114, 121, 189-190, 197, 460, 466
nipple confusion, 79, 89, 215-216, 231, 411
nitrates, 269-271, 277, 383
nontoxic environment, creating a, xii, 168, 181, 494
nosebleeds, xiii, 318, 419-421
nosodes 299, 304, *See* homeopathic vaccines
nutrition
allergenic preservatives, 271
allergies (*See* allergies, food) artificial sweeteners, 274
cage-free eggs, 252, 268
carbohydrates, 269, 272, 276, 365, 436, 451
chemicals, additives, and preservatives, 269, 277
choking hazards, 107, 254, 258, 442
dairy, 102, 205-206, 227, 230, 234-236, 242,

247, 253, 258, 262-267, 272, 275, 334, 336, 365, 369, 371, 385, 423, 436, 446, 451
fats and lipids, 238, 276
food storage, 125, 253
food temperature, 252
genetically modified organisms (GMO), 277
grocery shopping, 250
hydrogenated fats, 234, 241, 275-276
junk food, xiii, 115, 122, 124, 131-132, 135, 143, 205, 273, 311, 313, 451
monosodium glutamate (MSG), 270
natural food, preparing, xiii, 248, 276
nitrates, 269, 270-271, 276,
proteins and amino acids, 236, 276
saturated fats, 276, 405
standard American diet, xiii, 234, 274, 275
starches and fibers (complex carbohydrates), 237
stevia, 273
sugars (simple carbohydrates), 234, 237, 365
unsaturated fats, 238
USDA food pyramid, 235
vegetarian diets, 274-275
vitamins and minerals (*See* vitamins and minerals) 224, 230, 241-242, 269, 275-276
xylitol, 273, 274
Nux vomica, xiv, 151, 337, 347, 381, 398, 423, 429, 437, 439, 452, 481, 495, 499-502

O

oatmeal baths, 27, 386, 452. *See also* baths *and* family bath
obesity, childhood, 115, 122, 132, 134, 139-140, 203, 225, 241, 271, 314
obsessive-compulsive disorder (OCD), 321
onion, 27, 29, 155, 159-161, 167, 247, 251, 264, 325, 237, 336, 339, 351, 366, 460-461, 499, 500
onion poultice, 29, 161, 325, 327, 339, 366, 500
Opthalmia neonatorum, 343
organic headaches, 382-383
Oriental medicine, 32
Oriental Plane Tree (Platanus orientalis), 490
Oscillococcinum, xiv, 373, 482, 495, 499, 500, 506
Osgood-Schlatter disease, xiii, 129, 377, 421
Osteopathic Manipulative Technique (OMT), 33
osteopathy, vii, 2, 6, 14, 27, 33, 104, 187, 317, 365, 390, 393, 503-504
otitis media. *See* ear infections, 362

P

pacifiers, use of, 168-169, 446
pain, 50, 69, 125, 127, 140, 150, 192, 208, 225, 230, 287, 295-296, 324, 335
palmar grasping reflex, 41
Palmer, D.D., 32
pantothenic acid (vitamin B5), 244
parable, 309
parasites, 101, 281, 361, 492, 500
parasomnias, 113
parent practitioner, 148, 497
pediatric wellness, 11
Pediculus capitis. *See* lice penicillium notatum, 20
peppermint tea, 384, 435, 451, 501
persistent or worsening symptoms, 152
pertussis (whooping cough), xiii, 283, 285, 289-290, 347, 350-351, 353, 430, 439, 455, 470, 476, 485, 499
Petroleum, 56, 65, 178-179, 182, 312, 357, 414, 502
pharyngitis, xiii, 301, 430-431, 433
phenylketonuria (PKU) blood test, 47
Phosphoricum acidum, 376, 378, 500-501
Phosphorus, 202, 225, 230, 246-247, 331, 370, 421, 441, 499
phototherapy, 51-52, 399
physicial plane, xiv, 129, 320, 490,
physiotherapy, 32
Phytolacca, 406, 418, 434, 502
phytomedicine, 30
pinkeye, xiii, 101, 158, 342-343, 422
pinworm, xiii, 422-424, 501
Pitta, 35

plant bud therapy, 30
plantar warts, 453-454
Platanus orientalis. *See* Oriental Plane Tree
playtime, role of, 490
PMS, xiii, 22, 127, 244, 408-411, 424
pneumococcus (PCV), 291
pneumonia, xiii, 57, 202-203, 289-292, 294-295, 300, 338, 347-350, 407, 424-443, 461
Podophyllum, 361-362, 500
poison ivy, xiii, 320, 424-426, 483, 501
poison oak, xiii, 320, 424-426, 483
poison sumac, xiii, 320, 424-426
polio, 278, 283-284, 286-288, 292, 303
Polybrominated Diphenyl Ethers (PBDEs), 169
post-traumatic stress disorder (PTSD), 321
potatoes, 162, 167, 234, 237, 243, 251, 255-257, 269-270, 335, 339, 346, 451
poultices, 34, 154-155, 157, 160-162, 167, 327, 339, 351, 495
practitoners, xi, choosing conventional and holistic, 22
premature baby, breastfeeding, 212, 231
premenstrual syndrome. *See* PMS preteens. *See* puberty, 127
Prim Wort (Ligustrum vulgare), 490
print, 28, 222, 241, 311
private schools, 118, 122
proteins and amino acids, 236, 276
puberty acne, 128, 142, 320
advertising, impact of, 53, 135-136, 228
birth control pills, 128-129, 409, 491
cell phones, xii, 136-137, 143
competitive sports, participation in, 116, 129, 143
developmental milestones, xi, xii, 5, 40, 63, 66, 88, 91, 106, 109, 118, 121, 123, 142
eating disorders, xii, 130-131, 143
in boys, 418
in girls, 112, 124-125, 142, 324, 382, 402, 418, 422
Internet, xii, 23, 81, 83, 133, 135-138, 140, 143, 151, 511
junk food, xii, 115, 122, 124, 131-132, 135, 143, 205, 273, 311, 313, 451
menstrual cramps, xiii, 125, 127, 142, 154, 158, 355, 408-411, 424, 469, 478-479, 490, 499
menstruation, xii, 124, 126-127, 142, 383, 408-409
premenstrual syndrome (PMS), 127
television and video games, xii, 133-134, 137, 143, 313
public schools, 118
Pulsatilla nigricans (*Pulsatilla*), xiv, 482
pumping, breast, xiii, 102, 108, 204, 214, 216, 218-221, 231, 404, 412
pyloric stenosis, 450
pyridoxine (vitamin B6), 244

R

Ranunculus bulbosa, 333
rash, xiii, 5, 12-13, 21, 28, 31, 52-57, 65, 78, 101, 153,190, 244, 260, 277, 281, 291-294, 297, 332-333, 354-358, 368, 385-387, 389, 393, 399, 402, 406, 408, 415, 424-427, 431, 437, 445, 447, 492, 502
Raspberry (Rubus idaeus), 491
raw potato slices, 162, 327
Red Spruce (Abies pectinata), 491
reflux, xiii, 347, 374, 449-451
relactation, xiii, 217, 231
reproductive technology, 315-317
Rescue Remedy, 31, 323, 376, 387, 392, 412, 495, 499, 501, 506
resistance to antibiotics, 20
Resource for Infant Educators (RIE), 87, 514
respiratory syncytial virus (RSV), xiii, 347-348, 427
Rhus diversiloba, 425, 483
Rhus toxicodendron, xiv, 333, 373, 387, 391, 425, 483-484, 495, 499, 501
Ribes nigrum. *See* Black Currant riboflavin (vitamin B2), 486
Ricinus communis, 411

righting reflex, 41
rooting reflex, 41, 254
Rosa canina. *See* Briar Rose, 487
Rosemary (Rosmarinus officinalis), 491
roseola, 426-427
Rosmarinus officinalis. *See* Rosemary rotavirus, 491
rubella (German measles), xiii, 426-427
Rubus idaeus. *See* Raspberry, 491
Ruta graveolens, xiv, 392, 484

S

Sabadilla, 381, 423,
safe shot strategy, xiii, 299, 301, 304, 449,
salmonella, 268, 299, 360,
Sambucas nigra, 439, 502,
Sanguinaria, 384, 501,
Sarsaparilla, 326,
saturated fats, 238, 239, 274, 276, 405,
Scarlet Fever, 431, 433,
schools, public and private, 115117
Sears, William, 62, 65, 508, 511,
selective vaccination, 298, 303,
self-limiting illnesses, 18, 147, 318,
separation anxiety, 68, 88, 92, 94, 106, 107, 321, 499
Sepia, 335, 414, 501, 502,
Sever's Disease, xiii, 130, 377, 428,
Shigella, 360,
Silica, 323, 328, 344, 345, 347, 406, 499,
side effects of vaccines, preventing and treating,18, 102, 371,
side lying position, 211, 212, 230,
sinus infection, xiii, 20, 101, 156, 157, 295, 338, 343, 428, 429, 438, 439, 477, 487,
slap cheek syndrome, 427,
sleep bedtime rituals, 188, 189, 197,
conventional sleep training methods, xii, 190, 197,
developing sleep patterns, xii, 82, 184, 190, 191, 197,
family bed, xii, 3, 81, 83, 192, 193, 198, 224, 510,
napping, xii, 187, 196, 197,
poor sleep, xii, 114, 190, 196, 197, 397,
requirements, sleep, 87, 286,
sleeping tips, xii, 196, 198,
sleep training. *See* sleep
sleepwalking, xi 111, 113, 121, 190,
sling, 58, 59, 60, 65, 67, 80, ,
smallpox, 283, 296, 296, 297, 303,
social phobia, 321,
soft tissue manipulation, 33,
sore throat, xiii, 12, 20, 156, 157, 159, 162, 281, 288, 338, 339, 340, 341, 348, 406, 407, 414, 415, 428, 430, 431, 432, 433, 434, 438, 460, 462, 465, 473, 483, 487, 491, 495, 502,
Spigelia, 385, 423, 501,
spiritual life of children, xiii, 305, 316,
spondylolisthesis, 60,
Spongia tosta, xiv, 352, 353, 485, 495, 499,
supplemental nursing system, 27,
St. John's wort, 30, 331, 474,
Staphysagria, 326, 441, 502,
Star of Bethlehem, 376, 501,
starches and fibers (complex carbohydrates), 234, 237, 238, 451,
Steiner, Rudolf, 34, 119,
stevia, 273,
Still, Andrew Taylor, 33,
stomachache, xiii, strep throat, xiii, 20, 382, 415, 430, 431, 432, 433, 438, 502,
stuffed nose, xiii, 320, 341, 379, 428, 429, 430, 438, 439, 477, 481, 482,
substances to avoid, 152,

Sudden Infant Death Syndrome (SIDS), xii, 81, 90, 193,
sugars (simple carbohydrates), 234, 237, 365
Sulphur, xiv, 15, 16, 160, 271, 327, 328, 333, 341, 352, 353, 355, 358, 362, 406, 408, 426, 429, 433, 437, 444, 473, 495, 499, 500, 501, 502
sun safety, xii, 180, 182, 329
surgery, xiii, 14, 33, 46, 50, 166, 212, 214, 301, 329, 333, 343, 355, 390, 391, 421, 428, 432, 440, 441, 450, 463

swaddling, xi, 57, 58, 59, 65, 69, 263, 336,
Symphytum officinale, 392,

T

Tabacum, 414, 502,
Tantrums, xii, 93, 96, 97, 98, 99, 106, 107, 108, 141, 423,
tea tree oil (Melaleuca alternifolia), 392,
teething, xii, xiii, 12, 28, 67, 69, 71, 72, 79, 88, 89, 92, 100, 114, 122, 161, 163, 167, 169, 184, 190, 197, 256, 339, 340, 359, 361, 362, 363, 366, 369, 396, 398, 441, 442, 443, 452, 467, 468, 500, 506, 508,
Teflon, 74, 170,
television and video games, xii, 133, 134, 137, 143, 313,
tension headaches, 382, 385, 489,
TENS (transcutaneous electrical nerve stimulation), 34,
tetanus, xiii, 278, 284, 285, 286, 288, 289, 290, 299, 303, 330, 350, 443, 444, 475,
Teucrium, 424
thiamine (vitamin B1), 242,
three-day measles, 242
thrush, xiii, 21, 28, 57, 215, 216, 357, 405, 417, 444, 445, 446, 447, 490, 501,
Thuja, 448, 454,
thumbsucking, xii, 79, 80, 89,
Tilia tomentosa. *See* Lime Tree toddlers
babyproofing, xii, 94, 95, 107,
birth order, xii, 104, 105, 108,
daycare and preschool germs,xii, 100, 108,
developmental milestones five years, xii, 5, 40, 63, 66, 88, 91, 106, 109, 118, 121, 123, 142,
four years,
one and a half years, 92, 106, one year, 89–90
three years, 119,
two years, 6, 40, 41, 66, 72, 93, 106, 117, 134, 185, 186, 220, 223, 224, 254, 258, 277, 359, 384, 394, 413, 426, 435, 451,
learning disabilities, xii, 33, 103, 108, 169, 291, 313, 401,
meal planning, xiii, 254, 277,
tantrums, xii, 93, 96, 97, 98, 99, 106, 107, 108, 141, 313, 423
toilet training, xii, 55, 93, 99-100, 106, 108
toilet training, xii, 55, 93, 99-100, 106, 108
tongue-thrust reflex, 41, 75, 255
tonic neck reflex (fencer's position), 41
toys, role of, 81, 92, 93, 96, 106-107, 120, 135, 169, 181, 311-313, 317
traditions, importance of, 9, 16, 34, 49, 64, 86, 116, 207, 308, 310, 316, 512
twins, breastfeeding of, xiii, 205, 212-214, 231

U

Ulmus campestre. *See* English Elm umbilical cord care, 487,
unsaturated fats, 238, 239, 276,
Upledger, Dr. John, 33
upright baby carriers, 60, 65,
urination, 51, 55, 324, 325, 326, 359, 449, 468, 473, 502,
Urtica urens, 331, 387, 396, 501,
USDA food pyramid, 235

V

Vaccines advantages
anthrax, 296,
chickenpox (varicella), 303, 332, 333, 334, 415, 426, 483, 489, 501,
considerations, 174, 212, 218, 225, 253, 311, 317,
diphtheria, 278, 283, 285, 286, 288, 289, 299, 303, 350, 443,
disadvantages, 22, 87, 228,
DTaP (diphtheria, tetanus, and pertussis), 286,
functions of, germ theory, 280,
German measles (rubella), 293,
haemophilus influenza type B (HIB), 290,
hepatitis A, 295, 299,
hepatitis B, 242, 278, 284, 286, 287, 291, 295, 298, 303,
homeopathic vaccines (nosodes), 299,
humoral or adaptive immune system, 281,

influenza, 284, 286, 290, 294, 303,
innate immune system, 281, 284,
measles (rubeola), 292, 426,
MMR (measles, mumps, and rubella), 407,
mumps, xiii, 283, 284, 286, 292, 292, 293, 294, 303, 407, 417, 418,
no vaccinations, electing, 297, 303,
pertussis (whooping cough), 289,
pneumococcus (PCV), 291,
polio (paralytic polio), 287,
safe shot strategy, xiii, 299, 301, 304, 449,
selective vaccination, 298, 303,
side effects, preventing and treating, 18, 102,
smallpox, 283, 296, 297, 303,
standard vaccination schedule, 286, 297, 299, 303,
tetanus, xiii, 278, 284, 285, 286, 288, 289, 290, 299, 303, 330, 350, 443, 444, 475,
travel vaccinations, 299,
Vaccinum vitis idaea. *See* Wineberry varicella. *See* chickenpox
Vata, 35,
vegetarian diets, 274, 275,
Veratrum album, 362, 500,
Verbascum thapsus. *See* Mullein
Verruca plana, 453
Verruca vulgaris, 453,
Viburnum Lantana. See Lithy tree video games. *See* television and video games
Viola tricolor, 502,
viral infection, 20, 21, 101, 281, 293, 342, 348, 349, 350, 351, 416, 417, 426, 430, 431, 500,
visual tracking problems, 104,
vitamin A, 246,
vitamin C (ascorbic acid), 245,
vitamin D, 180, 240, 241, 246, 247,
vitamin E, 246, 335,
vitamin K, xi, 46, 47, 63, 64, 241, 247,
vitamins and minerals
biotin (vitamin H, vitamin B7), 244,
calcium, 189, 201, 205, 225, 227, 230, 235, 246, 247, 266, 267, 270, 275, 378, 401, 466, 491
cyanocobalamin (vitamin B12), 245,
folic acid (vitamin B9), 245,
iron, 68, 69, 170, 182, 202, 225, 227, 232, 248, 249, 256, 275, 329, 401, 415, 471,
niacin (vitamin B3), 243,
pantothenic acid (vitamin B5), 244,
pyridoxine (vitamin B6), 244
riboflavin (vitamin B2), 243,
thiamine (vitamin B1), 242,
vitamin A, 246,
vitamin C (ascorbic acid), 245
vitamin D, 180, 240, 241, 246, 247,
vitamin E, 246, 335,
vitamin K, xi, 46, 47, 63,
Vitis vinifera. *See* European Grapevine vomiting, 488,

W

Waldorf Schools, 34, 119, 120, 514,
walking or stepping reflex, 41,
warts, xiii, 453, 454, 455, 487, 488, 489,
weakness, 44, 105, 243, 245, 287, 296, 297, 301, 338, ,373, 392, 401, 420, 421, 464, 467, 472, 473, 480, 500,
weaning, xiii, 79, 80, 193, 222, 223, 224, 232, 406, 511,
whooping cough. *See* pertussis Wineberry (Vaccinum vitis idaea), 492,
wraps, 52, 65, 154, 155, 159, 399, 495,
Wyethia, 382,

X

xylitol, 273, 274,

Z

zinc oxide, 57, 65, 180, 357,